78-99

369 024042   D1766526

This book is due for return on or before the last date shown below.

Chronic Medical Disease and Cognitive Aging

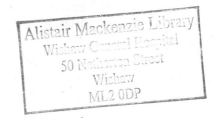
Chronic Medical Disease and Cognitive Aging

TOWARD A HEALTHY BODY AND BRAIN

EDITED BY

KRISTINE YAFFE, MD

Roy and Marie Scola Endowed Chair in Psychiatry
Professor, Departments of Psychiatry, Neurology, and Epidemiology
University of California, San Francisco
Director, Memory Disorders Clinic and
Chief of Geriatric Psychiatry
San Francisco Veterans Affairs Medical Center
San Francisco, CA

OXFORD
UNIVERSITY PRESS

OXFORD
UNIVERSITY PRESS

Oxford University Press is a department of the University of Oxford.
It furthers the University's objective of excellence in research, scholarship,
and education by publishing worldwide.

Oxford   New York
Auckland   Cape Town   Dar es Salaam   Hong Kong   Karachi
Kuala Lumpur   Madrid   Melbourne   Mexico City   Nairobi
New Delhi   Shanghai   Taipei   Toronto

With offices in
Argentina   Austria   Brazil   Chile   Czech Republic   France   Greece
Guatemala   Hungary   Italy   Japan   Poland   Portugal   Singapore
South Korea   Switzerland   Thailand   Turkey   Ukraine   Vietnam

Oxford is a registered trademark of Oxford University Press in the UK and certain other
countries.

Published in the United States of America by
Oxford University Press
198 Madison Avenue, New York, NY 10016

Library of Congress Cataloging-in-Publication Data
Chronic medical disease and cognitive aging: toward a healthy body and brain / [edited by]
Kristine Yaffe.
  p. ; cm.
  Includes bibliographical references and index.
  ISBN 978-0-19-979355-6 (hardcover: alk. paper)
  I. Yaffe, Kristine.
  [DNLM: 1. Chronic Disease. 2. Aging—physiology. 3. Cognition—physiology. WT 500]
612.6'7—dc23
2012040835

9 8 7 6 5 4 3 2 1
Printed in the United States of America
on acid-free paper

To my family, both here and there

Contents

Contributors

José Alejandro Luchsinger, MD, MPH
Associate Professor of Medicine and
  Epidemiology
Columbia University Medical Center
New York, New York

Sonia Ancoli-Israel, PhD
Professor Emeritus of Psychiatry and
Medicine Professor of Research
  Department of Psychiatry
University of California San Diego
San Diego, California

Laura D. Baker, PhD
Associate Professor of Internal
  Medicine and of Public Health
  Sciences
Wake Forest University School of
  Medicine
Winston-Salem, North Carolina

Pascale Barberger-Gateau, MD, PhD
Professor, University of Bordeaux
  Segalen and Director Nutritional
  Epidemiology
Univ. Bordeaux, ISPED
Centre INSERM U897-
  Epidemiologie-Biostatistique
F-33000 Bordeaux, France
INSERM, ISPED, Centre INSERM
  U897-Epidmiologie-Biostatistique
F-33000 Bordeaux, France

Deborah E. Barnes, PhD, MPH
Associate Professor of Psychiatry and
  Epidemiology & Biostatistics
University of California, San
  Francisco and
San Francisco Veterans Affairs
  Medical Center
San Francisco, California

Brenna Cholerton, PhD
Department of Psychiatry and
  Behavioral Science
University of Washington School of
  Medicine and
Geriatric Research, Education, and
  Clinical Center
Veterans Affairs Puget Sound Health
  Care System
Seattle, Washington

Suzanne Craft, PhD
Professor of Gerontology and
  Geriatric Medicine Co-Director
Roena B. Kulyncyh Center for
  Cognition and Memory Research
  Director
Sticht Center on Aging
Department of Internal Medicine
Wake Forest University School of
  Medicine
Winston-Salem, North Carolina

Catherine Feart, PhD
Univ. Bordeaux, ISPED
Centre INSERM U897-
  Epidemiologie-Biostatistique
F-33000 Bordeaux, France
INSERM, ISPED, Centre INSERM
  U897-Epidmiologie-
  Biostatistique
F-33000 Bordeaux, France

Cherie M. Falvey, MPH
Department of Psychiatry
University of California San
  Francisco and
San Francisco Veteran's
  Administration Medical Center
San Francisco, California

Róisín Gallinagh Smith, MB BCh
Centre for Public Health
The Queen's University Belfast
Belfast, United Kingdom

Deborah R. Gustafson, MS, PhD
Professor – Department of
  Neurology
State University of New York -
  Downstate Medical Center
Brooklyn, NY
and
docent, University of Gothenburg
Neuropsychiatric Epidemiology
  Research Unit
Gothenburg, Sweden

Tiffany L. Tsai
Research Assistant
Department of Anesthesia/
  Perioperative Care
University of California, San
  Francisco
San Francisco, California

Angela L. Jefferson, PhD
Associate Professor of Neurology
Vanderbilt Memory and Alzheimer's
  Center, Department of
  Neurology
Vanderbilt University Medical Center
Nashville, Tennessee

Miia Kivipelto, MD, PhD
Professor of Clinical Geriatric
  Epidemiology Aging
Research Center and Alzheimer
  Disease Research Center
Karolinska Institute
Sweden Institute of Clinical Medicine
  / Neurology
University of Eastern Finland
Finland Department of Chronic
  Disease Prevention
National Institute for Health and
  Welfare
Finland

Manjula Kurella Tamura, MD, MPH
Associate Professor
Division of Nephrology
Stanford University School of
 Medicine and
Geriatrics Research Education &
 Clinical Center
Veterans Affairs Palo Alto Health Care
 System
Palo Alto, California

Lenore J. Launer, PhD
Senior Investigator Chief,
 Neuroepidemiology Section
Laboratory of Epidemiology and
 Population Sciences
Intramural Research Program
National Institute on Aging
Bethesda, Maryland

Nicola T. Lautenschlager, MD
Professor of Psychiatry of Old Age
Academic Unit for Psychiatry of Old
 Age, St. Vincent's Health
Department of Psychiatry
University of Melbourne
Melbourne, Victoria, Australia

Luc Letenneur, PhD
Univ. Bordeaux, ISPED
Centre INSERM U897-
 Epidemiologie-Biostatistique
F-33000 Bordeaux, France
INSERM, ISPED, Centre INSERM
 U897-Epidmiologie-
 Biostatistique
F-33000 Bordeaux, France

Jacqueline M. Leung, MD, MPH
Professor of Anesthesia and
 Perioperative Care
Department of Anesthesia/
 Perioperative Care
University of California, San
 Francisco
San Francisco, California

Peter A. Passmore, MD
Professor of Ageing and Geriatric
 Medicine
Centre for Public Health
Queen's University Belfast
Belfast, United Kingdom

Cecilia Samieri, PhD
Univ. Bordeaux, ISPED
Centre INSERM U897-
 Epidemiologie-Biostatistique
F-33000 Bordeaux, France
INSERM, ISPED, Centre INSERM
 U897-Epidmiologie-
 Biostatistique
F-33000 Bordeaux, France

Alina Solomon, MD, PhD
Postdoctoral researcher
Aging Research Center and Alzheimer
 Disease Research Center
Karolinska Institute
Sweden Institute of Clinical Medicine
 / Neurology
University of Eastern Finland
Finland

Adam P. Spira, PhD
Assistant Professor Department of
 Mental Health
Johns Hopkins Bloomberg School of
 Public Health
Baltimore, Maryland

Melissa Thompson, DVM
Department of Neurology and
 Alzheimer's Disease Center and
Department of Pharmacology and
 Experimental Therapeutics
Boston University School of Medicine
Boston, Massachusetts

Stephen Todd, MD
Centre for Public Health
The Queen's University Belfast
Belfast, United Kingdom

Victor Valcour, MD
Professor of Medicine, Division of
    Geriatrics and Department of
    Neurology
UCSF Memory and Aging Center
San Francisco, California

Lauren Wendelken, MS
Project Analyst
UCSF Memory and Aging Center
San Francisco, California

Rachel A. Whitmer, PhD
Research Scientist II, Division of
    Research
Epidemiology, Etiology, and
    Prevention
Kaiser Permanente Northern
    California
Oakland, California

Kristine Yaffe, MD
Departments of Neurology and
    Epidemiology & Biostatistics
University of California, San
    Francisco and
San Francisco Veterans Affairs
    Medical Center
San Francisco, California

Introduction

The expansion of life expectancy over the past century coupled with the aging of the baby boom generation has created a shift in demographics to that of an aging population. As individuals are living longer, the incidence and prevalence of dementia and mild cognitive impairment is anticipated to grow exponentially. In the United States, Alzheimer's disease (AD) is now the fifth leading cause of death for adults ages 65 years and older (Alzheimer's Association, 2012). Cognitive function is one of the main predictors of independence in late-life (Fiocco, 2010). It not only is involved in planning, communication, and decision making but is critical for effective disease management. This is particularly important among elderly individuals who have a higher incidence of acute and chronic medical conditions. In addition, chronic medical diseases often increase risk of cognitive impairment, suggesting a reciprocal relationship may exist where medical disease impacts cognition that, in turn, may exacerbate physical health.

Research into the role of chronic medical diseases, such as cardiovascular and metabolic diseases, as well as lifestyle factors such as diet and physical inactivity, on the risk of cognitive impairment and dementia has recently garnered much interest. Evaluating the complex interactions of biological and lifestyle risk factors on cognition is important for three reasons, as it can (1) help us to disentangle the mechanisms associated with cognitive impairment, (2) lead to improved prevention and treatment options, and (3) enhance our ability to identify those who may be at risk for cognitive decline.

The etiology of cognitive impairment and dementia remains only partially understood. Evaluating the association between chronic medical disease and cognitive impairment may advance our knowledge of the biological processes involved in the pathogenesis of cognitive impairment, potentially leading the way for effective therapeutic interventions. For example, associations with midlife hypertension, obesity, and diabetes provide evidence that vascular disease, especially subclinical, may play a role in brain aging and cognitive impairment (Launer, 2009). Associations with diabetes and other metabolic disorders may point to a role of such factors as glucose dysregulation, insulin resistance, or inflammation in contributing to neurodegeneration (Yaffe, 2007; Yaffe et al., 2012). Understanding how such mechanisms influence brain health may help illuminate pathways that lead to brain damage. By targeting these pathways it may be possible to reduce or prevent cognitive impairment.

Because current pharmaceutical treatment of dementia has not yet proven to prevent the progression of the disease and can only modestly improve symptoms, risk factor modification continues to be a promising strategy to reduce the incidence of dementia. Recent studies have suggested that treatment of chronic medical diseases and lifestyle factors associated with dementia could lead to a reduction in the incidence of dementia (Ritchie et al., 2010; Barnes, 2011). One recent study projected that up to half of AD cases worldwide and in the United States may be attributable to seven potentially modifiable risk factors. These included low education, current smoking, physical inactivity, depression, midlife obesity, midlife hypertension, and diabetes (Barnes, 2011). By addressing modifiable risk factors, it may be possible to delay or prevent the occurrence of dementia.

Finally, determining which chronic medical diseases and lifestyle factors confer the greatest risk for cognitive impairment can help improve our efforts to identify and target those who my benefit the most from intervention. Neurodegeneration may begin years to decades before clinical symptoms of cognitive impairment and dementia appear (Lopez et al., 2011). If we can better distinguish those at greatest risk for cognitive impairment, then we may be able to intervene at an earlier point in disease progression, perhaps before neurodegeneration occurs, to maintain or improve cognitive health.

In this book, we explore current research and knowledge on the effects of chronic medical conditions and lifestyle factors on cognitive health and discuss promising strategies for prevention of cognitive decline and optimization of cognitive health in old age. Each chapter explores current research, mechanisms, and future directions for a chronic medical condition or lifestyle factor. The ultimate goal of this book is to promote awareness of the important connection between physical and cognitive health.

References

Alzheimer's Association. (2012). 2012 Alzheimer's disease facts and figures. *Alzheimers Dement,* 8(2), 131–168.

Barnes DE, & Yaffe K. (2011). The projected effect of risk factor reduction on Alzheimer's disease prevalence. *Lancet Neurol 10*(9), 819–828.

Fiocco AJ, & Yaffe K. (2010). Defining successful aging: the importance of including cognitive function over time. *Arch Neurol,* 67(7), 876–880.

Launer, L. (2009). Diabetes:vascular or neurodegenrative:an epidemiological perspective *Stroke* 40(3 Suppl), S53–S55.

Lopez OL, McDade E, Riverol M, & Becker JT. (2011). Evolution of the diagnostic criteria for degenerative and cognitive disorders. *Curr Opin Neurol 24*(6), 532–541.

Ritchie K, Carrière I, Ritchie CW, Berr C, Artero S, & Ancelin ML. (2010). Designing prevention programmes to reduce incidence of dementia: prospective cohort study of modifiable risk factors. *BMJ, 341.*

Yaffe, K. (2007). Metabolic syndrome and cognitive disorders: is the sum greater than its parts? *Alzheimer Dis Assoc Disord, 21*(2), 167–171.

Yaffe K, Falvey C, Hamilton N, Schwartz AV, Simonsick EM, Satterfield S, et al. (2012). Diabetes, glucose control, and 9-year cognitve decline among older adults without dementia. *Arch Neurol*(12), 1–6.

Chronic Medical Disease and Cognitive Aging

1

Epidemiologic Insights Into Blood Pressure and Cognitive Disorders

LENORE J. LAUNER, PHD

Introduction

Elevated systolic and diastolic blood pressure (SBP; DBP) increase the risk for clinical cardiovascular (CV) disease, including stroke, coronary disease, and kidney disease. As shown in an analysis of 1 million subjects from 61 cohort studies, the risk for CV diseases doubles with every 20/10 mmHg increase starting at or below 115/75 mmHg (Lewington, Clarke et al., 2002). In addition to being a strong risk factor for clinical stroke events, elevated levels of BP are associated with subclinical disease, such as ischemic and hemorrhagic lesions in the brain, and with more brain atrophy. These cerebral pathologies have functional consequences and increase the risk for future clinical events, as described below.

DEFINITION OF HIGH BLOOD PRESSURE

The Seventh Report of the Joint National Committee on Prevention, Detection, Evaluation, and Treatment of High Blood Pressure (JNC-7) (Chobanian, Bakris et al., 2003) provides guidelines for classifying BP by levels of risk for related morbidity and mortality. The last revision included three categories: hypertension (SBP/DBP) greater than 140/90, prehypertension (120–139/80–89), and normal (<120/80). The JCNC-7 redefined the normal category to include the prehypertension classification to better classify the continuous increase in risk as BP levels increase. This prehypertension group includes individuals who would benefit from an early intervention to reduce BP, or to slow down or prevent progression to hypertensive levels. The JNC-7 also concluded SBP is the most potent risk factor for CV disease in people older than age 50 years.

In 2001 to 2004, the prevalence of hypertension was 54.4% and 67.1% in men ages 65 to 74 years and men ages 75 years and older, respectively; similarly in women, the prevalence was 72.9% and 82.0%, respectively. National Health and Nutrition Examination Survey NHANES data also show mean levels of SBP and DBP have increased over calendar time, is higher in men than women, and is higher among African-Americans compared to Hispanics and Caucasians (Health United States, 2007; Table 1.1; see Table 1). Although over time the number of people using anti-hypertensive medications has increased, the prevalence of unsuccessful treatment is high, and a significant portion of the population is not aware of being hypertensive or is aware but not treated (Egan, Zhao et al., 2010).

Cerebral Lesions and Structural Changes that Are Associated With Elevated Blood Pressure

VASCULAR CEREBRAL SISEASE (MACRO- AND MICROVASCULAR CEREBRAL DISEASE)

In general, macrovascular clinical stroke can cause focal impairment, depending on the location and size of the infarct. More diffuse impairment can result if the stroke is so located that it disrupts neurocognitive networks in the brain. Disruption can also occur with the far more prevalent small vessel disease (SVD) caused by hypertension. Small vessel disease manifests as small focal lesions in the white matter (lacunaes) or diffuse white matter lesions resulting mainly from ischemia (Debette & Markus, 2010). Small vessel disease increases with age; for example, in a community-based sample mean age 48 years, 38% had at least one medium-size subcortical white matter lesion (Kruit, van Buchem et al., 2004); in another community study sample with mean age 62 years, approximately (Liao, Cooper et al., 1996) 86% had such lesions. Small vessel disease has been associated with cognitive impairment and decline and has been shown to be more frequent in persons with dementia (Vermeer, Prins et. al., 2003).

High BP is also the most consistently reported risk factor for microvascular disease. Cerebral microbleeds (CMBs) are hemosiderin deposits from minor hemorrhages or blood leaking through small vessels. Taking into account detection of CMBs depends on the MRI protocol, the prevalence of CMBs range from 5% in younger to approximately 20% in older subjects (Greenberg, Vernooij et al., 2009). Cerebral microbleeds have been shown to increase the likelihood of impaired cognition, or dementia (Qiu, Cotch et al., 2009). Another manifestation of cerebral microvascular disease is microinfarcts. Microinfarcts are a pervasive and very prevalent pathology that differ from larger infarcts in size and spatial distribution; they are below the limits of resolution of today's clinical neuroimaging methods and can only be seen on microscopic examination of brain tissue. Increasing untreated SBP was associated with an increased likelihood of having two or more microinfarcts (Wang, Larson et al., 2009). Presence of these

Table 1.1 **Hypertension and Elevated Blood Pressure Among Persons Ages 20 Years and Older, by Sex and Age: United States, 1988–1994 and 2001–2004**

	Hypertension[2,3]		Elevated blood pressure[2]	
	1988–1994	*2001–2004*	*1988–1994*	*2001–2004*
Male				
20–34 years..........................	7.1	7.0	6.6	6.1
35–44 years..........................	17.1	19.2	15.2	11.9
45–54 years..........................	29.2	35.9	21.9	23.0
55–64 years..........................	40.6	47.5	28.4	25.7
65–74 years..........................	54.4	61.7	39.9	30.2
75 years and over................	60.4	67.1	49.7	45.0
Female				
20–34 years..........................	2.9	2.7*	2.4*	*
35–44 years..........................	11.2	14.0	6.4	6.8
45–54 years..........................	23.9	35.2	13.7	22.3
55–64 years..........................	42.6	54.4	27.0	29.6
65–74 years..........................	56.2	72.9	38.2	48.3
75 years and over................	73.6	82.0	59.9	58.5

* Estimates are considered unreliable. Data preceded by an asterisk have a relative standard error of 20%–30%. Data not shown have an RSE greater than 30%.

Data are based on interviews and physical examinations of a sample of the civilian noninstitutionalized population

Source: Centers for Disease Control and Prevention, National Center for Health Statistics, National Health and Nutrition Examination Survey, Table 70.

microinfarcts has been associated with poorer ante-mortem cognitive function, particularly in those who died without a diagnosis of dementia (Launer, Hughes et. al., 2011).

NEURODEGENERATIVE PROCESSES

Elevated BP is also associated with brain atrophy. Although atrophy to some extent reflects the reabsorption of necrotic tissue caused by infarction, inflammatory processes, and demyelization, the major cause of atrophy in late age is neurodegeneration. There is evidence that elevated BP may directly or indirectly compromise neuronal viability, leading to neurodegeneration. Studies have shown elevated BP or hypertension is associated with smaller total brain (Strassburger, Lee et al., 1997; Heijer, Skoog et al., 2003) and hippocampal volumes (Korf, White et al., 2004) as well as higher Alzheimer's disease (AD) lesion load—that is, neurofibrillary tangles and neuritic plaques (Petrovitch, White et al., 2000). It is possible that the effect of hypertension on brain volume is increased in the presence of comorbidities or genetic susceptibility. For example, studies have shown having hypertension and T2D or hypertension and an Apolipoprotein E ε4 allele is associated with a higher risk for atrophy than having none or only one condition (Korf, White et al., 2004; Schmidt, Launer et al., 2004).

Pathophysiology: Why Elevated Blood Pressure Causes Brain Problems

There are several pathways through which elevated levels of BP can result in physiologic and pathologic changes that alter neuropsychologic functioning (Figure 1.1). Reflecting the findings in brain structure studies, experimental studies have suggested that hypertension can affect both vascular and neurodegenerative changes. Although the pathways leading to multiple pathologies may be independent of each other, the neuron and vessel thrive together, as described by the neurovascular (N-V) unit, and damage in one may result in

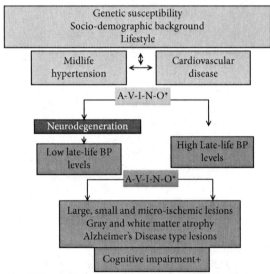

*Amyloid, vascular injury, inflammation, nutrition, oxidation

Figure 1.1 Pathways to high and low blood pressure (BP) in old age

damage in the other (Iadecola, 2004). Hypertension can lead to vascular damage through hypoxia, thrombosis, inflammation, oxidative stress, or atherosclerosis (Touyz & Briones, 2011; Girouard & Iadecola, 2006). Mechanical damage to the vessels can occur in the presence of aortic stiffness, excessive pressure, and when flow pulsatility is transferred to the carotids and cerebral microvasculature [Mitchell, van Buchem et al., 2011]. Hypertension also has a relatively unexplored link with β-amyloid metabolism, which is thought to initiate or be involved in the cascade leading to neurodegeneration (Hardy & Selkoe, 2002). Elevated BP may modulate or be modulated by Aβ1–40 and Aβ1–42 peptides by enhancing vasoconstriction. Aβ peptides may also contribute to cerebral vascular pathology and dysfunction when deposited in microvessels (Suo, Humphrey et al., 1998; Arendash, Su et al., 1999). Further, as encompassed in the N-V unit, hypertension can destroy neuronal cells by perturbing the interaction between vasoactive and metabolic factors controlling vascular health with neuronal and glial cells that maintain normal cerebral blood flow (Iadecola, 2004).

Thus hypertension may initiate or promote the cascade of inflammatory and oxidative responses (Tanzi, Moir et al., 2004) that lead to neurodegeneration. It should be noted that although most current and past research investigates β-amyloid toxicity, some forms of β-amyloid may also have a neuroprotective rescue function. It has been hypothesized this function becomes dysregulated in the presence of chronic hypertension (Cullen, Kocsi et al., 2006; Hardy & Cullen, 2006).

In addition to acting independently, or as a unit, there may be an interaction between the neuronal and vascular damage caused by elevated BP, such that vascular disease provides a local environment, such as one that is inflammatory or ischemic—that enhances the development and deposition of AD pathology or vice versa. Under this model, one would expect there to be more neuronal damage when there is vascular damage than in the absence of vascular damage. To date, studies suggest the two lesions have an additive effect on cognitive status (Snowdon, Greiner et al., 1997; Launer, Petrovitch et al., 2008). However, these analyses are limited to global measures of both the vascular and neurodegenerative measures, and data on a plaque level are scarce.

Risk for Cognitive Disorders Associated With Elevated Levels of Blood Pressure

Studies have suggested that elevated levels of BP are associated with impaired neuropsychologic functioning. The functions typically affected are in executive function domains, such as slowed information processing, trouble shifting from one task to another, and holding and manipulating information for further processing (Hachinski, Iadecola et al., 2006). These impairments are typical of a vascular-related cognitive disorder, of which hypertension is a major contributor. However, hypertension is also associated with impairment in other functions, such as verbal and nonverbal memory, which are typically affected in AD (Reed, Mungas et al., 2007). Hypertension has been associated with decline in test scores of these functions, as well as an increase in the occurrence of mild to severe levels of amnestic and multiple-domain mild cognitive impairment (Reitz, Tang et al., 2007). In addition to variability in function, the sequence of presentation and the relative dominance of impairment in specific cognitive functions are also variable (Hachinski, Iadecola et al., 2006). This clinical heterogeneity creates challenges to defining specific and sensitive phenotypes of vascular cognitive impairment (VCI) associated with hypertension specifically, and vascular disease in general (Reed, Mungas et al., 2007). Thus, to date there are no accepted standardized criteria for VCI. However, there are ongoing efforts to define the concept and characteristics of VCI and to harmonize and standardize definitions and tests used to assess VCI. The National Institute of Neurologic Disorders and Stroke-Canadian Stroke Network-sponsored publication (Hachinski, Iadecola et al., 2006) recommends several test batteries that vary in administration time, thus providing options depending on the context. Recently, the American Heart Association/American Stroke Association published a statement for healthcare providers summarizing the most recent evidence on diagnosis, as well as on pathology, treatment, and risk factors for VCI (Gorelick, Scuteri et al., 2011).

There is still controversy about whether dementia *per se* is more likely to occur in hypertensive compared to normotensive subjects. Studies of the association between hypertension and dementia are conflicting, particularly when the interval between the measure of BP and dementia diagnosis is not taken into account. Studies with short intervals between measures show increased risk, no risk, and risk in those with lower BP, only in treated individuals, or only in untreated patients (Qiu, Winblad et al., 2005). There are many reasons that could explain these inconsistencies, such as differences in prevailing medical practice to treat hypertension, subject access to health care, or other socioeconomic, lifestyle, and medical history factors. In addition, one confounding factor shown in studies with a long follow-up is the tendency for people close to converting to dementia to experience a significantly greater drop in BP than those not dementing (Stewart, Xue et al., 2009). This trend results in some studies with short intervals between BP and dementia measures showing higher BP protects against dementia. In general, these paradoxes and inconsistencies do not emerge in studies where BP was measured long before (i.e., middle age) dementia onset in late age. Several studies have robustly shown higher levels of midlife BP increases the risk for late-age dementia. These studies suggest high

BP increases the risk not only for vascular dementia, as would be expected, but also for AD (Qiu, Winblad et al., 2005).

Anti-Hypertensive Drugs and Cognition

OBSERVATIONAL STUDIES

Observational studies combined with experimental studies have identified several BP-regulating pathways and therapeutic targets that may be directly or indirectly active in processes leading to Alzheimer's pathology. Some studies (Haag, Hofman et al., 2009) have found treatment *per se* reduces the risk for AD, but have not found particular drug classes to be differentially associated with risk. In an analysis of the Leiden 85+ study, taking calcium-channel blockers reduced the risk for cognitive decline (Trompet, Westendorp et al., 2008), consistently with their effect on calcium homeostasis in reducing AD pathology (Hanon & Forette, 2004). To date, the most intensively investigated mechanisms have been within the renin–angiotensin system (RAS). The angiotension-converting enzyme 1 (ACE-1) can cleave the β-amyloid that is deposited in cerebral vessels and in extracellular space where neuritic plaques form (Kehoe & Wilcock, 2007). The RAS pathway is also an attractive therapeutic candidate based on evidence from meta-analyses that an insertion/deletion polymorphism in the ACE gene is associated with an increased risk for AD (Prince, Bird et al., 1996; Lehmann, Cortina-Borja et al., 2005). However, no single-nucleotide polymorphisms (SNPs) in this gene reached genome-wide significance in recent genome-wide association studies of AD, although there may be associations with relevant SNPs that were less than genome-wide significant (Seshadri, Fitzpatrick et al., 2010). Although several studies have suggested positive associations of anti-hypertensive medications (Li, Lee et al., 2010; Sink, Leng et al., 2009), these studies always need to be interpreted with the possibility of confounding by indication (the tendency for some drugs to be preferentially prescribed to persons who for other reasons have a reduced risk for AD or the tendency not to prescribe certain drugs to people who are cognitively impaired) in mind. Thus, some anti-hypertensive drugs could statistically look protective against AD, but it turns out they are not prescribed to people with cognitive impairment.

Clinical Trials

Several randomized clinical trials have investigated the efficacy of different anti-hypertensive medication versus placebo to reduce the occurrence of cognitive impairment or dementia. Several different classes of medications have been tested, including β-blockers (Prince, Bird et al., 1996; Prince, Rabe-Hesketh et al., 1998; Gurland, Teresi et al., 1988), ACE alone (Bosch, Yusuf et al. 2002) or with calcium-channel blockers (Forette, Seux et al., 2002) or diuretics (Tzourio, Anderson et al., 2003), angiotensin receptor blockers (ARBs) alone (Lithell, Hansson et al., 2003) or in combinations (Anderson, Teo et al., 2011; Diener, Sacco et al., 2008), or a diuretic (Peters, Beckett et al., 2008). In general the most frequently used cognitive measure in these trials is a measure of global cognitive impairment (Mini-Mental State Examination MMSE); the eligible participants have hypertension or CV disease and were provided treatment for 2 years to 4 years. A recent Cochrane Review of four of these studies did not find strong evidence that treatment of hypertension with any specific drug reduced the risk for cognitive impairment or dementia (McGuinness, Todd et al., 2009). However, exploratory subanalyses of trial data have provided clues about groups that may benefit most from an intervention. For example, after an extended (5-year) follow-up of Syst Eur trial participants, there was a statistically significant reduction in the risk for dementia (Forette, Seux et al., 2002). In subanalyses of other trials, some subgroups of the patient population seemed to benefit cognitively more than others. In the SCOPE trial, those with low baseline cognitive function seemed to benefit from the intervention (Skoog, Lithell et al., 2005). In PROGRESS, the Syst Eur trial and in the ONTARGET/TRANSCEND trial, those with the lowest BP declined the least in the MMSE, regardless of treatment (Anderson, Teo et al., 2011).

There are several reasons why clinical trials may not have shown overall benefit, including age of the cohort, cohort medical history, where the cohort is in the trajectory toward pathologic cognitive decline, baseline BP, the achieved BP differences between placebo and treatment group, the duration of treatment, and, in many trials, the sensitivity and number of cognitive outcome measures

There is a new National Heart Lung and Blood Institute hypertension trial (SPRINT) that takes a novel approach; rather than testing one or two medications against a placebo control group, SPRINT is designed to compare two theraputic strategies with two different treatment goals. The intensive strategy aims to lower SBP to less than 120 mmHG, and the standard therapy aims to lower SBP to 140 mmHG. Eligible individuals are at least 55 years old, with SBP of 130 mmHg to 180 mmHg on no or one medication or 130 mmHg to 170 mmHg on up to two medications, and 130 mmHg to 160 mmHg on up to three medications. Targeted subgroups are those with chronic kidney disease (eGFR 25–59 mL/min/1.73 m^2), presence of clinical or subclinical CV disease other than stroke and diabetes, a Framingham Risk Score for 10-year CV disease risk 15% or greater, and age older than 75 years. The trial is currently recruiting with a goal of 9250. This trial has a substantial cognitive component (SPRINT MIND), which includes all respondents getting a three-test cognitive screening battery and a neuropsychologic battery on a random sample and on individuals who "fail" the screening criteria. To reach an adjudicated diagnosis of dementia, proxies of screen positives subjects are administered a questionnaire. In addition, a subsample will undergo magnetic resonance imaging with structural and functional sequences. Subjects will be followed 4 years to 6 years (http://clinicaltrials.gov/ct2/show/NCT01206062).

Prevention

Based on these studies, the question arises: Will a shift in the population distribution of midlife BP to lower levels be associated with lower rates of dementia in the population? The population attributable risk (PAR) describes the proportion of cases that could be prevented if a specific exposure were eliminated in a target population (Launer, Hughes et al., 2010). In the context of BP level, the PAR measures the potential impact on cognitive impairment and dementia rates of reducing elevated levels of BP in the population. Based on a systematic review of published articles on midlife BP and cognitive end-points, it has been estimated that worldwide, about 5.1% (1.4–9.9) (1.7 million) of AD cases are potentially attributable to midlife hypertension (Barnes & Yaffe, 2011).

A more in-depth estimation of PAR taking into account competing risk for death and control for comorbidity and other factors that covary with hypertension found 27% (95% CI 8.9%, 42.1%) of dementia cases can be attributed to untreated midlife levels of systolic BP greater than120 mmHG. This translates into 17 excess cases per 1000. Of these, there are 17.7% (95% CI 4.6%–29.1%) of cases that are attributable to prehypertensive levels (SBP 120 mmHg to <140 mmHG) of BP, regardless of treatment status, which translates into 11 excess cases per 1000. These estimates are based on a combination of risk and number of cases in the HAAS cohort (Launer, Hughes et al., 2010). In this cohort, the PAR for hypertension is lower than for prehypertension. This reflects the fact that this hypertensive group includes the smallest proportion of the sample and is at significantly increased risk for death compared to others, and the *prehypertension* group has a moderately raised risk for dementia, a similar risk for death compared to normotensives, and a higher number of prehypertensive men and cases. Because the population distributions of SBP vary by sex, race/ethnic group, socio-economic status, diet, the force of mortality associated with elevated BP, as well as other factors (Launer, Hughes et al., 2010), as for any PAR, separate calculations are needed for subgroups in the population.

Summary

There is an extensive body of experimental, clinical, and epidemiologic data supporting the hypothesis that elevated levels of BP increase the risk for cognitive disorders in late life. For reasons described above, to date there is no consistent randomized trial data supporting the use of BP control to reduce the occurrence of cognitive disorders. Because the effects of elevated BP on late-life cognitive disorders may take a long time, longitudinal observational study results, especially with a life-course approach, in addition to clinical trials are an important source of information on the impact of elevated BP on reducing cognitive impairment. In the interim there are many other reasons for treating elevated BP.

References

Anderson, C., K. Teo, et al.(2011) Renin-angiotensin system blockade and cognitive function in patients at high risk of cardiovascular disease: analysis of data from the ONTARGET and TRANSCEND studies. *Lancet Neurol 10*(1): 43–53.

Arendash, G. W., G. C. Su, et al. (1999). Intravascular beta-amyloid infusion increases blood pressure: implications for a vasoactive role of beta-amyloid in the pathogenesis of Alzheimer's disease. *Neurosci Lett 268*(1): 17–20.

Barnes, D. E. & K. Yaffe "The projected effect of risk factor reduction on Alzheimer's disease prevalence. *Lancet Neurol 10*(9): 819–828.

Bosch, J., S. Yusuf, et al. (2002). Use of ramipril in preventing stroke: double blind randomised trial. *BMJ 324*(7339): 699–702.

Chobanian, A. V., G. L. Bakris, et al. (2003). Seventh report of the Joint National Committee on Prevention, Detection, Evaluation, and Treatment of High Blood Pressure. *Hypertension 42*(6): 1206–1252.

Cullen, K. M., Z. Kocsi, et al. (2006). Microvascular pathology in the aging human brain: evidence that senile plaques are sites of microhaemorrhages. *Neurobiology of Aging 27*(12): 1786–1796.

Debette, S. & H. S. Markus (2010) "The clinical importance of white matter hyperintensities on brain magnetic resonance imaging: systematic review and meta-analysis." *BMJ 341*: c3666.

Diener, H. C., R. L. Sacco, et al. (2008). Effects of aspirin plus extended-release dipyridamole versus clopidogrel and telmisartan on disability and cognitive function after recurrent stroke in patients with ischaemic stroke in the Prevention Regimen for Effectively Avoiding Second Strokes (PRoFESS) trial: a double-blind, active and placebo-controlled study. *Lancet Neurol 7*(10): 875–884.

Egan, B. M., Y. Zhao, et al. (2010) US trends in prevalence, awareness, treatment, and control of hypertension, 1988–2008. *JAMA 303*(20): 2043–2050.

Forette, F., M. L. Seux, et al. (2002). The prevention of dementia with antihypertensive treatment: new evidence from the Systolic Hypertension in Europe (Syst-Eur) study. *Archives of Internal Medicine 162*(18): 2046–2052.

Girouard, H. & C. Iadecola (2006). Neurovascular coupling in the normal brain and in hypertension, stroke, and Alzheimer disease. *J Appl Physiol 100*(1): 328–335.

Gorelick, P. B., A. Scuteri, et al. (2011) Vascular Contributions to Cognitive Impairment and Dementia: A Statement for Healthcare Professionals From the American Heart Association/American Stroke Association. *Stroke 42*(9): 2672–2713.

Greenberg, S. M., M. W. Vernooij, et al. (2009). Cerebral microbleeds: a guide to detection and interpretation. *Lancet Neurol 8*(2): 165–174.

Gurland, B. J., J. Teresi, et al. (1988). Effects of treatment for isolated systolic hypertension on cognitive status and depression in the elderly. *Journal of the American Geriatrics Society 36*(11): 1015–1022.

Haag, M. D., A. Hofman, et al. (2009). Duration of antihypertensive drug use and risk of dementia: A prospective cohort study. *Neurology 72*(20): 1727–1734.

Hachinski, V., C. Iadecola, et al. (2006). National Institute of Neurological Disorders and Stroke-Canadian Stroke Network vascular cognitive impairment harmonization standards. *Stroke* 37(9): 2220–2241.

Hanon, O. & F. Forette (2004). Prevention of dementia: lessons from SYST-EUR and PROGRESS. *J Neurol Sci* 226(1-2): 71–74.

Hardy, J. & K. Cullen (2006). Amyloid at the blood vessel wall. *Nat Med* 12(7): 756–757.

Hardy, J. & D. J. Selkoe (2002). The amyloid hypothesis of Alzheimer's disease: progress and problems on the road to therapeutics. *Science* 297(5580): 353–356.

Heijer, T., I. Skoog, et al. (2003). Association between blood pressure levels over time and brain atrophy in the elderly. *Neurobiology of Aging* 24(2): 307–313.

Iadecola, C. (2004). Neurovascular regulation in the normal brain and in Alzheimer's disease. *Nat Rev Neurosci* 5(5): 347–360.

Kehoe, P. G. & G. K. Wilcock (2007). Is inhibition of the renin-angiotensin system a new treatment option for Alzheimer's disease? *Lancet Neurol* 6(4): 373–378.

Korf, E. S., L. R. White, et al. (2004). Midlife blood pressure and the risk of hippocampal atrophy: the Honolulu Asia Aging Study. *Hypertension* 44(1): 29–34.

Kruit, M. C., M. A. van Buchem, et al. (2004). Migraine as a risk factor for subclinical brain lesions. *JAMA* 291(4): 427–434.

Launer, L. J., T. Hughes, et al. (2010) Lowering midlife levels of systolic blood pressure as a public health strategy to reduce late-life dementia: perspective from the Honolulu Heart Program/Honolulu Asia Aging Study. *Hypertension* 55(6): 1352–1359.

Launer L. J., Hughes T. M., White L. R. (2011) Microinfarcts, brain atrophy, and cognitive function: the Honolulu Asia Aging Study Autopsy Study. *Ann Neurol.* 70(5):774–780.

Launer, L. J., H. Petrovitch, et al. (2008). AD brain pathology: vascular origins? Results from the HAAS autopsy study. *Neurobiology of Aging* 29(10): 1587–1590.

Lehmann, D. J., M. Cortina-Borja, et al. (2005). Large meta-analysis establishes the ACE insertion-deletion polymorphism as a marker of Alzheimer's disease. *American Journal of Epidemiology* 162(4): 305–317.

Lewington, S., R. Clarke, et al. (2002). Age-specific relevance of usual blood pressure to vascular mortality: a meta-analysis of individual data for one million adults in 61 prospective studies. *Lancet* 360(9349): 1903–1913.

Li, N. C., A. Lee, et al. (2010) Use of angiotensin receptor blockers and risk of dementia in a predominantly male population: prospective cohort analysis. *BMJ* 340: b5465.

Liao, D., L. Cooper, et al. (1996). Presence and severity of cerebral white matter lesions and hypertension, its treatment, and its control. The ARIC Study. Atherosclerosis Risk in Communities Study. *Stroke* 27(12): 2262–2270.

Lithell, H., L. Hansson, et al. (2003). The Study on Cognition and Prognosis in the Elderly (SCOPE): principal results of a randomized double-blind intervention trial. *J Hypertens* 21(5): 875–886.

McGuinness, B., S. Todd, et al. (2009). Blood pressure lowering in patients without prior cerebrovascular disease for prevention of cognitive impairment and dementia. *Cochrane Database Syst Rev*(4): CD004034.

Mitchell GF, van Buchem MA, et al. (2011). Arterial stiffness, pressure and flow pulsatility and brain structure and function: the Age, Gene/Environment Susceptibility—Reykjavik study. *Brain.* 134(Pt 11):3398–3407.

Peters, R., N. Beckett, et al. (2008). Incident dementia and blood pressure lowering in the Hypertension in the Very Elderly Trial cognitive function assessment (HYVET-COG): a double-blind, placebo controlled trial. *Lancet Neurol* 7(8): 683–689.

Petrovitch, H., L. R. White, et al. (2000). Midlife blood pressure and neuritic plaques, neurofibrillary tangles, and brain weight at death: the HAAS. Honolulu-Asia aging Study. *Neurobiology of Aging.* 21(1): 57–62.

Prince, M., S. Rabe-Hesketh, et al. (1998). Do antiarthritic drugs decrease the risk for cognitive decline? An analysis based on data from the MRC treatment trial of hypertension in older adults. *Neurology* 50(2): 374–379.

Prince, M. J., A. S. Bird, et al. (1996). Is the cognitive function of older patients affected by antihypertensive treatment? Results from 54 months of the Medical Research Council's trial of hypertension in older adults. *BMJ 312*(7034): 801–805.

Qiu, C., M. F. Cotch, et al. (2009) Cerebral microbleeds, retinopathy, and dementia: the AGES-Reykjavik Study. *Neurology 75*(24): 2221–2228.

Qiu, C., B. Winblad, et al. (2005). The age-dependent relation of blood pressure to cognitive function and dementia. *Lancet Neurol 4*(8): 487–499.

Reed, B. R., D. M. Mungas, et al. (2007). Profiles of neuropsychological impairment in autopsy-defined Alzheimer's disease and cerebrovascular disease. *Brain 130*(Pt 3): 731–739.

Reitz, C., M. X. Tang, et al. (2007). Hypertension and the risk of mild cognitive impairment. *Archives of Neurology 64*(12): 1734–1740.

Schmidt, R., L. J. Launer, et al. (2004). Magnetic resonance imaging of the brain in diabetes: the Cardiovascular Determinants of Dementia (CASCADE) Study. *Diabetes 53*(3): 687–692.

Seshadri, S., A. L. Fitzpatrick, et al. (2010) Genome-wide analysis of genetic loci associated with Alzheimer disease. *JAMA 303*(18): 1832–1840.

Sink, K. M., X. Leng, et al. (2009). Angiotensin-converting enzyme inhibitors and cognitive decline in older adults with hypertension: results from the Cardiovascular Health Study. *Archives of Internal Medicine 169*(13): 1195–1202.

Skoog, I., H. Lithell, et al. (2005). Effect of baseline cognitive function and antihypertensive treatment on cognitive and cardiovascular outcomes: Study on COgnition and Prognosis in the Elderly (SCOPE). *Am J Hypertens 18*(8): 1052–1059.

Snowdon, D. A., L. H. Greiner, et al. (1997). Brain infarction and the clinical expression of Alzheimer disease. The Nun Study. *JAMA 277*(10): 813–817.

Stewart, R., Q. L. Xue, et al. (2009). Change in blood pressure and incident dementia: a 32-year prospective study. *Hypertension 54*(2): 233–240.

Strassburger, T. L., H. C. Lee, et al. (1997). Interactive effects of age and hypertension on volumes of brain structures. *Stroke 28*(7): 1410–1417.

Suo, Z., J. Humphrey, et al. (1998). Soluble Alzheimers beta-amyloid constricts the cerebral vasculature in vivo. *Neurosci Lett 257*(2): 77–80.

Tanzi, R. E., R. D. Moir, et al. (2004). Clearance of Alzheimer's Abeta peptide: the many roads to perdition. *Neuron 43*(5): 605–608.

Touyz, R. M. and A. M. Briones (2011). Reactive oxygen species and vascular biology: implications in human hypertension. *Hypertens Res 34*(1): 5–14.

Trompet, S., R. G. Westendorp, et al. (2008). Use of calcium antagonists and cognitive decline in old age. The Leiden 85-plus study. *Neurobiology of Aging 29*(2): 306–308.

Tzourio, C., C. Anderson, et al. (2003). Effects of blood pressure lowering with perindopril and indapamide therapy on dementia and cognitive decline in patients with cerebrovascular disease. *Archives of Internal Medicine 163*(9): 1069–1075.

Vermeer S. E., N. D. Prins, et al. (2003). Silent brain infarcts and the risk of dementia and cognitive decline. *N Engl J Med. 348*(13):1215–1222.

Wang, L. Y., E. B. Larson, et al. (2009). Blood pressure and brain injury in older adults: findings from a community-based autopsy study. *Journal of the American Geriatrics Society 57*(11): 1975–1981.

2

Cholesterol, Statins, and Late-Life Cognitive Disorders

ALINA SOLOMON, MD, PHD, AND MIIA KIVIPELTO, MD, PHD

Introduction

The brain is the most cholesterol-rich organ of the human body yet, compared to circulating cholesterol, little is known about brain cholesterol metabolism or about the interactions between the two cholesterol pools. Cholesterol research has long been dominated by the associations with atherosclerosis and heart disease, the topic of numerous debates throughout most of the twentieth century (Steinberg, 2004). While the roles of circulating lipoproteins were being defined, the possibility of cholesterol influencing central nervous system (CNS) functions also received some attention. It was suggested, for example, that plasma cholesterol levels in the new born infant might affect brain development and even intelligence (Dietschy, 2004). But the fact that brain cholesterol metabolism was different from sterol metabolism in the rest of the body did not become clear until the end of the 1960s (Dietschy, 2004). Nearly 30 years later, the first interactions between the two cholesterol pools were shown (Björkhem, 2004).

This chapter provides an overview of current research on cholesterol and lipid-lowering drugs in the prevention and treatment of dementia-related diseases, particularly Alzheimer's disease (AD) and vascular dementia (VaD). A first glance at the literature on cholesterol and late-life cognitive disorders reveals many conflicting findings that emphasize several important problems within the dementia research field. Alzheimer's disease, the main cause of dementia, has a long preclinical phase before symptoms start to appear (Jack et al., 2011). However, because current diagnostic criteria and most trials are focused on dementia, a later stage in the pathophysiology of AD, the window of opportunity for effective interventions may be missed. In addition, the Alzheimer-vascular diagnostic dichotomy has delayed the recognition of vascular factors as modifiable risk factors for AD, as well as the recognition of cognitive symptoms as important manifestations of cerebrovascular disease.

In this chapter, we focus on potential sources of contradictions between studies, methodological adjustments, and future investigations that are needed for translation of research findings from bench to bedside. It has become clear that cholesterol alone will not provide an easy solution to such complex problems. Rather, a change of research strategy is needed, with a life-course perspective and a more integrative, transdisciplinary approach to late-life cognitive disorders.

Genetic Risk Factors and Cholesterol

Although the link between cholesterol and VaD was suggested several decades ago (i.e., Mumenthaler, 1975), plasma lipids were initially thought to be useful mainly in separating VaD from AD (i.e., Muckle, 1985, Erkinjuntti, 1988), as the underlying mechanisms for these disorders were believed to be unrelated. The main studies reporting an association between AD and cholesterol were published in the beginning of the 1990s. The ε4 allele of the cholesterol transporter apolipoprotein E (APOE ε4) was reported as a major risk factor for AD (Corder, 1993; Poirier, 1993), and abundant senile plaques were described in the brains of non-demented patients with coronary artery disease (Sparks, 1990).

The APOE–AD association has been confirmed in several studies worldwide, and to date the APOE ε4 allele is the only genetic risk factor for AD of established general significance (www.alzgene.org). The APOE ε4 allele appears to be a risk factor for stroke and VaD as well (Schmidt, 2002), although conflicting results have been reported in some studies (Tonk, 2007; Kim, 2008). Problems with outcome definitions caused by the heterogeneity of both stroke and VaD are a likely cause of differences in results. Apolipoprotein E has a central role in lipid metabolism, and the APOE ε4 allele is associated with increased plasma total and low-density lipoprotein (LDL) cholesterol levels, atherosclerosis, and coronary heart disease (Hooijmans, 2008). However, the mechanisms relating different apolipoprotein E isoforms to AD pathophysiology are not completely understood. Within the brain, apolipoprotein E has many functions: being involved in cholesterol and phospholipid redistribution during development, regeneration after brain injury, and synaptic plasticity; deposition and clearance of β-amyloid (Aβ); inflammatory processes; aggregation of tau proteins; neurotransmission; neuronal survival, and sprouting (Hooijmans, 2008).

Genetic and environmental risk factors are most often considered separately, but their interactions in relation to the risk of cognitive impairment need more attention. APOEε4 carriers, for example, may be more vulnerable to environmental factors (e.g., physical inactivity, saturated fat intake, alcohol drinking, diabetes, high blood pressure, low B12/folate) and thus may benefit more from lifestyle changes and pharmacological interventions (Kivipelto, 2008). Apart from APOE, more than 100 additional genes related to cholesterol metabolism have been linked to AD (Carter, 2007). However, the individual role of other such genes is unclear because of different results in different populations. More answers may be found by studying genetic synergies and interactions rather than individual genes (Carter, 2007). An interesting approach is to calculate aggregate cholesterol-related genetic risk scores. Such scores have been associated with, for example, PET measurements of hypometabolism in AD-affected brain regions (Reiman, 2008).

Circulating Cholesterol in Epidemiological Studies: What Happens Between Midlife and Late Life?

Table 2.1 (midlife cholesterol), Table 2.2 (late-life cholesterol), and Table 2.3 (life-course approach) summarize the main longitudinal population-based studies investigating the association between cholesterol and dementia/cognition. This grouping of studies provides important keys to making sense of the large and confusing research literature on cholesterol and late-life cognition.

Of the long-term follow-up studies on total cholesterol at midlife (Table 2.1), the Finnish Cohort of the Seven Countries Study (Notkola, 1998) and the Cardiovascular Risk Factors, Aging and Incidence of Dementia (CAIDE) study (Kivipelto 2001) in Finland, as well as the Kaiser Permanente Medical Care Program of Northern California in the United States (Whitmer, 2005; Solomon, 2009) reported elevated cholesterol as a risk factor for subsequent dementia, AD, VaD, or mild cognitive impairment (MCI). The 2002 Adult Treatment Panel (ATP) III guidelines define total cholesterol levels as desirable (<200 mg/dL or <5.2 mmol/L), borderline (200–239 mg/dL or 5.2–6.2 mmol/L), or high (≥240 mg/dL or ≥6.2 mmol/L). Not only high cholesterol but also levels within the borderline range seemed to increase the risk of AD and VaD (Solomon, 2009).

In the Honolulu-Asia Aging Study (HAAS), clustered cardiovascular risk factors (including cholesterol) were associated with increased risk of dementia, VaD, or AD with cerebrovascular disease but not AD alone (Kalmijn, 2000). No significant associations between midlife cholesterol and dementia were reported in the Israeli Ischemic Heart Disease Study (Beeri, 2004) or the Prospective Population Study of Women in Gothenburg, Sweden (Mielke, 2010). Differences between populations and outcome definitions in these studies could explain the differences in results.

In the Framingham study in the United States, with more than 40 years of follow-up and cholesterol measurements from several occasions starting at midlife, a different approach was used in the analyses (averaging total cholesterol levels

Table 2.1 **Observational Studies of Mid-Life Total Cholesterol (TC) and Risk of Subsequent Cognitive Impairment/Dementia**

Study	Population and follow-up time	Cognitive impairment/ dementia
Notkola et al. (*Neuroepidemiology* 1998; 17:14–20)	*n* = 444 men Baseline age: 40–59 years Follow-up: 15–25 years	Elevated TC and OR (95% CI) for AD: 3.1 (1.2–8.5)
Kalmijn et al. (*Arterioscler. Thromb. Vasc. Biol.* 2000;*20*:2255–2260)	*n* = 3734 men Mean baseline age: 53 years Mean follow-up: 25 years	Clustered cardiovascular risk factors (including TC) and RR (95% CI) for: – Dementia 1.05 (1.02–1.09) – AD 1.00 (0.94–1.05) – AD with CVD 1.06 (0.97–1.15) – VaD 1.11 (1.05–1.18) TC and RR (95% CI) for dementia: 1.10 (0.95–1.26)
Kivipelto et al. (*BMJ* 2001; 322 (7300):1447–1451)	*n* = 1449 Mean baseline age: 50 years Mean follow-up: 21 years	Elevated TC and OR (95% CI) for AD: 2.1 (1.0–4.4)
Kivipelto et al. (*Neurology* 2001; *56*(12):1683–1689)	*n* = 1352 Mean baseline age: 50 years Mean follow-up: 21 years	Elevated TC and OR (95% CI) MCI: 1.9 (1.2–3.0)
Tan et al. (*Arch. Intern. Med.* 2003; *163*:1053–1057)	*n* = 1026 Mean baseline age: 66 years TC averaged more than 30 years Follow-up: 10 years	Elevated TC and HR (95% CI) for AD: 0.95 (0.87–1.04)
Beeri et al. (*Neurology* 2004; *63*:1902–1907)	*n* = 1892 men Mean baseline age: 44.8 years Follow-up: 36 years	Elevated TC and OR (95% CI) for dementia: 1.00 (0.99–1.01)

(*continued*)

Table 2.1 **(Continued)**

Study	Population and follow-up time	Cognitive impairment/ dementia
Whitmer et al. (*Neurology* 2005;64: 277–281)	n = 8845 Baseline age: 40–44 years Mean follow-up: 27 years	Elevated TC and HR (95% CI) for dementia: 1.42 (1.22–1.66)
Elias et al. (*Psychosom. Med.* 2005; 67:24–30)	n = 1894 Mean baseline age = 66 years TC averaged over 16–18 years Follow-up: 4–6 years	Lower TC and OR (95% CI) for lower cognitive test performance: 1.49 (1.02–2.18)
Solomon et al. (*Dement. Geriatr. Cogn. Disord.* 2009;28:75–80)	n = 9,844 Baseline age: 40–45 years Follow-up: 30 years	Elevated TC and HR (95% CI) for: – AD 1.57 (1.23–2.01) – VaD 1.50 (1.01–2.23)
Mielke et al. (*Neurology* 2010;75: 1888–1895)	n = 1,462 women Baseline age: 38–60 years Follow-up: 32 years	Elevated TC and HR (95% CI) for dementia: 1.68 (0.80–3.52 Elevated TC and HR (95% CI) for AD: 2.82 (0.94–8.43)

over 30 years; Tan, 2003; Elias, 2005). This approach does not allow conclusions on the relation between midlife cholesterol and subsequent dementia/cognitive impairment.

The relation between late-life cholesterol levels and cognitive impairment/ dementia is less straightforward. Shorter-term follow-up studies of older individuals (Table 2.2) report either no association or results that are opposite to those using midlife as a baseline (Table 2.1). These contradictions likely indicate that the effect of an adverse lipid profile does not remain constant with age. Several cross-sectional and longitudinal studies have shown that total cholesterol levels tend to increase with age in young- or middle-aged adults but later decrease as individuals get older (Abbott, 1997). This pattern can be partly explained by physiological aging, unintentional or voluntary changes in lifestyle (i.e., cardiovascular prevention programs meant to lower cholesterol levels), or selective mortality. However, there is another explanation that must be considered. The relationship between cholesterol and health status may be bidirectional, as lower cholesterol levels are frequently observed in association with clinical and subclinical diseases (Ferrara, 1997), and a decrease in cholesterol levels, although beneficial for other age groups, may reflect early or occult disease or a gradual decline in the overall health of older persons. Chronic diseases with a long preclinical phase (such as AD or even cerebrovascular disease) pose

Table 2.2 Observational Studies of Late-Life Cholesterol and Risk of Cognitive Impairment/Dementia

Study	Population and follow-up time	Risk of cognitive impairment/dementia
Yoshitake et al. (*Neurology* 1995; 45(6):1161–1168)	n = 828 Mean age: 73.6 years Follow-up: 7 years	Elevated TC and RR (95% CI) for: - AD 1.10 (0.80–1.51) - VaD 0.89 (0.66–1.21)
Hyman et al. (*Ann. Neurol.* 1996;40:55–66)	n = 1899 Mean age: 79.1 Follow-up: 4–7 years	Elevated TC and OR (95% CI) for cognitive impairment: 0.997 (0.993–0.999)
Kalmijn et al. (*Stroke* 1996;27:2230–2235)	n = 353 men Mean age: 74.6 years Follow-up: 3 years	Elevated TC and OR (95% CI) for cognitive decline: 1.0 (0.4–2.6) Elevated HDL-C and OR (95% CI) for cognitive decline: 2.0 (0.6–7.1)
Kuusisto et al. (*BMJ* 1997; 315(7115):1045–1049)	n = 980 Mean age: 73–74 years Follow-up: 3.5 years	Elevated TC and OR (95% CI) for AD 0.69 (0.52–0.92)
Wada et al. (*J. Am. Geriatr. Soc.* 1997; 45:1411–1412)	n = 93 Mean age: 79.4 years Follow-up: 3 years	Decline in MMSE scores more pronounced in the low TC group (p = 0.0178)
Romas et al. (*Neurology* 1999;53:517–521)	n = 987 Mean age: 73 years Follow-up: 2.5 years	Lower TC and OR (95% CI) for AD: 1.3 (0.8–2.1)
Slooter et al. (*Neurology* 2000; 54:2356–2358)	n = 6435 Mean age: 69.5 years Follow-up: 5.8 years	Elevated TC and OR (95% CI) for: - Dementia 0.95 (0.69–1.31) - AD 0.98 (0.66–1.45) - VaD 2.00 (0.85–4.70)

Reference	Demographics	Results
Karlamangla et al. (*J. Am. Geriatr. Soc.* 2004; 52:487–494)	$n = 267$ Mean age: 74 years Follow-up: 4.5 years	Elevated non-HDL-C and OR (95% CI) for cognitive decline 0.86 (0.73–1.02)
Reitz et al. (*Arch. Neurol.* 2004; 61:705–714)	$n = 1168$ Mean age: 78.4 years Follow-up: 4.8 years	Elevated TC and HR (95% CI) for – AD 0.48 (0.26–0.86) – VaD 1.05 (0.42–2.60) Elevated non-HDL-C and HR (95% CI) for – AD 0.60 (0.34–1.04) – VaD 2.01 (0.84–4.77) Elevated HDL-C and HR (95% CI) for – AD 0.70 (0.37–1.32) – VaD 0.81 (0.32–2.05) Elevated LDL-C and HR (95% CI) for – AD 0.80 (0.46–1.40) – VaD 2.07 (0.85–5.06)
Solfrizzi et al. (*Neurology* 2004; 63:1882–1891)	$n = 2963$ Mean age: 71.8 years Follow-up: 3.5 years	Elevated TC and RR (95% CI) for MCI 0.67 (0.45–1.00)
Li et al. (*Neurology* 2005; 65:1045–1050)	$n = 2141$ Mean age: 74.9 years Follow-up: 5.6 years	Elevated TC and HR (95% CI) for: – Dementia 1.16 (0.81–1.67) – AD 1.00 (0.61–1.62) Lower HDL-C and HR (95% CI) for: – Dementia 1.04 (0.69–1.55) – AD 1.23 (0.71–2.15)

(*continued*)

Table 2.2 **(Continued)**

Study	Population and follow-up time	Risk of cognitive impairment/dementia
Mielke et al. (*Neurology* 2005; 64:1689–1695)	*n* = 382 Age: 70 years Follow-up: up to 18 years	Elevated TC at different ages and HR (95% CI) for dementia between ages 79–88 years: – at age 70: 0.77 (0.61–0.96) – at age 75: 0.70 (0.52–0.93) – at age 79: 0.73 (0.55–0.98)
Reitz et al. (*Neurology* 2005; 64:1378–1383)	*n* = 1147 Mean age: 76.3 years Follow-up: 7 years	Elevated TC and HR (95% CI) for low cognitive performance 1.0 (0.9–1.1) Elevated HDL-C and HR (95% CI) for low cognitive performance 0.9 (0.9–1.1) Elevated LDL-C and HR (95% CI) for low cognitive performance 1.0 (0.9–1.0)
Vanhanen et al. (*Neurology* 2006; 67(5):843–847)	*n* = 959 Mean age: 73 years Follow-up: 3.5 years	Elevated TC and OR (95% CI) for AD: 0.68 (0.51–0.91)
Reitz et al. (*Dement. Geriatr. Cogn. Disord.* 2008; 25(3):232–237)	*n* = 854 Mean age: 76 years Follow-up: about 5 years	Elevated TC and HR (95% CI) for MCI: 0.8 (0.57–1.11) Elevated HDL-C and HR (95% CI) for MCI: 0.9 (0.65–1.20) Elevated LDL-C and HR (95% CI) for MCI: 0.8 (0.54–1.04)
Reitz et al. (*Arch. Neurol.* 2010; 67(12):1491–1497)	*n* = 1130 Mean age: 75.7 years Follow-up: 4469 person-years	Elevated TC and HR (95% CI) for AD: 0.8 (0.4–1.5) Elevated HDL-C and HR (95% CI) for AD: 0.5 (0.3–0.9) Elevated non-HDL-C and HR (95% CI) for AD: 0.7 (0.4–1.3) Elevated LDL-C and HR (95% CI) for AD: 0.9 (0.5–1.7)

inherent difficulties in risk factor identification. Because disease onset cannot be pinpointed, it is difficult to disentangle true risk relationships (factors increasing the probability of getting the disease) and reverse causality (the effects of the disease itself on various factors). Most populations in late life will be a mixture of individuals without the disease and individuals who have the disease, although clinically silent and undiagnosed. Therefore, midlife is more suitable as a start point when looking for risk factors, because the disease is not so likely to already be present.

More recent epidemiological studies are taking these issues into account by investigating not only cholesterol at specific time-points over the life-course but also the pattern of change in cholesterol levels from midlife to late life in relation to cognition and dementia (Table 2.3). There are several reports that cholesterol levels decline over time—particularly in people who develop dementia or cognitive impairment. Interestingly, similar patterns have been reported for other risk factors such as blood pressure or body mass index. In predicting dementia, midlife profiles are clearly different from profiles at older ages (Kivipelto, 2006; Barnes, 2009).

Minding the Blood–Brain Barrier

Epidemiological studies have focused mainly on circulating total cholesterol levels, and very little is known about the links between brain cholesterol and dementia-related diseases. As the blood–brain barrier (BBB) separates the brain from the circulation, brain cholesterol homeostasis is mostly independent from the periphery (Björkhem, 2004). The human brain accounts for only 2% of the total body mass but contains 25% of the total cholesterol in the body. Most brain cholesterol (about 70%–80%) is in myelin, and another pool is represented by neurons and glial cells. Because about 90% of brain cells are glial cells, neurons contribute to only a small fraction of the total brain cholesterol (Vance, 2005). In cells, cholesterol is mainly found in the cell membrane—particularly in lipid rafts—but it is also part of the membranes of intracellular organelles performing specialized tasks.

Cellular cholesterol homeostasis is maintained by the balance of synthesis, transport, storage, and degradation, with important differences in the brain compared to the rest of the body. Synthesis in the developing CNS is relatively high but declines to a very low level in the adult because of efficient recycling (Björkhem, 2004). Brain cholesterol thus has an extremely long half-life, estimated to be at least 5 years (Björkhem, 2004). Oligodendrocytes have a clear role in myelin formation, but the roles of neurons and astrocytes in cholesterol synthesis are poorly understood. Brain cholesterol homeostasis is not uniform,

Table 2.3 **Observational Studies of Cholesterol at Different Ages and Time-Points in Relation to Cognition**

Study (reference)	Population and follow-up time	Main results
Stewart et al. (*Arch. Neurol.* 2007; 64:103–107)	1027 Japanese American men Study baseline: midlife Follow-up: 26 years	Cholesterol levels in men with dementia/AD declined at least 15 years before diagnosis.
Solomon et al. (*Neurology* 2007; 68:751–756)	1449 Finnish men and women Study baseline: midlife Follow-up: 21 years	Decline in TC and OR (95%CI) for more impaired cognition (MCI or dementia): 3.5 (1.5–8.0)
Solomon et al. (*Neurobiol Aging* 2009; 30:1006–1009)	1382 non-demented Finnish men and women Study baseline: midlife Follow-up: 21 years	A more pronounced decrease in total cholesterol from midlife to late life was related to poorer late-life episodic memory and psychomotor speed but not if subjects used statins.
Mielke et al. (*Neurology* 2010; 75:1888–1895)	1,462 Swedish women Study baseline: midlife Follow-up: 32 years	Decline in TC and HR (95% CI) for dementia: 2.35 (1.22–4.58)
van Vliet et al. (*J. Neurol. Neurosurg. Psychiatry* 2010;81: 1028–1032)	599 women and men Study baseline: late life (>85 years) Follow-up: 5 years	In old age, cognitive decline preceded declines in total cholesterol and HDL levels.
Reynolds et al. (*J. Am. Geriatr. Soc.* 2010; 58:501–509)	819 men and women Study baseline: all age groups (range: 50–96 years) Follow-up: 16 years	High lipid levels may constitute a more important risk factor for cognitive decline before age 65 years than after. Findings for women were consistent with clinical recommendations. In men there were earlier age-associated shifts in lipid profiles.
Beydoun et al. (*J Epidemiol Community Health.* 2011; 65(11):949–955)	1604 men and women Study baseline: all age groups >50 years Follow-up: 25 years	Decline in TC and HR (95% CI) for dementia: 4.21 (1.28–13.85)

but the cholesterol content and expression level of specific enzymes show strong regional variation (Pfrieger, 2003).

The main cholesterol transporter in the brain is apolipoprotein E, compared to the periphery where apolipoprotein B and apolipoprotein AI are predominant. Brain apolipoprotein E is synthesized primarily by glial cells, especially astrocytes (Vance, 2005). Astrocytes secrete cholesterol bound to apolipoprotein E in the form of HDL-like particles, which are internalized by neurons (Björkhem, 2004). Other proteins involved in transporting cholesterol in lipoproteins in the circulation are also present in the CNS (e.g., apolipoproteins AI, D and J, several members of the LDL receptor family, and membrane transporters of the ABC family) (Vance, 2005). Their relative importance for the transport and recycling of cholesterol within CNS is still unknown, and there is probably redundancy in these systems.

The links between circulating and brain cholesterol are not entirely clarified, but oxysterols (particularly 24- and 27-hydroxycholesterol) can cross the BBB (Björkhem, 2006). Oxysterols are mono-oxygenate derivatives of cholesterol (or cholesterol precursors) that are important as intermediates and end-products in cholesterol excretion pathways. They are typically found in conjunction with cholesterol in almost all biological locations but at significantly lower concentrations (10- to 100,000-fold less) and unevenly distributed across different tissues. 24-hydroxycholesterol (24OHC) is formed almost exclusively in the brain, where it is present in greater amounts than in any other organ (Björkhem, 2006). There is a daily flux of about 6 to 7 mg of 24OHC from the brain into the circulation, and the majority of this efflux occurs as direct transport across the BBB (Lütjohann, 1996). An estimated 1% of the 24OHC produced in the brain is transported to the circulation through the cerebrospinal fluid (CSF). 27-hydroxycholesterol (27OHC) is formed from cholesterol in most extrahepatic organs, as an important mechanism for the daily elimination of cholesterol by the body. There is also a flux of 27OHC from the circulation into the brain (Leoni, 2005).

Cholesterol, Neurodegenerative, and Vascular Pathologies: Some Mechanisms of Association

INTERACTIONS BETWEEN ALZHEIMER'S DISEASE-TYPE AND VASCULAR PATHOLOGY

That the two types of pathologies can interact with each other was clearly shown by findings from the Nun Study (Snowdon, 1997), in which elderly nuns could have typical AD changes in their brains without having cognitive impairment as long as they did not additionally have cerebrovascular lesions (CVLs). Cerebrovascular lesions thus have the potential to tip the balance so that persons with AD pathology express a dementia syndrome. A high proportion of individuals fulfilling the neuropathological criteria for AD also have significant CVLs, just like VaD cases diagnosed by current criteria can have AD pathology at autopsy (Kalaria & Skoog, 2002).

Alzheimer's disease patients can show atherosclerosis in both intracranial and extracranial vessels. Moreover, atherosclerosis has been associated with increased frequency of neuritic plaques (Honig, 2005). One possible mechanism is through cerebral infarcts that influence β-amyloid processing, although additional mechanisms may exist. People with AD also frequently have cerebral amyloid angiopathy (CAA), which has been associated with microbleeds. Cerebral amyloid angiopathy is not uncommon in VaD, where it is related to cortical microinfarcts. APOE ε4 allele is associated with increased vascular β-amyloid deposition (Kumar-Singh, 2008). Although CAA related to capillaries and smaller arterioles (a type more closely linked with AD) is related to APOE ε4, larger vessel CAA seems to be associated with APOE ε2 (Kumar-Singh, 2008).

In addition to its neurotoxic and proinflammatory properties, β-amyloid seems to be involved in cerebral blood flow (CBF) dysregulation. In turn, ischemia may upregulate amyloid precursor protein (APP) and β-amyloid cleavage. Vascular dysfunction can affect β-amyloid trafficking across the BBB, reducing the rate of β-amyloid clearance from the brain (Girouard, 2006). Thus, these two processes reinforce each other. It remains to be established whether neurofibrillary tangles also contribute to vascular dysregulation.

Cholesterol, Alzheimer's Disease-Type and Vascular Pathology

The most obvious connection between increased plasma cholesterol and dementia is through vascular mechanisms. Cholesterol is involved in atherosclerosis, and several cardio- and cerebrovascular conditions have been reported to increase the risk of both AD and VaD. Increased plasma total cholesterol (especially at midlife) has also been linked to AD-type pathology in autopsy studies (Launer, 2001; Pappolla, 2003). In addition, several population-based imaging studies using MRI have documented a positive correlation between the number of cortical infarcts and white matter lesions (WMLs) with plasma cholesterol levels (Amarenco, 2006). Cholesterol-rich diets in rabbits or mice were associated with increased cerebral accumulation of β-amyloid (Sparks, 1994) and tau hyperphosphorylation (Rahman, 2005). Interestingly, in a mouse model of AD pathology, the effects of cholesterol-rich diet on vascular parameters (i.e., relative cerebral blood volume) were observed before effects on β-amyloid load were noted (Hooijmans, 2009).

Less data are available on LDL and high-density lipoprotein (HDL). Higher LDL was found to increase the risk of VaD or dementia with stroke (Reitz, 2004) and was also associated with WMLs (Amarenco, 2006). A dose–response relationship between plasma HDL and number of neuritic plaques and neurofibrillary tangles has been reported (Launer, 2001), whereas low HDL levels were associated with lower hippocampal volumes in some, but not all, studies. High-density lipoprotein is particularly interesting, as only HDL-like lipoproteins are found in the CSF, and CSF HDL levels correlate with plasma HDL levels (there is no such correlation between total cholesterol and LDL in plasma and CSF).

Findings on brain cholesterol levels vary depending on which brain cholesterol pool is investigated (reviewed in Solomon, 2009). An increase in brain cholesterol levels as well as decreased cholesterol in the white matter of AD patients have been reported. The temporal cortex from AD patients showed loss of lipid rafts, whereas hippocampi showed reduced cholesterol content in the rafts. Changes in the distribution of cholesterol in neuronal cell membranes have been suggested as more important in β-amyloid production than total cholesterol.

The relationship between cholesterol and β-amyloid seems to be bidirectional. Cholesterol is a major component of lipid rafts, which are involved in modulating cellular structures and cellular function, including APP processing. It has been hypothesized that APP is located in two different compartments in the membrane and that non-amyloidogenic α-cleavage occurs outside the lipid rafts, whereas APP within rafts is processed by β- and γ-secretases, leading to the formation of β-amyloid (Hartmann, 2007). Very little is known about a physiological function of β-amyloid besides its pathological AD-related aspects, but there is evidence that APP processing, and especially β-amyloid, influence lipid metabolism. β-amyloid can inhibit cholesterol synthesis by inhibiting 3-hydroxy-3-methylglutaryl-coenzyme A reductase (HMG-CoA), although it is not clear how this regulation is mediated (Hartmann, 2007). A negative feedback cycle can thus be hypothesized: When increased cholesterol increases β-amyloid production, β-amyloid acts to inhibit cholesterol synthesis. The difficulty consists in determining where and how this balance becomes disrupted. There is evidence that increased cholesterol could be a determinant for switching APP processing toward the amyloidogenic pathway, and some studies have shown that soluble oligomers of β-amyloid impair cholesterol synthesis and finally reduce cholesterol levels in neurons. Besides their involvement in β-amyloid production, lipid rafts seem to be involved in β-amyloid aggregation and toxicity but may also be involved in β-amyloid clearance.

The ratio between free and total cellular cholesterol may also be important in APP processing (Björkhem, 2004), but the exact role of free and esterified cholesterol is unclear. Apart from cell membrane cholesterol, mitochondrial cholesterol is beginning to receive attention in relation to dementia. Mitochondria are cholesterol-poor organelles, including about 0.5% to 3% of the content found in other cellular membranes. However, mitochondrial cholesterol fulfills vital physiological functions, and its accumulation may be important in pathophysiological processes leading to dementia.

A connection between cholesterol and tauopathy is suggested by Niemann-Pick disease models, where there is cholesterol accumulation with development of NFT that are essentially identical to those observed in AD. It has been reported that the state of tau phosphorylation is modulated not so much by total cellular cholesterol levels as by cholesterol levels in specific compartments such as lipid rafts, with reduced cholesterol promoting phosphorylation (Michikawa, 2006).

24- AND 27-HYDROXYCHOLESTEROL IN ALZHEIMER'S DISEASE AND VASCULAR DEMENTIA

Plasma 24OHC levels seem to be increased in the early stages of AD, possibly reflecting ongoing demyelinization, but they are reduced in advanced AD as a consequence of the loss of neurons containing the enzyme producing 24OHC (Björkhem, 2006). Decreased plasma levels of 24OHC and 27OHC have been reported in patients with AD or VaD compared to non-demented controls, and plasma 24OHC has also been linked to hippocampal size in middle-aged normal individuals (reviewed in Solomon, 2009).

Increased 27OHC levels were found in CSF in patients with advanced AD who are believed to have BBB disturbances (Björkhem, 2006). Autopsy studies in AD patients showed that the levels of 24OHC were decreased in most brain areas, whereas the levels of 27OHC were increased.

It has been shown that 24OHC is an efficient inhibitor of the formation of β-amyloid peptides under in vitro conditions, whereas 27OHC has a much lower capacity to inhibit the reactions. It is possible that 27OHC "translates" circulating high total cholesterol into AD-related changes in the brain (Björkhem, 2009).

Effects of Statins on Cholesterol, β-Amyloid, and Brain Vascular Lesions

Statins are HMG-CoA reductase inhibitors, interfering with cholesterol synthesis at its rate-limiting step and reducing the production of both cholesterol and its isoprenoid intermediates. In addition, statins have several cholesterol-independent (pleiotropic) effects: reduction of endothelial dysfunction, atherosclerotic plaque stabilization, anti-inflammatoy and antioxidant effects, effects on coagulation, immunomodulation, and reduced cell proliferation.

In plasma, statin treatment decreases LDL and may slightly increase HDL. The effects of statins on the human brain are however more difficult to study. Depending on their solubility in lipid solvents or water, statins can be more lipophilic or hydrophilic, and this characteristic influences their crossing of the BBB (Höglund, 2007). Also, the BBB may be affected in dementia, which may influence drug levels in the brain. It is currently unclear whether statins need to enter the brain and act directly on disease processes or whether a more indirect action on the brain should be desirable.

Experimental studies are not easy to translate into a human context, especially as the statin dosages are usually much higher than therapeutic dosages in patients. Data are conflicting regarding the effects of statins on brain cholesterol in animal models as well as data from in vitro studies of neuronal structures and immune cells (reviewed in Solomon, 2009). Either decrease or no change in total brain cholesterol levels in animal studies has been reported.

Several studies have shown that statin treatment lowers β-amyloid production, but conflicting results exist as well (Solomon, 2009). β-secretase is affected by statins, and the effect on β-amyloid could be cholesterol-dependent. Statins also reduce β-amyloid-mediated microglial neurotoxicity in vitro independently of cholesterol lowering. Other pleiotropic effects may be important as well.

Several clinical studies have investigated the effects of statins on β-amyloid production and cholesterol metabolism in various populations, from adult healthy controls to patients with hypercholesterolemia or AD (Höglund, 2007). Whereas in vitro studies interpret reduced β-amyloid levels in cell media as reduced β-amyloid production, studies in humans measure β-amyloid in blood and CSF, where reduced levels are considered a pathological finding. It is not clear whether statin treatment should be expected to lead to lowered or increased β-amyloid or how the changes should be interpreted. With two exceptions, most clinical studies reported no effect of statins on β-amyloid levels in blood or CSF (Höglund, 2007). However, it seems that statin treatment can reduce cholesterol synthesis in the CNS.

The potential role of statins in dementia of vascular origin has been less explored. Such actions of statins may be partly independent of their cholesterol-lowering effect. For example, both atorvastatin and pitavastatin attenuated L-Methionine-induced endothelial dysfunction-associated memory deficits in rat models of VaD (Koladiya, 2008). Statins also reversed L-Methionine-induced rise in brain oxidative stress and serum cholesterol (Koladiya, 2008). Acute protection by simvastatin in transient cerebral ischemia in rats has been reported (Nagaraja, 2006), and statins may reduce the risk of ischemic stroke in humans (Heart Protection Study, 2002).

Statins and Prevention of Cognitive Impairment/Dementia

The National Lipid Association (NLA) Statin Safety Assessment Task Force in the United States has concluded that statin treatment is safe with respect to cognition (McKenney, 2006). Although several studies have suggested that statins may have beneficial effects in preventing cognitive impairment/dementia, a recent report from the National Institutes of Health (NIH) (http://www.ahrq. gov/clinic/tp/alzcogtp.htm) stated that the evidence is currently insufficient. In this evaluation, the evidence rating was low for observational studies and high for randomized controlled trials (RCTs). The conclusions were not surprising considering the lack of adequate RCTs designed specifically for prevention of cognitive impairment or dementia.

Tables 2.4 and 2.5 summarize the main longitudinal studies related to statins or other lipid-lowering agents (LLAs) and prevention of dementia/cognitive impairment. The established effects of statins on cardiovascular outcomes raise ethical questions that make the planning of RCTs with cognitive outcomes more difficult. Thus, the data come mainly from observational studies.

An initial wave of mostly cross-sectional studies resulted in optimism toward the role of statins in dementia prevention. At present the attitude is more neutral after many longitudinal studies heterogeneous in design, populations, outcomes, and drug exposure evaluation. It is still unclear when statin treatment should be started and what duration it should have to demonstrate an effect on the incidence of cognitive impairment or dementia. It is also unclear whether there is a difference between types of LLAs—that is, more lipophilic versus more hydrophilic statins. Regarding LLAs other than statins, current data do not indicate any effect in cognitive impairment/dementia prevention.

Table 2.5 shows the RCTs of statins in prevention of cognitive decline or dementia. The largest are the Heart Protection Study (HPS) and PROSPER, reporting no effects. However, the add-on design (with cognition/dementia as tertiary outcomes in studies focused on prevention of cardiovascular events) and the possible lack of power (too few dementia cases) question these results. The HPS included only a telephone interview of cognitive status (TICS) at the end of the study, and PROSPER had only a mini-mental state examination (MMSE) at the last clinical visit, without any information on baseline cognitive performance.

Statins in Patients With Dementia

Some observational studies have reported a slower cognitive decline in memory clinic patients with AD treated with LLAs (Masse, 2005); lower risk of

Study	Design	Source	Findings
Parale et al. (*Eur. J. Clin. Pharmacol.* 2006;62(4):259–265)	Before and after comparison study with controls 97 subjects (49 atorvastatin, 48 placebo) Age ≥40 years Duration: 6 months	Atorvastatin 10 mg/day vs placebo	Beneficial effects of atorvastatin on performance in cognitive tests
Wolozin et al. (*BMC Med* 2007; 5:20)	1290071 patients: 841963 statins; 394739 cardiovascular and 53369 warfarin comparator Age: ≥65 years Follow-up: 2 years	Pharmacy database	Simvastatin and HR (95% CI) for dementia: 0.46 (0.44–0.48) Atorvastatin and HR (95% CI) for dementia: 0.91 (0.80–1.02) Lovastatin and HR (95% CI) for dementia: 0.95 (0.86–1.05)
Li et al. (*Neurology* 2007; 69(9):878–885)	Cohort (community) 110 subjects Mean age: 74 years; mainly Caucasian Follow-up: about 7 years	Pharmacy database	Statins and OR (95% CI) for typical AD pathology (Braak stage > or = IV and CERAD rating > or = moderate): 0.20 (0.05–0.86).
Rockwood et al. (*Neuroepidemiology* 2007;29(3–4):201–207)	Case–control (community) 347 cases, 693 controls Age: ≥65 years Follow-up: 5 years	Self-reported	Statins and OR (95% CI) for Cognitive Impairment No Dementia (CIND): 0.37 (0.16–0.84) Other LLAs and OR (95% CI) for CIND: 0.43 (0.09–2.02)
Szwast et al. (*Neurology* 2007; 69(19):1873–1880)	Cohort (community) 1146 subjects Mean age: 77 years; African-American Follow-up: 3 years	Self-reported	Statins and risk of dementia: OR = 0.32; *p* = 0.0673

(continued)

Tabel 2.4 **(Continued)**

Study (reference)	*Design and population*	*Assessment of LLA use*	*Results*
Arvanitakis et al. (*Neurology* 2008; 70 (19 Pt 2):1795–1802)	Cohort 929 subjects; autopsy data: 262 subjects Mean age: 75 years Follow-up: up to 12 years	Direct visual inspection of containers	Statins and HR (95% CI) for AD: 0.93 (0.56–1.55) More lipophilic statins and HR (95% CI) for AD: 1.05 (0.57–1.95) Less lipophilic statins and HR (95% CI) for AD: 0.71 (0.29–1.74) Statin users were less likely to have amyloid (*p* = 0.02). Statins were not related to tangles or infarction
Smeeth et al. (*Br. J. Clin. Pharmacol.* 2009;67(1):99–109)	Cohort (GP patients) The Health Improvement Network (THIN), UK 129288 statin users&matched sample of 600241 non-users Age: ≥40 years Median follow-up: 4.4 years	THIN database	Statins and HR (95% CI) for dementia: 0.81 (0.69, 0.96) Statins and HR (95% CI) for AD: 0.81 (0.49, 1.35) Statins and HR (95% CI) for non-AD dementia: 0.82 (0.69, 0.97)
Sparks et al. (*Curr. Alzheimer Res.* 2008;5(4):416–421)	Elective statin use in a RCT cohort Alzheimer's Disease Anti-inflammatory Prevention Trial (ADAPT) 2233 subjects Mean age: 74 years Follow-up: up to 4 years	LLA use recorded at each scheduled RCT visit	Statins and HR (95% CI) for AD: 0.33 (0.11–0.98)

Study	Design / Subjects	Method	Results
Reitz et al. (*Dement. Geriatr. Cogn. Disord.* 2008; 25(3):232–237)	Cohort (community) Medicare recipients (northern Manhattan) 854 subjects Mean age 76 years; multi-ethnic Follow-up: about 5 years	Self-reported	LLAs and HR (95% CI) for MCI: 1.0 (0.75–1.37) LLAs and HR (95% CI) for amnestic MCI: 1.0 (0.66–1.58) LLAs and HR (95% CI) nonamnestic for MCI: 1.0 (0.67–1.52)
Cramer et al. (*Neurology* 2008; 71(5):344–350)	Cohort (community) 1674 subjects Mean age: 70 years; Mexican-Americans Follow-up: 5 years	Direct inspection of containers	Statins and HR (95%CI) for dementia/CIND: 0.52 (0.34–0.80).
Haag et al. (*J. Neurol. Neurosurg. Psychiatry* 2009; 80(1):13–17)	Cohort (community) 6992 subjects Mean age 69 years Follow-up: mean 9 years	Pharmacy databases	Statins and HR (95% CI) for AD: 0.57 (0.37–0.90) Lipophilic statins and HR (95% CI) for AD: 0.54 (0.32–0.89) Hydrophilic statins and HR (95% CI) for AD: 0.54 (0.26–1.11) Other LLAs and HR (95% CI) for AD: 1.05 (0.45–2.44)
Solomon et al. (*Neurodegenerative Dis.* 2010;7:180–182)	Cohort (community) 17597 subjects Age: >60 years Follow-up: mean 10 years	Drug reimbursement register	LLAs and HR (95% CI) for dementia: 0.42 (0.37–0.49)
Beydoun et al. (*J. Epidemiol. Community Health.* 2011; 65(11):949–957)	Cohort (community) 1604 subjects Age: >50 years Follow-up: median 25 years	Direct inspection of containers	Statins and HR (95% CI) for dementia: 0.41 (0.18–0.92)

Table 2.5 **Summary of Randomized Clinical Trials of Lipid-Lowering Agents in and Cognitive Impairment/Dementia Prevention**

Study (reference)	Population	Treatment	Results
Muldoon et al. (*Am. J. Med.* 2000; 108(7): 538–546)	Hypercholesterolemic adults, $n = 209$ Mean age: 46 years Duration: 6 months	Lovastatin 20 mg vs. placebo	No treatment effect
HPS Collaborative Group (*Lancet* 2002; 360(9326): 7–22)	Subjects with substantial 5-year risk of death from coronary heart disease, $n = 20536$ Age: 40–80 years Duration: mean 5 years	Simvastatin 40 mg vs. placebo	No treatment effect
Shepherd et al. (*Lancet* 2002; 360(9346): 1623–1630)	Elderly at risk of vascular disease, $n = 5804$ Mean age: 75 years Duration: mean 3.2 years	Pravastatin 40 mg vs. placebo	No treatment effect
Muldoon et al. (*Am. J. Med.* 2004; 117(11):823–829)	(hypercholesterolemic adults) 283 subjects Mean age: 54 years Duration: 6 months	Simvastatin 10 mg or 40 mg vs. placebo	No treatment effect
Carlsson et al. (*J. Alzheimers Dis.* 2008; 13(2):187–197)	57 middle-aged asymptomatic children of AD patients Duration: 4 months	Simvastatin 40 mg vs. placebo	Individuals randomized to simvastatin had greater improvements in some measures of verbal fluency ($p = 0.024$) and working memory ($p = 0.015$)

Study (reference)	Design and population	Assessment of LLA use	Results
Jick et al. (*Lancet* 2000; 356:1627–1631)	Nested case–control (GP patients) UK-based General Practice Research Database 284 cases, 1080 controls Age ≥50 (85.6% 70–89 years old) Follow-up: mean 5.5 years	Pharmacy database	Statins and RR (95% CI) for dementia: 0.29 (0.13–0.63) Other LLAs and RR (95% CI) for dementia: 0.96 (0.47–1.97)
Rockwood et al. (*Arch. Neurol.* 2002; 59:223–227)	Case–control (community and institutions) 492 cases (326 AD), 823 controls Age ≥65 years Follow-up: up to 5 years	Self-reported	Statins and other LLAs and OR (95% CI) for dementia/AD: – 0.26 (0.08–0.88) at ages <80 years – 0.50 (0.13–1.88) at ages >80 years
Yaffe et al. (*Arch. Neurol.* 2002; 59(3):378–384)	Prospective study of 1037 post-menopausal women Mean age: 71 years Duration: 4 years	Self-reported	Statins and OR (95% CI) for cognitive impairment: 0.67 (0.42–1.05)
Zamrini et al. (*Neuroepidemiology* 2004:23:94–98)	Nested case–control 309 cases, 3088 controls Mean age: 73 years; males only; multi-ethnic Follow-up: up to 4 years	Pharmacy database	Statins and OR (95% CI) for AD: 0.61 (0.42–0.87) Protective effect especially in subjects with cardio/cerebrovascular conditions
Reitz et al. (*Arch. Neurol.* 2004; 61:705–714)	Prospective, Medicare recipients, Manhattan, NY 1168 subjects Mean age: 78 years; multi-ethnic Follow-up: mean 4.8 years	Self-reported	LLAs and HR (95% CI) for AD: 0.88 (0.44–1.76) LLAs and HR (95% CI) for VaD: 1.45 (0.65–3.28)

(continued)

Table 2.4 **(Continued)**

Study (reference)	Design and population	Assessment of LLA use	Results
Li et al. (*Neurology* 2004; 63:1624–1628)	Prospective, cohort (community) 2356 subjects Mean age: 75 years; multi-ethnic Follow-up: up to 8 years	Pharmacy database	Statins and HR (95% CI) for dementia: 1.19 (0.82–1.75) Statins and HR (95% CI) for AD: 0.82 (0.46–1.46)
Zandi et al. (*Arch. Gen. Psychiatry* 2005; 62:217–224)	Prospective, cohort (community and institutions) 3308 subjects Mean age: about 73–75 years Follow-up: 3 years	Direct visual inspection of containers; physician and nursing home records	Statins and HR (95% CI) for dementia: 1.19 (0.53–2.34) Statins and HR (95% CI) for AD: 1.19 (0.35–2.96)
Rea et al. (*Arch. Neurol.* 2005; 62: 1047–1051)	Prospective Cohort (community) 2798 subjects; mean age: 75 years; multi-ethnic Follow-up: 5 years	Self-reported	Statins and HR (95% CI) for dementia: 1.08 (0.77–1.52) Statins and HR (95% CI) for AD: 1.21 (0.76–1.91) Statins and HR (95% CI) for mixed AD and VaD: 0.87 (0.44–1.72) Statins and HR (95% CI) for VaD: 1.36 (0.61–3.06)
Bernick et al. (*Neurology* 2005; 65(9):1388–1394)	Cohort (community) 3334 subjects Mean age: 73–75 years; multi-ethnic Follow-up: average 7 years	Self-reported	Rate of cognitive decline was lower in subjects taking statins compared to untreated subjects (*p* = 0.009)
Li et al. (*Alzheimer Dis. Assoc. Disord.* 2006; 20(Suppl 2):S103–S104)	Cohort (community) 2356 subjects Age: ≥65 years Follow-up: up to 8 years	Pharmacy database	Statins and HR (95% CI) for AD: – 0.41 (0.20–0.82) at ages <80 years – 1.96 (0.89–4.33) at ages >80 years

deterioration with statin use in AD patients from the community (Ellul, 2007); delay of cognitive decline with statin use in subjects with AD from the Dementia Progression Study of the Cache County Study on Memory, Health, and Aging (Rosenberg, 2008); and reduced risk of hospitalization with dementia among statin users (Horsdal, 2008). However, a *post hoc* analysis conducted on data pooled from three RCTs of galantamine in patients with AD showed no significant effects of statin treatment (Winblad, 2007).

Four RCTs have investigated the effects of statin treatment in persons who already have AD. The first study involved a 26-week treatment with 80 mg simvastatin versus placebo in 44 patients with mild and moderate AD (MMSE: 12–26). Slower progression of cognitive decline as measured with MMSE (but not ADAS-Cog) was reported (Simons, 2002). Some beneficial effects were also reported for atorvastatin (80 mg vs. placebo) in the Alzheimer's Disease Cholesterol-Lowering Treatment (ADCLT) study, a 1-year RCT of 63 patients with mild-to-moderate AD (MMSE: 12–28) (Sparks, 2005). Secondary assessment indicated that the ADCLT subjects who had the greatest benefit from atorvastatin therapy in terms of their 6-month ADAS-cog score were those with higher cholesterol levels at trial entry, those with the APOE ɛ4 allele, and those less affected by AD at trial entry (i.e., with higher entry MMSE scores) (Sparks, 2006). The Atorvastatin/Donepezil in Alzheimer's Disease Study (LEADe), a large-scale international, multicenter, 72-week RCT investigated atorvastatin 80 mg/day versus placebo in 640 patients with mild-to-moderate AD (MMSE: 13–25) receiving background therapy of donepezil 10 mg/day (Feldman, 2010). Results indicated that cholesterol lowering in patients with already established AD dementia, without elevated LDL levels, and at low risk of ischemic events was not associated with better preservation of cognition or global functioning.

A meta-analysis of these three RCTs concluded that there was insufficient evidence to recommend statins for the treatment of dementia, and no evidence that statins were detrimental to cognition (McGuinness, 2010). A fourth RCT, the large multicenter Cholesterol Lowering Agent to Slow Progression of AD (CLASP) study, has investigated the effects of 18 months of simvastatin treatment (20 mg/day for 6 weeks, then 40 mg/day) versus placebo in 406 subjects with mild-to-moderate AD (mean MMSE: 20). Detailed results have not been published, although preliminary results seem to indicate a lack of effect of simvastatin in AD treatment (Sparks, 2009).

Because current clinical guidelines recommend statin treatment for patients with hypercholesterolemia or high vascular risk factor burden, statin RCTs in treatment of dementia-related diseases have been restricted to patients without indications for statins. It is thus possible that patients suffering from AD with high cholesterol levels and/or cardiovascular risk factors might have responded better to statin treatment. In addition, current diagnostic criteria for AD focus on the end-stage of the disease (dementia), which may be too late to see any treatment benefits.

Cholesterol, Statins, and the New Generation of Cognitive Impairment Prevention Trials

The 2010 NIH report on AD prevention (http://www.ahrq.gov/clinic/tp/alzcogtp.htm), presented by an independent panel of health professionals and public representatives from outside the AD research field, has provided an unbiased perspective on the current state of evidence. Two main conclusions point out the directions to be followed in future research: the importance of adopting a life-course perspective, with long-term population-based studies starting already at midlife, and the need for RCTs to be multidimensional, combining interventions for multiple risk factors. Cholesterol is only one piece of a complex puzzle and must be addressed together with other risk factors.

The first RCTs integrating several prevention approaches have already been started. A 2-year multidomain intervention study aiming to delay cognitive impairment and disability among 1,200 high-risk individuals is currently ongoing in Finland (Finnish Geriatric Intervention Study to Prevent Cognitive Impairment and Disability; FINGER). The intervention has four main components: nutrition, exercise, cognitive and social activity, and monitoring and management of metabolic and vascular risk factors (including cholesterol). There is one intervention group receiving all four components, whereas the placebo group receives general health advice on lifestyle and vascular risk factors. Three other ongoing multidomain RCTs are Prevention of dementia by intensive vascular care (PreDIVA) in the Netherlands, Multi-domain Alzheimer Prevention Trial (MAPT) in France, and Austrian Polyintervention Study to Prevent Cognitive Decline After Ischemic Stroke (ASPIS). Within a few years, results will hopefully lead to much-needed public health and clinical recommendations for preventing late-life cognitive impairment.

Conclusions

Epidemiological, genetic, and experimental evidence links cholesterol to dementia-related disorders, particularly neurodegenerative and vascular pathologies. However, the complexity of these relationships makes it difficult to formulate specific cholesterol treatment guidelines for preventing cognitive impairment and dementia. Existing guidelines for cardiovascular and cerebrovascular disease prevention may also be effective for dementia prevention. Cholesterol alone will certainly not provide a solution, and multifactorial prevention approaches are more likely to succeed. Two main directions are particularly important for future research: further investigating brain cholesterol metabolism and conducting large international RCTs with multifactorial preventive measures.

References

Abbott RD, Sharp DS, Burchfiel CM, et al. Cross-sectional and longitudinal changes in total and high-density-lipoprotein cholesterol levels over a 20-year period in elderly men: the Honolulu Heart Program. *Ann Epidemiol* 1997;7:417–424.

Amarenco P, Labreuche J, Elbaz A, et al. Blood lipids in brain infarction subtypes. *Cerebrovasc Dis* 2006;22:101–108.

Barnes DE, Covinsky KE, Whitmer RA, Kuller LH, Lopez OL, Yaffe K. Predicting risk of dementia in older adults: the late-life dementia risk index. *Neurology* 2009;73:173–179.

Björkhem I. Crossing the barrier: oxysterols as cholesterol transporters and metabolic modulators in the brain. *J Intern Med.* 2006;260(6):493–508.

Björkhem I, Cedazo-Minguez A, Leoni V, Meaney S. Oxysterols and neurodegenerative diseases. *Mol Aspects Med.* 2009;30(3):171–179.

Björkhem I, Meaney S. Brain cholesterol: long secret life behind a barrier. *Arteriosclr Thromb Vasc Biol.* 2004; 24:806–815.

Carter CJ. Convergence of genes implicated in Alzheimer's disease on the cerebral cholesterol shuttle: APP, cholesterol, lipoproteins, and atherosclerosis. *Neurochem Int.* 2007;50(1):12–38.

Corder EH, Saunders AM, Strittmatter WJ, et al. Gene dose of apolipoprotein E type 4 allele and the risk of Alzheimer's disease in late onset families. *Science* 1993;261(5123):921–923.

Dietschy JM, Turley SD. Cholesterol metabolism in the central nervous system during early development and in the mature animal. *J. Lipid Res.* 2004;45:1375–1397.

Ellul J, Archer N, Foy CM, et al. The effects of commonly prescribed drugs in patients with Alzheimer's disease on the rate of deterioration. *J Neurol Neurosurg Psychiatry.* 2007;78(3):233–239.

Erkinjuntti T, Sulkava R, Tilvis R. Is determination of plasma lipids useful in the differentiation of multi-infarct dementia from Alzheimer's disease? *Compr Gerontol* 1988;2(1):1–6.

Feldman HH, Doody RS, Kivipelto M, et al.; LEADe Investigators. Randomized controlled trial of atorvastatin in mild to moderate Alzheimer disease: LEADe. *Neurology.* 2010;74(12):956–964.

Ferrara A, Barrett-Connor E, Shan J. Total, LDL, and HDL cholesterol decrease with age in older men and women. The Rancho Bernardo Study 1984–1994. *Circulation* 1997;96:37–43.

Girouard H, Iadecola C. Neurovascular coupling in the normal brain and in hypertension, stroke, and Alzheimer disease. *J Appl Physiol* 2006;100(1):328–335.

Hartmann T, Kuchenbecker J, Grimm MO. Alzheimer's disease: the lipid connection. *J Neurochem.* 2007;103 Suppl 1:159–170.

Höglund K, Blennow K. Effect of HMG-CoA reductase inhibitors on beta-amyloid peptide levels: implications for Alzheimer's disease. *CNS Drugs.* 2007;21(6):449–462.

Honig LS, Kukull W, Mayeux R. Atherosclerosis and AD. Analysis of data from the US National Alzheimer's Coordinating Center. *Neurology* 2005;64; 494–500.

Hooijmans CR, Kiliaan AJ. Fatty acids, lipid metabolism and Alzheimer pathology. *Eur J Pharmacol.* 2008;585(1):176–196.

Hooijmans CR, Van der Zee CE, Dederen PJ, et al. DHA and cholesterol containing diets influence Alzheimer-like pathology, cognition and cerebral vasculature in APPswe/PS1dE9 mice. *Neurobiol Dis* 2009;33(3):482–498.

Horsdal HT, Olesen AV, Gasse C, Sørensen HT, Green RC, Johnsen SP. Use of Statins and Risk of Hospitalization With Dementia: A Danish Population-based Case-control Study. *Alzheimer Dis Assoc Disord.* 2009; 23(1):18–22..

Jack CR Jr, Albert MS, Knopman DS, et al. Introduction to the recommendations from the National Institute on Aging-Alzheimer's Association workgroups on diagnostic guidelines for Alzheimer's disease. *Alzheimers Dement.* 2011;7(3):257–262.

Kalaria RN, Skoog I. Overlap with Alzheimer's disease. In: T Erkinjuntti T and S Gauthier (Eds),, *Vascular Cognitive Impairment.* The Livery House, London, UK: Martin Dunitz Ltd, 2002; 145–166.

Kim KW, Youn JC, Han MK, et al. Lack of association between apolipoprotein E polymorphism and vascular dementia in Koreans. *J Geriatr Psychiatry Neurol* 2008;21(1):12–17.

Kivipelto M, Ngandu T, Laatikainen T, Winblad B, Soininen H, Tuomilehto J. Risk score for the prediction of dementia risk in 20 years among middle aged people: a longitudinal, population-based study. *Lancet Neurol* 2006;5:735–741.

Kivipelto M, Rovio S, Ngandu T, et al. Apolipoprotein E epsilon4 Magnifies Lifestyle Risks for Dementia: A Population Based Study. *J Cell Mol Med* 2008; 12(6B):2762–2771.

Koladiya RU, Jaggi AS, Singh N, Sharma BK. Ameliorative role of Atorvastatin and Pitavastatin in L-Methionine induced vascular dementia in rats. *BMC Pharmacol.* 2008;8:14.

Kumar-Singh S. Cerebral amyloid angiopathy: pathogenetic mechanisms and link to dense amyloid plaques. *Genes Brain Behav* 2008;7 (Suppl 1):67–82.

Launer LJ, White LR, Petrovitch H, Ross GW, Curb JD. Cholesterol and neuropathologic markers of AD: a population-based autopsy study. *Neurology* 2001;57:1447–1452.

Leoni V. On the possible use of oxysterols for the diagnosis and evaluation of patients with neurological and neurodegenerative diseases. Doctoral thesis, Karolinska Institutet, Stockholm, Sweden. 2005. http://diss.kib.ki.se/2005/91-7140-255-1/thesis.pdf

Lütjohann D, Breuer O, Ahlborg G, et al. Cholesterol homeostasis in human brain: evidence for an age-dependent flux of 24S-hydroxycholesterol from the brain into the circulation. *Proc Natl Acad Sci USA.* 1996;93(18):9799–9804.

Masse I, Bordet R, Deplanque D, et al. Lipid lowering agents are associated with a slower cognitive decline in Alzheimer's disease. *J Neurol Neurosurg Psychiatry.* 2005;76(12):1624–1629.

McGuinness B, O'Hare J, Craig D, Bullock R, Malouf R, Passmore P. Statins for the treatment of dementia. *Cochrane Database Syst Rev.* 2010;(8):CD007514.

McKenney JM, Davidson MH, Jacobson TA, Guyton JR; National Lipid Association Statin Safety Assessment Task Force. Final conclusions and recommendations of the National Lipid Association Statin Safety Assessment Task Force. *Am J Cardiol.* 2006;97(8A):89C–94C.

Michikawa M. Role of cholesterol in amyloid cascade: cholesterol-dependent modulation of tau phosphorylation and mitochondrial function. *Acta Neurol Scand Suppl.* 2006;185:21–26.

Muckle TJ, Roy JR. High-density lipoprotein cholesterol in differential diagnosis of senile dementia. *Lancet* 1985;1(8439):1191–1193.

Mumenthaler M. Cerebral sclerosis. Diagnostic criteria and differential diagnostic consideration in practice. *Schweiz Med Wochenschr* 1975;105(12):353–361.

Nagaraja TN, Knight RA, Croxen RL, Konda KP, Fenstermacher JD. Acute neurovascular unit protection by simvastatin in transient cerebral ischemia. *Neurol Res.* 2006;28(8):826–830.

National Cholesterol Education Program Expert Panel on Detection, Evaluation and Treatment of High Blood Cholesterol in Adults (Adult Treatment Panel III): Final Report (NIH Publication No. 02-5215). Bethesda, National Heart, Lung and Blood Institute, National Institutes of Health, 2002.

Pappolla MA, Bryant-Thomas TK, Herbert D, et al. Mild hypercholesterolemia is an early risk factor for the development of Alzheimer amyloid pathology. *Neurology* 2003;61(2):199–205.

Pfrieger FW. Cholesterol homeostasis and function in neurons of the central nervous system. *Cell Mol Life Sci.* 2003;60(6):1158–1171.

Poirier J, Davignon J, Bouthillier D, Kogan S, Bertrand P, Gauthier S. Apolipoprotein E polymorphism and Alzheimer's disease. *Lancet* 1993;342(8873):697–699.

Rahman SMA, Akterin S, Flores-Morales A, et al. High cholesterol diet induces tau hyperphosphorylation in apolipoprotein E deficient mice. *FEBS Lett.* 2005;579(28): 6411–6416.

Reiman EM, Chen K, Caselli RJ, et al. Cholesterol-related genetic risk scores are associated with hypometabolism in Alzheimer's-affected brain regions. *Neuroimage.* 2008;40(3):1214–1221.

Reitz C, Tang MX, Luchsinger J, et al. Relation of plasma lipids to Alzheimer disease and vascular dementia. *Arch Neurol* 2004; *61*:705–714.

Rosenberg PB, Mielke MM, Tschanz J, et al. Effects of cardiovascular medications on rate of functional decline in Alzheimer disease. *Am J Geriatr Psychiatry.* 2008;*16*(11):883–892.

Schmidt H, Schmidt R. Genetic factors. In: T Erkinjuntti T and S Gauthier (Eds.), *Vascular Cognitive Impairment.* The Livery House, London, UK: Martin Dunitz Ltd, 2002; 85–100.

Simons M, Schwärzler F, Lütjohann D, et al. Treatment with simvastatin in normocholesterolemic patients with Alzheimer's disease: A 26-week randomized, placebo-controlled, double-blind trial. *Ann Neurol.* 2002;*52*(3):346–350.

Snowdon DA, Greiner LH, Mortimer JA, et al. Brain infarction and the clinical expression of Alzheimer disease. *JAMA* 1997; *277*:813–817.

Solomon A, Kivipelto M. Cholesterol-modifying strategies for Alzheimer's disease. *Expert Rev Neurother.* 2009;*9*(5):695–709.

Sparks DL, Connor DJ, Sabbagh MN, Petersen RB, Lopez J, Browne P. Circulating cholesterol levels, apolipoprotein E genotype and dementia severity influence the benefit of atorvastatin treatment in Alzheimer's disease: results of the Alzheimer's Disease Cholesterol-Lowering Treatment (ADCLT) trial. *Acta Neurol Scand Suppl.* 2006;*185*:3–7.

Sparks DL, Hunsaker JC 3rd, Scheff SW, Kryscio RJ, Henson JL, Markesbery WR. Cortical senile plaques in coronary artery disease, aging and Alzheimer's disease. *Neurobiol Aging* 1990; *11*(6):601–607.

Sparks DL, Sabbagh MN, Connor DJ, et al. Atorvastatin for the treatment of mild to moderate Alzheimer disease: preliminary results. *Arch Neurol.* 2005;*62*(5):753–757.

Sparks DL, Scheff SW, Hunsaker JC 3rd, Liu H, Landers T, Gross DR. Induction of Alzheimer-like beta-amyloid immunoreactivity in the brains of rabbits with dietary cholesterol. *Exp Neurol.* 1994;*126*(1):88–94.

Sparks L. Statins and cognitive function. *J Neurol Neurosurg Psychiatry* 2009;*80*(1):1–2.

Steinberg D. An interpretive history of the cholesterol controversy: part I. *J. Lipid Res* 2004;*45*:1583–1593.

Tonk M, Haan J. A review of genetic causes of ischemic and hemorrhagic stroke. *Journal of the Neurological Sciences* 2007; *257*:273–279.

Vance JE, Hayashi H, Karten B. Cholesterol homeostasis in neurons and glial cells. *Semin Cell Dev Biol.* 2005;*16*(2):193–212.

Winblad B, Jelic V, Kershaw P, Amatniek J. Effects of statins on cognitive function in patients with Alzheimer's disease in galantamine clinical trials. *Drugs Aging.* 2007;*24*(1):57–61.

3

Cardiovascular Disease and Cognitive Aging

ANGELA L. JEFFERSON, PHD AND MELISSA THOMPSON, DVM

Introduction

This chapter reviews the complex processes involved in the pathogenesis of cognitive aging associated with clinically common forms of prevalent cardiovascular disease (CVD), including atrial fibrillation, atherosclerotic disease (e.g., myocardial infarction, coronary artery bypass grafting [CABG]), heart failure, and cardiac arrest. For our purposes, abnormal cognitive aging will encompass pathological aspects of the cognitive aging spectrum, including subclinical cognitive impairment (i.e., cognitive difficulties that exist prior to the onset of clinical diagnosis), mild cognitive impairment (MCI), and dementia, especially Alzheimer's disease (AD). We summarize literature from a combination of basic science, animal, post mortem, clinical referral, and epidemiological studies. In an effort to better understand the connection between CVD and cognitive aging, we review pathways associated with a cardiovascular hypothesis for abnormal cognitive aging, which posits that abnormalities in cerebral blood flow, endothelium dysfunction, compromised blood brain barrier integrity, and inflammatory processes contribute to microvascular injury, AD-related neuropathological processes, and neurodegeneration, as outlined in Table 3.1 and illustrated in Figure 3.1.

Consideration of Shared Risk Factors for Cardiovascular Disease and Cognitive Aging

Vascular disease plays a critical role in cognitive decline; however, common shared risk factors between CVD and cognitive aging pose a challenge in fully understanding the independent or mediating role that CVD plays in the etiology

Table 3.1 **Mechanisms Associated With Cardiovascular Disease and Brain Aging**

Cardiovascular event	Purported mechanism for brain aging/insult
Atrial fibrillation	Reduced cardiac output and increased risk of stroke; subsequent cerebral hypoperfusion and ischemic insults may increase APP and BACE1 expression
Atherosclerosis	Inflammation increases risk for stroke and promotes endothelial cell dysfunction, compromising blood–brain barrier integrity
Myocardial infarction	Arrhythmia and reduced cardiac output contribute to microembolism and reduced cerebral perfusion
Coronary artery bypass grafting (CABG)	Peri-operative mechanisms: Hypotension reduces cerebral perfusion; manipulation of vessels causes cerebral microembolism; anesthesia increases APP and amyloid-β Postoperative mechanisms: Atrial fibrillation; inflammation and oxidative stress
Heart failure	Reduced cardiac function contributes to reduced cerebral perfusion
Cardiac arrest	Reduced cerebral perfusion leads to cerebral glucose deficiency and neuronal death; ischemia causes cell death and secondary cerebral reperfusion injury (e.g., glutamate excitotoxicity, cardiotoxic potassium levels)

and progression of abnormal cognitive aging. In particular, shared environmental risk factors for CVD and dementia include hypertension (Kivipelto et al., 2005; Hayden et al., 2006), diabetes mellitus (Borenstein et al., 2005; Luchsinger et al., 2005; Hayden et al., 2006), cigarette smoking (Luchsinger et al., 2005; Yusuf et al., 2004), and inflammation (Aviles et al., 2003; Vasan et al., 2003; Ridker et al., 2002). As an example, inflammation is associated with atrial fibrillation (Aviles et al., 2003), heart failure (Vasan et al., 2003), and myocardial infarction (Ridker et al., 2002) and has been related to neurological compromise, including clinical stroke (Tarkowski et al., 1995) and dementia (Tarkowski et al., 2003; Yasojima et al., 2000). More recently, inflammation has been related to imaging and cognitive markers of preclinical brain changes associated with stroke (van Dijk et al., 2005) and dementia (Jefferson et al., 2011; Jefferson, Massaro et al., 2007; Yaffe et al., 2003). Despite compelling evidence that shared risk factors exist between CVD and cognitive aging, statistically accounting for these risks (assessed at a single time point) is a challenge in multivariable models (Wilson

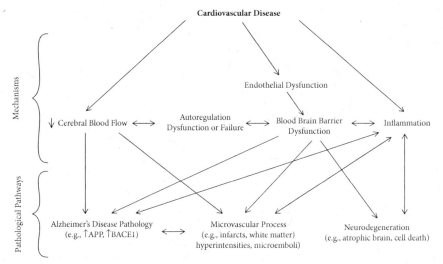

Figure 3.1 Theoretical model for complex association between cardiovascular disease and cognitive aging.

et al., 1997) and complicates our understanding of the individual effects on cognitive aging.

In addition to shared environmental risk factors, animal and clinical studies have suggested genetic links between CVD and pathology underlying abnormal cognitive aging, such as AD. For example, genes associated with familial early onset AD (i.e., presenilin 1 and 2) are expressed in murine myocardium (Hebert et al., 2004) and are associated with cardiomyopathy in humans (Li et al., 2006). Possession of the apolipoprotein E (APOE) ε4 allele, which increases the risk for MCI (Boyle et al., 2010) and late-onset AD (Corder et al., 1994), is associated with impaired cholesterol transport in the body, predisposing individuals to severe coronary atherosclerosis (Kosunen et al., 1995) and increasing the risk of cardiac ischemia and ventricular dysfunction (van der Cammen et al., 1998). The etiological link between the APOE ε4 allele and both CVD and AD is not well understood. Although only speculation, a serial mechanism may include cardiac and brain injury as manifestations of end-organ damage subsequent to atherosclerotic disease (Tabas, 2011; Muller et al., 2011). Alternatively, in an intermediary pathway it is possible that the impaired cholesterol transport function associated with APOE ε4 (Dupuy et al., 2001) may mediate distinct vascular effects in the cerebral and peripheral circulation (Mahley, Weisgraber, & Huang 2009). As an example, APOE ε4 is an established risk factor for cerebral amyloid angiopathy (CAA), which is characterized by Aβ deposits in vessel walls (Greenberg et al., 1996). Although impaired cholesterol transport may mediate the development of atherosclerotic lesions globally, APOE ε4 may also specifically contribute to cerebrovascular dysfunction through its relationship to CAA.

Furthermore, CAA-induced vascular inflammation, which is strongly associated with APOE ε4 homozygosity, may directly contribute to cognitive symptoms (Kinnecom et al., 2007). Yet despite these strong links, systematic studies are needed to determine whether the relationship between APOE ε4 and CAA is independent of APOE ε4's contribution to overall amyloid burden. Collectively, these animal, clinical, and neuropathological data suggest that CVD and abnormal cognitive aging share genetic risk factors. However, many of these subtle genetic effects depend on other premorbid conditions (i.e., gene–environment interactions) as well as the entire genetic context (i.e. gene–gene interactions).

Atrial Fibrillation

Atrial fibrillation is a cardiac arrhythmia that involves an irregular rhythm that results from asynchronous and ineffectual atrial contraction. In the normal heart, the majority of ventricular filling occurs with active, energy-dependent relaxation of the ventricular myocardium, which creates a pressure difference across the atrioventricular valve, thus allowing blood to flow passively down its pressure gradient from the atria to the ventricles. A portion of the remaining ventricular filling results from atrial contraction, commonly referred to as "atrial kick," which forcibly expels the remaining blood from the atrium to the ventricle (Alpert, Petersen, & Godtfredsen, 1988).

Epidemiologic data link atrial fibrillation to cognitive decline. In the Rotterdam Study, the incidence of vascular dementia and AD in participants with atrial fibrillation was double that of participants without atrial fibrillation, even after adjustment for prevalent CVD (Ott et al., 1997). Atrial fibrillation is also associated with cognitive impairment in the absence of clinical dementia. For example, in one Italian population study, a history of atrial fibrillation was more common in people with a diagnosis of "cognitive impairment no dementia" (Di Carlo et al., 2000). Similarly, Framingham Heart Study data indicated that men with atrial fibrillation had poorer cognitive performance across multiple domains (Elias et al., 2006). In clinical series of patients with existing cognitive impairment, data have supported an association between atrial fibrillation and conversion to dementia. For example, in longitudinal studies of people with MCI, atrial fibrillation was more common in those subjects who converted to dementia over an average of 3 years to 4 years (Ravaglia et al., 2006; Forti et al., 2006). However, in the absence of any pre-existing dementing condition, atrial fibrillation is not associated with cross-sectional cognitive impairment (Park et al., 2005), longitudinal cognitive decline (Park et al., 2007), or conversion to dementia (Forti et al., 2006). A recent meta-analysis has provided some evidence that may help explain the conflicting data within the literature on atrial fibrillation and dementia (Kwok et al., 2011). Participants with baseline atrial fibrillation (compared to controls) had a higher risk of dementia at follow-up (OR = 2.0); however, when the sample was limited to participants with recent stroke and prevalent atrial fibrillation, the OR for dementia increased (OR = 2.4) (Kwok et al., 2011). These data suggest cerebrovascular disease may act as an intermediary between atrial fibrillation and cognitive decline.

There are several mechanisms that are thought to account for the association between atrial fibrillation and cognitive aging. First, because there is a direct relation between the end-diastolic volume of the ventricle and cardiac stroke volume (which is a principal determinant of cardiac output), the loss of effectual atrial contraction reduces cardiac efficiency and results in reduced cardiac output and cerebral blood flow (Petersen et al., 1989). Second, atrial fibrillation is associated with increased thromboembolic risk (Barber et al., 2004) as well as silent (Ezekowitz et al., 1995) and clinical stroke (Wolf, Abbott, & Kannel, 1987). Furthermore, chronic cerebral hypoperfusion and ischemic insults, resulting either directly from cardiac output reductions or indirectly from the associated increased thromboembolic risk, may contribute to increased expression of amyloid precursor protein (APP; Kalaria, 2000) and β secretase (BACE1; Zhiyou et al., 2009), which are both important in the pathogenesis of AD (Kalaria, 2000). Finally, just as the meta-analysis described above suggests that atrial fibrillation's link to stroke may account for the association with dementia, it is possible that because atrial fibrillation is often a consequence of other existing heart disease, that pre-existing CVD is a key determinant of cognitive aging. Future studies are needed to better establish the temporal relations for the development of atrial fibrillation and dementia as well as to investigate how the efficacy of intervention in atrial fibrillation—particularly control of thromboembolic risk through anticoagulation—impacts incidence of dementia.

Atherosclerosis and Myocardial Infarction

Atherosclerosis occurs when fatty material accumulates along the vessel walls and thickens or hardens to form plaques. Common complications from plaque formation and subsequent obstruction of blood flow include myocardial infarction (MI) and surgical interventions, such as coronary artery bypass grafting (CABG) described in a separate section below. Myocardial infarction refers to the acute limitation of coronary blood flow that may occur following the rupture and embolism of vulnerable atherosclerotic plaques within the coronary arterial circulation, leading to coronary ischemia and, in severe cases, myocardial necrosis.

Animal models suggest that acute MI is followed by neurobiological changes, including apoptotic events in the prefrontal cortex and hypothalamus (Wann et al., 2007). In humans, a history of MI is more common in patients with multi-infarct dementia as compared to patients with AD (Tresch et al., 1985) and associated with a five-time increase in all-cause dementia incidence among women (Aronson et al., 1990). Even in the absence of clinical dementia, individuals with cognitive impairment have a higher prevalence of past MI compared to cognitively normal individuals, as evidenced by a population-based Italian study (Di Carlo et al., 2000).

Atherosclerosis in the absence of MI may also impact the brain. Neuritic plaques are associated with atherosclerosis (i.e., large-vessel cerebrovascular disease) but not arteriosclerosis (i.e., small vessel cerebrovascular disease; Honig, Kukull, & Mayeux, 2005), and post mortem measures of intracranial atherosclerosis are significantly more severe in individuals with clinical dementia (Beach et al., 2007). Atherosclerosis grade is clinically associated with incidence of AD and vascular dementia (Hofman et al., 1997), and severe atherosclerosis confers a threefold increase in the risk of developing clinical dementia (Hofman et al., 1997; Grammas, 2011). In a clinical series of Japanese individuals, Watanabe et al. (2004) demonstrated greater atherosclerotic plaque burden and increased carotid artery intima-media thickness in patients with vascular dementia as compared to patients with AD or their dementia-free peers (Ban et al., 2006). Among Japanese-American men in the Honolulu-Asia Aging Study, coronary heart disease was associated with an increased risk for vascular dementia (Ross et al., 1999). Cross-sectional epidemiological data from the Rotterdam Study have linked increased carotid and leg vessel atherosclerosis to the presence of dementia (Hofman et al., 1997) and identified a positive correlation between increasing atherosclerotic burden and risk for both AD and vascular dementia (Hofman et al., 1997). Over a mean follow-up period of 5 years, data from the Cardiovascular Health Study suggest common carotid arterial wall thickness is associated with incident dementia (Newman et al., 2005).

Taken together, these findings suggest that both the presence of vascular atherosclerosis and a history of MI are associated with increased risk for cognitive impairment. Myocardial infarction promotes arrhythmogenesis, and infarction is thought to contribute to reduced cardiac function (e.g., low cardiac output), reduction in cerebral blood flow, and microembolism. However, relations between MI and dementia may be partially mediated by the systemic burden of atherosclerosis that led to the initial MI. For example, low-grade chronic inflammation is associated with atherosclerosis (Lee et al., 2011) and coronary artery disease (Hansson, 2005). Such inflammation can promote endothelial cell dysfunction (Picchi et al., 2006; Gao et al., 2007), increase stroke risk (Hallenbeck, 2002), and contribute to inflammation in both stable and unstable atherosclerotic plaques (Hansson, 2005). In the absence of MI, atherosclerosis may also impact the brain through shared genetic factors (Slooter et al., 2004) or other mechanisms of CNS injury, such as lipid peroxidation (Napoli & Palinski, 2005), inflammation (Napoli & Palinski, 2005), oxidative stress (Napoli & Palinski, 2005), and cerebrovascular compromise.

Coronary Artery Bypass Grafting

Clinicians and researchers have been interested in neurological injury secondary to cardiac surgery for many decades (Samuels, 2006). Coronary artery bypass grafting, the most common cardiac surgery in the United States, is used to treat coronary artery disease. Coronary artery disease involves narrowing of the arteries supplying blood to the heart, secondary to atherosclerosis. Surgical grafts provide a conduit for blood to flow around arterial blockages using either an on-pump procedure (i.e., stopping the heart and relying on a heart-lung machine to perform the mechanics of heart and lung function) or an off-pump procedure (i.e., performing the procedure while the heart is still beating).

Although patients undergoing CABG experienced neurological complications immediately following cardiac surgery, these complications were thought to resolve over time (Savageau et al., 1982). However, longer follow-up intervals with cardiac surgical patients have suggested that late cognitive impairments can manifest several years post-surgery. For example, although a series from Newman et al. (2001) found that cognitive difficulties post-CABG resolved within 6 months, nearly half of study patients had cognitive impairment 5 years post-surgery. Variables predicting cognitive impairment at follow-up included older age, lower education levels, and cognitive impairment at hospital discharge (Newman et al., 2001). One criticism of the literature examining cognitive correlates of CABG is that "control" groups with comparable coronary artery disease are rarely included. McKhann et al. (2005) addressed this shortcoming when they compared CABG patients to off-pump cardiac surgery patients, medically treated cardiac patients, and healthy adults without cardiovascular disease. At baseline, there were significant between-group differences in cognitive performance for all coronary heart disease groups as compared to the heart-healthy control group. However, at follow-up 1 year later, the slope of change in cognitive performance was comparable among all four groups. The worsening of atherosclerotic disease with age may explain the cognitive decline observed over the longer follow-up intervals. Coronary artery bypass grafting has also been linked to increased risk for dementia, yet this is controversial. One case–control series found no difference in history of CABG between patients with dementia and age-matched control participants (Knopman et al., 2005). In contrast, data from a larger cohort of CABG patients followed over a 6-year period have suggested CABG is a risk factor for dementia (Lee et al., 2005). See Table 3.2 for an overview of CABG studies.

There are several purported mechanisms accounting for postsurgical cognitive decline, including both peri- and post-operative factors. Much of the research to date has focused on peri-operative factors. First, reductions in cerebral blood flow have been proposed as a primary underlying mechanism for cognitive changes seen post-CABG (Patel et al., 1993). Such blood flow reductions hypothetically result from intra-operative hypotension associated with cardiopulmonary bypass (Sendelbach et al.,

Table 3.2 **Summary of Coronary Artery Bypass Grafting Studies**

Citation	Sample size	Mean age (years)	Type of study	Sample description	Summary of findings
Dijk et al., 2007	Off-pump=142 On-pump = 139	Off-pump = 61.7 On-pump = 60.8	Randomized control trial	Patients were recruited in three centers in the Netherlands. All subjects enrolled were low-risk CABG patients between 1998 and 2000.	First large randomized trial reporting long-term cognitive outcomes after off-pump versus on-pump CABG surgery. Findings suggest that factors other than CABG may be responsible for cognitive decline as researchers were unable to demonstrate any benefit in cognitive outcome from avoiding CABG.
Knopman et al., 2005	Dementia Cases = 557 Matched controls = 557 AD cases = 438 Matched controls = 438	Dementia: 82 AD: 83	Case–control design	Authors used the infrastructure of the records-linkage system of the Rochester Epidemiology Project and the Mayo Clinic AD Patient Registry to ascertain incident cases of dementia for the years of Jan. 1990 to Dec.1994.	A population based case–control study finding CABG was not a major risk factor for overall dementia or AD.
Lee et al., 2005	CABG = 5,216	67.2	Cohort	VA patients undergoing CABG or PTCA between October 1, 1996 and September 30, 1997. Patients were followed from their surgery date until a diagnosis of AD, death, or the end of their follow-up period.	Retrospective cohort analysis of VA patients—results suggest that patients undergoing CABG surgery were at increased risk for the emergence of AD, supporting the hypothesis that CABG surgery is associated with a reduced neuronal reserve in an aging population.

Study	Sample	Mean Age	Design	Description	Findings
McKhann et al., 2005	CABG = 140 Off-pump coronary surgery = 72 NSCC w/ diagnosed coronary artery disease = 99 HHC = 69	CABG = 63.4 Off-pump coronary surgery = 65.9 NSCC w/ diagnosed coronary artery disease = 65.7 HHC = 62.5	Cohort	Patients who were native English speakers, not mechanically ventilated, able to sit upright, and able to give informed consent were enrolled. CABG = patients scheduled to undergo isolated on-pump CABG at Johns Hopkins were enrolled from eight surgeons between September 1997 and March 1999. Off-pump coronary surgery = Patients scheduled to undergo off-pump CABG surgery without the use of CPB were asked to participate enrolled from five sites. NSCC with diagnosed coronary artery disease = Patients diagnosed by cardiac catheterization with coronary artery disease and under medical management were recruited from four cardiologists at Johns Hopkins. HHC = Subjects were recruited via newspaper advertisements. Controls were selected to be comparable with the other groups in terms of age, sex, and education classification.	First study to compare the outcome of patients undergoing CABG with the outcome of other patients with coronary artery disease (another cardiac surgery group and a medically treated group) and with heart-healthy controls. Findings highlight the importance of appropriate control groups for interpreting changes in cognition after CABG. CABG patients, like similar patients with long-standing coronary artery disease, have some degree of cognitive dysfunction secondary to cerebrovascular disease before surgery.
Newman et al., 2001	261	60.9	Cohort	Patients undergoing elective CABG	Results confirm the relatively high prevalence and persistence of cognitive decline after CABG and suggest a pattern of early improvement followed by the presence of early postoperative cognitive decline.

(continued)

Table 3.2 **(Continued)**

Citation	Sample size	Mean age (years)	Type of study	Sample description	Summary of findings
Patel et al, 1993	Alpha-stat group = 35 pH-stat group = 35	Alpha-stat group: 56.9 pH-stat group: 57.6	Randomized control trial	Patient scheduled for elective CABS under the care of one surgical team. Patients were then randomized to undergo CPB managed by either alpha-stat or pH-stat acid-base management protocols	The cause of cerebral dysfunction following CPB is probably multifactorial. Results demonstrate that differing acid-base management protocols during bypass have a profound influence on CBF. Data from this study support modification of the acid-base protocol adopted during hypothermic CPB from the temperature-corrected method of pH from the temperature-corrected method of pH-stat to the temperature-uncorrected method of alpha-stat.
Ramlawi et al, 2006	NCD = 16 Without NCD = 24	NCD = 69.1 Without NCD = 66 Total *n* = 67.3	Cohort	Subjects from a single institution included patient scheduled for elective or urgent primary CABG, vascular surgery, or a combination of the two using CPB.	Neuron-specific enolase and tau are better associated with neurocognitive decline and less influenced by cardiotomy suction compared with S-100β. Inflammatory and oxidative stress is associated with neurocognitive decline post-CPB.
Savageau et al, 1982	245	54.7	Cohort	Patients undergoing CABG (75%), valve replacement (14%), or some combination of the two (11%)	Findings underscore the need for clinicians and investigators studying neuropsychological dysfunction following cardiac operations to take concurrent emotional and physical states account and make repeated measures well separated in time, before interpreting the presence or absence of residual neuropsychological problems. Findings demonstrate that sustained postoperative neuropsychological dysfunction 6 months after cardiac operations were rare in their specific sample. Suggested that causes of postoperative dysfunction are multifactorial (i.e. other pre-operative and postoperative variables)

Sendelbach et al, 2006	54	64.5	Cohort	Data were collected in cardiovascular units at Abbott Northwestern Hospital. All patients who were scheduled for an off-pump CABG surgery procedure were screened for eligibility for participation in the study	Older patients, anxious patients, and patients with new-onset atrial fibrillation are at risk for neurocognitive changes after off-pump CABG surgery.
Stanley et al, 2002	Atrial fibrillation = 69 No atrial fibrillation = 239	Atrial fibrillation = 66 No atrial fibrillation = 60	Cohort	Patients were individually examined with a battery of well-validated and established cognitive tests by experienced psychometricians blinded to the patient's cardiac rhythm status. Testing took place the day before CABG surgery (baseline) and 6 weeks postoperatively. All patients were operated on by the same team of surgeons. Patients were considered to have postoperative AFIB if telemetry displayed a sustained rhythm that was confirmed by a cardiologist interpreted 12-lead electrocardiogram and that did not convert spontaneously	Of patients undergoing CABG, authors showed that the occurrence of postoperative AFIB was associated with neurocognitive dysfunction at 6-week postoperative follow up.
Wityk et al, 2001	14	69	Cohort	Medical records were reviewed for patients who had DWI performed after cardiac surgery between March 1999 and January 2000 Of the 14 patients, 12 underwent CABG Of the 14 patients who underwent DWI studies, 13 had coronary artery disease; 9, hypertension; 6, hyperlipidemia; 5, diabetes; and 4 were current smokers.	Findings demonstrated the value of DWI and MRPI in patients with neurologic complications after cardiac surgery.

Note: AD = Alzheimer's disease; AFIB = atrial fibrillation; APP = amyloid precursor protein; CABG = coronary artery bypass graft; CABS = coronary artery bypass surgery; CBF = cerebral blood flow; CPB = cardiopulmonary bypass; CTF = C-terminal fragment; DWI = diffusion-weighted imaging; FL = full-length; HHC = heart healthy controls; MRPI = magnetic resonance perfusion imaging; NCD = neurocognitive decline; NSCC = nonsurgical cardiac controls; PTCA = percutaneous transluminal coronary angioplasty; VA = Veterans Affairs

2006). However, off-pump versus on-pump comparisons suggest comparable longitudinal cognitive decline, minimizing support for this hypothesis (van Dijk et al., 2007). A second peri-operative mechanism is based on diffusion-weighted and perfusion MRI data suggesting that peri-operative manipulation of major vessels causes cerebral microembolism (common with cardiac surgery), which contributes to cognitive decline (Wityk et al., 2001). A third peri-operative mechanism comes from basic science models suggesting that the use of general anesthetics may account for increased risk of cognitive decline and dementia postoperatively (Xie et al., 2006; Eckenhoff et al., 2004). For example, one popular general inhalation anesthetic is isoflurane, which has been shown to alter APP processing and increase β-amyloid protein (pathogenic feature of AD) in human cell cultures (Xie et al., 2006). In addition to peri-operative mechanisms, there are also several postoperative factors that may account for cognitive decline in CABG. First, atrial fibrillation incidence increases postsurgically and is associated with worse cognitive outcomes (Stanley et al., 2002). Second, circulating inflammatory markers and oxidative stress increase post-CABG. Patients who present post-CABG with cognitive decline have higher elevations of inflammatory markers than those patients without cognitive decline (Ramlawi et al., 2006).

In summary, clinical and epidemiological findings have linked CABG to cognitive impairment and dementia, although findings have been mixed regarding the long-term implications of CABG on cognition (McKhann et al., 2005; Lee et al., 2005). Mechanisms accounting for this association are likely multifactorial and include peri-operative (e.g., microembolism (Wityk et al., 2001), anesthesia (Xie et al., 2006) , postoperative variables (e.g., changes in cardiac function; Stanley et al., 2002), and inflammation (Ramlawi et al., 2006). In addition to post-CABG cognitive complications, there is a broader literature on postoperative cognitive dysfunction that has examined mechanisms underlying abnormal cognitive aging following surgical interventions (e.g., orthopedic cohorts). See Dr. Jacqueline Leung's Chapter 13 on postoperative cognitive dysfunction for more details.

Heart Failure

Heart failure occurs when the heart is unable to efficiently pump a sufficient volume of blood to meet the body's demand. Heart failure can result from impaired ventricular contractility (as seen in systolic heart failure) or relaxation (as seen in diastolic heart failure).

Heart failure has been linked to compromised cognitive function (Zuccala et al., 1997; Qiu et al., 2006). In clinical series of heart failure cases, measures of cardiac function, including lower left ventricular ejection fraction (Zuccala et al., 1997) and reduced cardiac output (Putzke et al., 1998), have been associated with poorer cognitive status. Collectively, these findings suggest that as the cardiac dysfunction worsens, cognitive status also worsens. When arterial hypotension co-occurs with heart failure, the risk of cognitive impairment appears to increase (Zuccala et al., 2001). Larger-scale epidemiological work supports the hypothesis that heart failure is associated with cognitive aging. In a large Italian cohort, individuals with cognitive impairment who were not yet demented had a higher frequency of heart failure compared to cognitively normal older adults (Di Carlo et al., 2000). In a Swedish cohort, heart failure was associated with an increased risk of dementia (and AD in particular) over a 9-year follow-up period (Qiu et al., 2006). The clinical and epidemiological evidence suggest that both subclinical (in the form of reduced cardiac output) and clinical (in the form of heart failure) cardiac dysfunction are associated with cognitive impairment and an increased risk for dementia.

There are several possible mechanisms linking heart failure to abnormal cognitive aging. The primary theoretical pathway is that reduced cardiac function contributes to reduced cerebral perfusion. Support for this pathway comes from the observation that there is a correlation between severity of heart failure and reductions in cerebral blood flow (Loncar et al., 2011), and reductions in cerebral blood flow increase when cardiac function is restored following cardiac transplant (Gruhn et al., 2001). Additional mechanistic pathways between heart failure and unhealthy brain aging include neurohumoral factors (Felder et al., 2003), thromboemboli (Freudenberger & Massie, 2005), and oxidative stress (Mariani et al., 2005).

Cardiac Arrest

Although cardiac arrest is less common, it involves the abrupt cessation of effective cardiac contraction, frequently caused by ventricular fibrillation or asystole. Given the difficulties in studying the neurological consequences of cardiac arrest, studies have used animal models to identify neuropathological features of AD following cardiac arrest. In one study, rats resuscitated after ten minutes of cardiac arrest had multifocal to diffuse deposition of amyloid β and increased APP in the hippocampus and entorhinal cortex (Pluta, 2000). The rats were followed from 2 days post-ischemic injury out to 1 year, and data indicated long-term effects from the short-term ischemic event (Pluta, 2000). These animal data suggest that the molecular events following acute ischemia-reperfusion are linked to the pathogenesis of AD. Although clinical series are subject to less experimental control, findings have been similar. In one series, 12 patients (ages 44–78 years) with no history of dementia were resuscitated within minutes of cardiac arrest (Wisniewski & Maslinska, 1996). All cases came to autopsy within 36 days with overexpression of β protein precursor. In a clinical series with a longer follow-up period, patients with cardiac arrest were more likely to be demented within 3 years as compared to patients with MI (Nielsen et al., 1983).

Taken together, these animal and clinical studies suggest cardiac arrest is associated both with clinical dementia and neuropathological features of AD.

There are several mechanisms that may account for these past observations. Because cerebral autoregulation exerts its effects within a defined range of blood pressure fluctuations (rather than a complete absence of blood pressure), cardiac arrest compromises cerebral perfusion homeostasis during and immediately following arrest. Such compromise in cerebral blood flow has multiple implications on brain health. First, the brain does not store glucose, has no active transport mechanism for glucose across the neuronal membrane, and has no capacity for anaerobic metabolism, so neuronal injury and death rapidly follow compromised cerebral blood flow and brain ischemia (Sierra, Coca, & Schiffrin 2011). Second, resuscitation can immediately restore heart function and blood flow; however, animal models of reperfusion suggest that following cardiac arrest, cardiac function and oxygen delivery to the brain is compromised (Oku et al., 1994). Third, ischemia-reperfusion injury plays a significant role in the impairment of brain function, so the longer the ischemic event, the more adverse the outcome. Ischemia results in cell death and subsequent release of intracellular contents into the systemic circulation, including the release of potassium from dying cells in the periphery and glutamate from neurons in the CNS. When blood flow is restored, further tissue injury occurs when high levels of circulating potassium reach the heart and exert arrhythmogenic and cardiotoxic effects (Bouchard, Jacquemet, & Vinet, 2011) while glutamate excitotoxicity occurs in the brain and causes cell death (Kato & Kogure, 1999). Collectively, cardiac arrest's adverse impact on the brain commences with an acute reduction in cerebral blood flow often followed by resuscitation and subsequent cerebral reperfusion injury with abnormal cerebral hemodynamics.

Theoretical Considerations

There are a number of mechanisms that may account for relations between cardiovascular disease and abnormal cognitive aging, as outlined in Table 3.1. The discussion below outlines some broad theoretical considerations that link possible mechanisms to multiple pathological processes associated with abnormal cognitive aging, including AD pathology, microvascular processes, and neurodegeneration. The complex interplay of these mechanisms and neuropathological processes is outlined in Figure 3.1; however, it is important to note that these theoretical considerations represent an overly simplistic explanation and are not meant to be exhaustive.

CEREBRAL BLOOD FLOW AND AUTOREGULATION

The brain is one of the most highly perfused organs in the body, and despite comprising roughly 2% of body weight, it receives 15% to 20% of resting cardiac output (Attwell et al., 2010). The principal determinants of cerebral blood flow are cardiac output, vessel diameter (i.e., determined by *structural-* and *neural-*mediated factors), blood viscosity, and perfusion pressure. The "neurovascular unit," which represents the relation between neural tissue and its blood supply, is both structurally and functionally complex, consisting of the endothelium and its basement membrane, pericytes (i.e., connective tissue cells associated with the vasculature), neurons, and glia or astrocytes (i.e., cells providing structural and metabolic support to the neurons) (Bonkowski et al., 2011; Fisher, 2009).

Cerebral autoregulation is a fundamental protective homeostatic function of the brain and involves the automatic adjustment of cerebrovascular tone in response to blood pressure changes. Such adjustments are coordinated through a complex interplay of neurogenic, myogenic, and metabolic mechanisms to maintain relatively constant blood flow to the brain over a wide range of systemic blood pressure. However, some debate exists regarding the mechanisms, robustness, and reliability of cerebral autoregulation during gradual versus acute blood pressure changes (Tzeng et al., 2010) and in healthy versus chronic disease states (Paulson, Strandgaard, & Edvinsson, 1990). Recent work suggests that *dynamic* cerebral autoregulation, which occurs in response to blood pressure changes that take place over seconds, is more effective in compensating for rising rather than falling blood pressure (Tzeng et al., 2010). This differential capacity to maintain cerebral blood flow at high versus low pressures may have important implications for maintenance of appropriate cerebral blood flow during acute intraoperative hypotension (as seen in CABG) and in a chronic heart failure state, which can co-occur with arterial hypotension (Zuccala et al., 2001). However, extrapolation of evidence from acute to chronic states is inexact, and there are few models that evaluate the efficacy of cerebral autoregulation in chronic hyper- and hypotensive states. Further, the integrity of cerebral autoregulation may be compromised in advanced age (Jefferson, 2010; Jefferson, Poppas et al., 2007; Jefferson, Tate et al., 2007), even in the absence of prevalent cardiovascular disease, but there are limited data examining autoregulatory capacity among aged adults.

Cardiovascular disease is thought to contribute to abnormal cognitive aging through cerebral blood flow reductions by promoting vascular or AD pathology. In cognitively normal aging samples, reductions in cerebral blood flow to the microvasculature is associated with white matter hyperintensities (WMHs) on structural imaging (Hatazawa et al., 1997; Marstrand et al., 2002), which are believed to reflect myelin or axonal loss (Udaka, Sawada, & Kameyama, 2002), rarefaction (Englund, 1998), gliosis (Englund, 1998), disruption of the ependymal lining (Fazekas et al., 1993; Thomas et al., 2003), and disruption in white matter fibers (Fazekas et al., 1993; Thomas et al., 2003). In addition to microvascular injury, decreased cerebral blood flow is associated with an increased risk of developing

AD (Maalikjy Akkawi et al., 2005). In post mortem examination, individuals with clinical dementia had a higher grade of atherosclerosis within the Circle of Willis than control subjects, and the atherosclerotic burden correlated with higher neuritic plaque density and Braak neurofibrillary tangle stage (Beach et al., 2007). These findings support a mechanistic pathway between reduced cerebral blood flow and AD pathology. Considering that atherosclerosis affects a vessel's ability to provide adequate blood supply to organs, these findings provide additional evidence that decreased cerebral blood flow secondary to vascular disease may contribute to the development or progression of cognitive decline.

THE BLOOD-BRAIN BARRIER AND ENDOTHELIAL DYSFUNCTION

Although rarely considered among the list of vascular risk factors for dementia, blood–brain barrier (BBB) and endothelial dysfunction are altered vascular states that may contribute to the pathology of cognitive impairment with age. The BBB is a physical and metabolic barrier that separates nervous tissue from the systemic circulation. Its major functions are to maintain brain parenchymal ion homeostasis and shield the brain from potentially harmful substances (Pasha & Gupta, 2010). Key constituents of the BBB are unfenestrated capillary endothelial cells closely adjoined by tight intercellular junctions, along with surrounding pericytes and astrocyte end feet separated from the endothelial cells by the basal lamina (Pasha & Gupta, 2010; Pahnke et al., 2009). The BBB's fundamental basis is a network of tight junctions located circumferentially around the perimeter of each endothelial cell, adjoining each cell to every other cell around it, thus forming zonula occludens. Under normal circumstances, these networks restrict paracellular diffusion (Pasha & Gupta, 2010), and astrocytes within the networks not only serve as physical participants in the barrier but may also modulate angiogenesis and tight junction formation in the brain (Lee et al., 2003).

Although often considered impenetrable, the BBB is dynamic and capable of responding to physiological stimuli (Bonkowski et al., 2011; Fisher, 2009; del Zoppo, 2010). In the absence of disease, numerous mechanisms facilitate transport across the BBB, including passive transcellular or paracellular diffusion of small lipophilic molecules, carrier-mediated transport, and ion channels (Huber, Egleton, & Davis, 2001). However, permeability can be increased when tight junction integrity is compromised, which occurs with central nervous system injury seen in AD (Bowman et al., 2007) or stroke (Jiao et al., 2011; Candelario-Jalil et al., 2011); in metabolic diseases, such as diabetes (Mogi & Horiuchi 2011); and with systemic inflammation (McColl, Rothwell, & Allan 2008). In fact, there is a reciprocal relation between BBB integrity and inflammation, as BBB dysfunction contributes to neuroinflammation and neurodegeneration (Palmer, 2011), whereas a pro-inflammatory environment leads to tight junction breakdown and subsequent BBB compromise. Perivascular inflammation and consequent gliosis may impair amyloid β clearance. Thus, not only does a breakdown of the tight junction network in disease states affect the physical barrier integrity and paracellular permeability of the BBB, but overall endothelial health also affects transcellular permeability through alterations in membrane integrity and transporter expression. Vascular inflammation is detrimental to endothelial health and is an important feature of AD. For example, microvessels of AD brains have higher levels of pro-inflammatory cytokines than non-AD brains (Grammas & Ovase, 2001). Vukic et al. (2009) found that exposure to amyloid β increased pro-inflammatory gene expression in cultured human brain endothelial cells, and this in vitro finding also correlated with similar upregulation in AD brains. Thus, it is plausible that inflammation may be a key mediator of the AD pathology associated with plaque deposition.

Whether vascular and BBB compromise precede AD pathology, coincide and subsequently exacerbate it, or are consequences of AD has not been well established, and it is possible that these three pathways converge in the complex matrix of AD etiopathogenesis. For example, a link between compromised microvascular integrity and neurodegeneration in AD is suggested by a study that documented collapsed or degenerated brain capillary endothelium in more than 90% of AD cases as compared to less than 30% of controls (Kalaria & Hedera 1995). However, there is evidence that in some individuals, loss of BBB integrity may occur early in the AD process and is an independent factor influencing progression. In a study of patients with mild to moderate AD, there was a significant correlation between cerebrospinal fluid-albumin index (i.e., a proxy for BBB permeability) and both clinical dementia rating and MRI indices of neurodegeneration, which could not be explained by age, sex, or APOE ε4 status (Bowman et al., 2007).

Aside from serving a barrier function, the endothelium is a highly synthetic bioreactive interface believed to be functionally altered in AD (Grammas, 2011). For example, markers of endothelial activation, such as E-selectin, are increased in patients with vascular dementia and AD (Zuliani et al., 2008). Evidence also suggests that impaired energy metabolism seen in AD brains occurs both at the level of the neuron and the endothelium. Specifically, AD brains exhibit decreased mitochondrial content in the endothelium of the cerebrovasculature (Stewart et al., 1992) and mitochondrial dysfunction at the level of the neuron (Manczak, Calkins, & Reddy, 2011; Yang, Askarova, & Lee, 2010). However, causal relations or mechanistic explanations for endothelial breakdown in AD have yet to be clearly established.

Summary and Future Directions

To better explain relations between cardiac disease and cognitive aging, this chapter reviews basic science, animal, post mortem, clinical, and epidemiological studies linking clinically common cardiovascular conditions (i.e., atrial fibrillation, atherosclerosis, myocardial infarction, CABG, heart failure, and cardiac arrest) with abnormal cognitive aging among older adults. We propose several plausible pathways to account for the complex relations between cardiovascular and neurological aging (*see* Fig. 3.1), and it is likely that clinical cardiac disease negatively impacts brain aging through a combination of these factors or pathways.

There are several key directions for future research in this area. First, additional work is warranted to better understand the mechanistic pathways between cardiovascular disease and abnormal cognitive aging. Such information would be important for developing future risk reduction and treatment studies. Second, future studies should identify subclinical disease states associated with early cognitive or neuroimaging changes prior to the onset of clinical dementia or stroke. For example, heart failure is associated with dementia (Qiu et al., 2006), but recent research suggests that in the absence of heart failure, markers of cardiac function, such as cardiac output (Jefferson et al., 2010) and ejection fraction (Jefferson et al., 2011), are associated with neuroimaging and cognitive markers of abnormal brain changes in a cohort free of clinical dementia or stroke. Therefore, future research should emphasize subclinical states or early markers of cardiovascular disease, which would yield important information for prevention purposes in the absence of effective disease-modifying therapeutics for dementia. Third, although older adults may not effectively manage their cardiovascular risk factors, such as hypertension (Hajjar & Kotchen, 2003) and hypercholesterolemia (Ford et al. 2003), recent research suggests that disclosing risk susceptibility information for future dementia does impact prevention behaviors among adults (Chao et al., 2008).

References

Alpert, J. S., P. Petersen, & J. Godtfredsen. (1988). Atrial fibrillation: natural history, complications, and management. *Annual Review of Medicine* 39:41–52.

Aronson, M. K., W. L. Ooi, H. Morgenstern, A. Hafner, D. Masur, H. Crystal, et al. (1990). Women, myocardial infarction, and dementia in the very old. *Neurology* 40(7):1102–1106.

Attwell, D., A. M. Buchan, S. Charpak, M. Lauritzen, B. A. Macvicar, & E. A. Newman. (2010). Glial and neuronal control of brain blood flow. *Nature* 468(7321):232–243.

Aviles, R. J., D. O. Martin, C. Apperson-Hansen, P. L. Houghtaling, P. Rautaharju, R. A. Kronmal, et al. (2003). Inflammation as a risk factor for atrial fibrillation. *Circulation* 108(24):3006–3010.

Ban, Y., T. Watanabe, A. Miyazaki, Y. Nakano, T. Tobe, T. Idei, et al. (2006). Impact of increased plasma serotonin levels and carotid atherosclerosis on vascular dementia. *Atherosclerosis* 195 (1):153–159.

Barber, M., R. C. Tait, J. Scott, A. Rumley, G. D. Lowe, & D. J. Stott. (2004). Dementia in subjects with atrial fibrillation: hemostatic function and the role of anticoagulation. *Journal of Thrombosis and Haemostasis* 2 (11):1873–1878.

Beach, T. G., J. R. Wilson, L. I. Sue, A. Newell, M. Poston, R. Cisneros, et al. (2007). Circle of Willis atherosclerosis: association with Alzheimer's disease, neuritic plaques and neurofi-brillary tangles. *Acta Neuropathologica (Berl)* 113(1):13–21.

Bonkowski, D., V. Katyshev, R. D. Balabanov, A. Borisov, & P. Dore-Duffy. (2011). The CNS microvascular pericyte: pericyte-astrocyte crosstalk in the regulation of tissue survival. *Fluids Barriers CNS* 8(1):8.

Borenstein, A. R., Y. Wu, J. A. Mortimer, G. D. Schellenberg, W. C. McCormick, J. D. Bowen, et al. (2005). Developmental and vascular risk factors for Alzheimer's disease. *Neurobiology of Aging* 26(3):325–334.

Bouchard, S., V. Jacquemet, & A. Vinet. (2011). Automaticity in acute ischemia: Bifurcation analysis of a human ventricular model. *Phys Rev E Stat Nonlin Soft Matter Phys* 83(1-1):011911.

Bowman, G. L., J. A. Kaye, M. Moore, D. Waichunas, N. E. Carlson, & J. F. Quinn. (2007). Blood-brain barrier impairment in Alzheimer disease: stability and functional significance. *Neurology* 68(21):1809–1814.

Boyle, P. A., A. S. Buchman, R. S. Wilson, J. F. Kelly, & D. A. Bennett. (2010). The APOE epsilon4 allele is associated with incident mild cognitive impairment among community-dwelling older persons. *Neuroepidemiology* 34(1):43–49.

Candelario-Jalil, E., J. Thompson, S. Taheri, M. Grossetete, J. C. Adair, E. Edmonds, et al. (2011). Matrix Metalloproteinases Are Associated With Increased Blood-Brain Barrier Opening in Vascular Cognitive Impairment. *Stroke* 42(5):1345–1350.

Chao, S., J. S. Roberts, T. M. Marteau, R. Silliman, L. A. Cupples, & R. C. Green. (2008). Health behavior changes after genetic risk assessment for Alzheimer disease: The REVEAL Study. *Alzheimer's Disease & Associated Disorders* 22(1):94–97.

Corder, E. H., A. M. Saunders, N. J. Risch, W. J. Strittmatter, D. E. Schmechel, P. C. Gaskell, Jr., et al. (1994). Protective effect of apolipoprotein E type 2 allele for late onset Alzheimer disease. *Nature Genetics* 7(2):180–184.

del Zoppo, G. J. (2010). The neurovascular unit in the setting of stroke. *J Intern Med* 267(2):156–171.

Di Carlo, A., M. Baldereschi, L. Amaducci, S. Maggi, F. Grigoletto, G. Scarlato, et al. (2000). Cognitive impairment without dementia in older people: prevalence, vascular risk factors, impact on disability. The Italian Longitudinal Study on Aging. *Journal of the American Geriatric Society* 48 (7):775–782.

Dupuy, A. M., E. Mas, K. Ritchie, B. Descomps, S. Badiou, J. P. Cristol, et al. (2001). The relationship between apolipoprotein E4 and lipid metabolism is impaired in Alzheimer's disease. *Gerontology* 47(4):213–218.

Eckenhoff, R. G., J. S. Johansson, H. Wei, A. Carnini, B. Kang, W. Wei, et al. (2004). Inhaled anesthetic enhancement of amyloid-beta oligomerization and cytotoxicity. *Anesthesiology* 101(3):703–709.

Elias, M. F., L. M. Sullivan, P. K. Elias, R. B. D'Agostino, R. S. Vasan, S. Seshadri, et al. (2006). Atrial fibrillation and cognitive performance in the Framingham offspring men. *International Journal of Stroke & Cardiovascular Disease* 15(5):214–222.

Englund, E. (1998). Neuropathology of white matter changes in Alzheimer's disease and vascular dementia. *Dement Geriatr Cogn Disord* 9(Suppl 1):6–12.

Ezekowitz, M. D., K. E. James, S. M. Nazarian, J. Davenport, J. P. Broderick, S. R. Gupta, et al. (1995). Silent cerebral infarction in patients with nonrheumatic atrial fibrillation. The Veterans Affairs Stroke Prevention in Nonrheumatic Atrial Fibrillation Investigators. *Circulation* 92(8):2178–2182.

Fazekas, F., R. Kleinert, H. Offenbacher, R. Schmidt, G. Kleinert, F. Payer, et al. (1993). Pathologic correlates of incidental MRI white matter signal hyperintensities. *Neurology* 43(9):1683–1689.

Felder, R. B., J. Francis, Z. H. Zhang, S. G. Wei, R. M. Weiss, & A. K. Johnson. 2003. Heart failure and the brain: new perspectives. *American Journal of Physiology. Regulatory, Integrative, & Comparative Physiology* 284(2):R259–R276.

Fisher, M. (2009). Pericyte signaling in the neurovascular unit. *Stroke* 40(3 Suppl):S13–S15.

Ford, E. S., A. H. Mokdad, W. H. Giles, & G. A. Mensah. (2003). Serum total cholesterol concentrations and awareness, treatment, and control of hypercholerolemia among US adults: findings from the National Health and Nutrition Examination Survey, 1999 to 2000. *Circulation* 107(17):2185–2189.

Forti, P., F. Maioli, N. Pisacane, E. Rietti, F. Montesi, & G. Ravaglia. (2006). Atrial fibrillation and risk of dementia in non-demented elderly subjects with and without mild cognitive impairment. *Neurological Research* 28(6):625–629.

Freudenberger, R. S., & B. M. Massie. (2005). Silent cerebral infarction in heart failure: vascular or thromboembolic? *Journal of Cardiac Failure* 11(7):490–491.

Gao, X., S. Belmadani, A. Picchi, X. Xu, B. J. Potter, N. Tewari-Singh, et al. (2007). Tumor necrosis factor-alpha induces endothelial dysfunction in Lepr(db) mice. *Circulation* 115(2):245–254.

Grammas, P. (2011). Neurovascular dysfunction, inflammation and endothelial activation: Implications for the pathogenesis of Alzheimer's disease. *J Neuroinflammation* 8:26.

Grammas, P., & R. Ovase. (2001). Inflammatory factors are elevated in brain microvessels in Alzheimer's disease. *Neurobiol Aging* 22(6):837–842.

Greenberg, S. M., M. E. Briggs, B. T. Hyman, G. J. Kokoris, C. Takis, D. S. Kanter, et al. (1996). Apolipoprotein E epsilon 4 is associated with the presence and earlier onset of hemorrhage in cerebral amyloid angiopathy. *Stroke* 27(8):1333–1337.

Gruhn, N., F. S. Larsen, S. Boesgaard, G. M. Knudsen, S. A. Mortensen, G. Thomsen, et al. (2001). Cerebral blood flow in patients with chronic heart failure before and after heart transplantation. *Stroke* 32(11):2530–2533.

Hajjar, I., & T. A. Kotchen. 2003. Trends in prevalence, awareness, treatment, and control of hypertension in the United States, 1988-2000. *The Journal of the American Medical Association* 290(2):199–206.

Hallenbeck, J. M. (2002). The many faces of tumor necrosis factor in stroke. *Nat Med* 8 (12):1363–1368.

Hansson, G. K. (2005). Inflammation, atherosclerosis, and coronary artery disease. *N Engl J Med* 352(16):1685–1695.

Hatazawa, J., E. Shimosegawa, T. Satoh, H. Toyoshima, & T. Okudera. (1997). Subcortical hypoperfusion associated with asymptomatic white matter lesions on magnetic resonance imaging. *Stroke* 28(10):1944–1947.

Hayden, K. M., P. P. Zandi, C. G. Lyketsos, A. S. Khachaturian, L. A. Bastian, G. Charoonruk, et al. (2006). Vascular risk factors for incident Alzheimer disease and vascular dementia: the Cache County study. *Alzheimer Disease and Associated Disorders* 20(2):93–100.

Hebert, S. S., L. Serneels, T. Dejaegere, K. Horre, M. Dabrowski, V. Baert, et al. (2004). Coordinated and widespread expression of gamma-secretase in vivo: evidence for size and molecular heterogeneity. *Neurobiology of Disease* 17(2):260–272.

Hofman, A., A. Ott, M. M. Breteler, M. L. Bots, A. J. Slooter, F. van Harskamp, et al. (1997). Atherosclerosis, apolipoprotein E, and prevalence of dementia and Alzheimer's disease in the Rotterdam Study. *Lancet* 349(9046):151–154.

Honig, L. S., W. Kukull, & R. Mayeux. (2005). Atherosclerosis and AD: analysis of data from the US National Alzheimer's Coordinating Center. *Neurology* 64(3):494–500.

Huber, J. D., R. D. Egleton, & T. P. Davis. (2001). Molecular physiology and pathophysiology of tight junctions in the blood-brain barrier. *Trends Neurosci* 24(12):719–725.

Jefferson, A. L. (2010). Cardiac output as a potential risk factor for abnormal brain aging. *Journal of Alzheimer's Disease* 20(3):813–821.

Jefferson, A. L., J. J. Himali, R. Au, S. Seshadri, C. DeCarli, C. J. O'Donnell, et al. (2011). Relation of left ventricular fraction to cognitive aging (from the Framingham Heart Study). *American Journal of Cardiology* 108(9):1346–1351.

Jefferson, A. L., J. J. Himali, A. S. Beiser, R. Au, J. M. Massaro, S. Seshadri, et al. (2010). Cardiac index is associated with brain aging: The Framingham Heart Study. *Circulation* 122:690–697.

Jefferson, A. L., J. M. Massaro, A. S. Beiser, S. Seshadri, M. G. Larson, P. A. Wolf, et al. (2011). Inflammatory biomarkers and neuropsychological functioning: The Framingham Heart Study. *Neurobiology of Aging* 37(1):21–30.

Jefferson, A. L., J.M. Massaro, M.G. Larson, P. A. Wolf, R. Au, R. B. D'Agostino, et al. (2007). Inflammatory biomarkers are associated with total brain volume: The Framingham Heart Study. *Neurology* 68 (13):1032–1038.

Jefferson, A. L., A. Poppas, R. H. Paul, & R. A. Cohen. (2007). Systemic hypoperfusion is associated with executive dysfunction in geriatric cardiac patients. *Neurobiology of Aging* 28(4):477–483.

Jefferson, A. L., D. F. Tate, A. Poppas, A. M. Brickman, R. H. Paul, J. Gunstad, et al. (2007). Lower cardiac output is associated with greater white matter hyperintensities in older adults with cardiovascular disease. *Journal of the American Geriatrics Society* 55(7):1044–1048.

Jiao, H., Z. Wang, Y. Liu, P. Wang, & Y. Xue. (2011). Specific Role of Tight Junction Proteins Claudin-5, Occludin, and ZO-1 of the Blood-Brain Barrier in a Focal Cerebral Ischemic Insult. *J Mol Neurosci* 44(2):130–139.

Kalaria, R. N. (2000). The role of cerebral ischemia in Alzheimer's disease. *Neurobiol Aging* 21(2):321–330.

Kalaria, R. N., & P. Hedera. (1995). Differential degeneration of the cerebral microvasculature in Alzheimer's disease. *Neuroreport* 6(3):477–480.

Kato, H., & K. Kogure. (1999). Biochemical and molecular characteristics of the brain with developing cerebral infarction. *Cell Mol Neurobiol* 19(1):93–108.

Kinnecom, C., M. H. Lev, L. Wendell, E. E. Smith, J. Rosand, M. P. Frosch, et al. (2007). Course of cerebral amyloid angiopathy-related inflammation. *Neurology* 68(17):1411–1416.

Kivipelto, M., T. Ngandu, L. Fratiglioni, M. Viitanen, I. Kareholt, B. Winblad, et al. (2005). Obesity and vascular risk factors at midlife and the risk of dementia and Alzheimer disease. *Archives of Neurology* 62(10):1556–1560.

Knopman, D. S., R. C. Petersen, R. H. Cha, S. D. Edland, & W. A. Rocca. (2005). Coronary artery bypass grafting is not a risk factor for dementia or Alzheimer disease. *Neurology* 65(7):986–990.

Kosunen, O., S. Talasniemi, M. Lehtovirta, O. Heinonen, S. Helisalmi, A. Mannermaa, et al. (1995). Relation of coronary atherosclerosis and apolipoprotein E genotypes in Alzheimer patients. *Stroke* 26(5):743–748.

Kwok, C. S., Y. K. Loke, R. Hale, J. F. Potter, & P. K. Myint. (2011). Atrial fibrillation and incidence of dementia: a systematic review and meta-analysis. *Neurology* 76 (10):914–922.

Lee, S., Y. Park, M. Y. Zuidema, M. Hannink, & C. Zhang. (2011). Effects of interventions on oxidative stress and inflammation of cardiovascular diseases. *World J Cardiol* 3(1):18–24.

Lee, S. W., W. J. Kim, Y. K. Choi, H. S. Song, M. J. Son, I. H. Gelman, et al. (2003). SSeCKS regulates angiogenesis and tight junction formation in blood-brain barrier. *Nat Med* 9 (7):900–906.

Lee, T. A., B. Wolozin, K. B. Weiss, & M. M. Bednar. (2005). Assessment of the emergence of Alzheimer's disease following coronary artery bypass graft surgery or percutaneous transluminal coronary angioplasty. *Journal of Alzheimer's Disease* 7(4):319–324.

Li, D., S. B. Parks, J. D. Kushner, D. Nauman, D. Burgess, S. Ludwigsen, et al. (2006). Mutations of presenilin genes in dilated cardiomyopathy and heart failure. *American Journal of Human Genetics* 79(6):1030–1039.

Loncar, G., B. Bozic, T. Lepic, S. Dimkovic, N. Prodanovic, Z. Radojicic, et al. (2011). Relationship of reduced cerebral blood flow and heart failure severity in elderly males. *Aging Male* 14(1):59–65.

Luchsinger, J. A., C. Reitz, L. S. Honig, M. X. Tang, S. Shea, & R. Mayeux. (2005). Aggregation of vascular risk factors and risk of incident Alzheimer disease. *Neurology* 65(4):545–551.

Maalikjy Akkawi, N., B. Borroni, C. Agosti, M. Magoni, M. Broli, A. Pezzini, et al. (2005). Volume cerebral blood flow reduction in pre-clinical stage of Alzheimer disease: evidence from an ultrasonographic study. *Journal of Neurology* 252(5):559–563.

Mahley, R. W., K. H. Weisgraber, & Y. Huang. 2009. Apolipoprotein E: structure determines function, from atherosclerosis to Alzheimer's disease to AIDS. *J Lipid Res* 50(Suppl):S183–S188.

Manczak, M., M. J. Calkins, & P. H. Reddy. (2011). Impaired Mitochondrial Dynamics and Abnormal Interaction of Amyloid Beta with Mitochondrial Protein Drp1 in Neurons from Patients with Alzheimer's Disease: Implications for Neuronal Damage. *Hum Mol Genet* 20(13):2495–2509.

Mariani, E., M. C. Polidori, A. Cherubini, & P. Mecocci. (2005). Oxidative stress in brain aging, neurodegenerative and vascular diseases: an overview. *Journal of Chromatography. B, Analytical Technologies in the Biomededical & Life Sciences* 827(1):65–75.

Marstrand, J. R., E. Garde, E. Rostrup, P. Ring, S. Rosenbaum, E. L. Mortensen, et al. (2002). Cerebral perfusion and cerebrovascular reactivity are reduced in white matter hyperintensities. *Stroke* 33(4):972–976.

McColl, B. W., N. J. Rothwell, & S. M. Allan. (2008). Systemic inflammation alters the kinetics of cerebrovascular tight junction disruption after experimental stroke in mice. *J Neurosci* 28(38):9451–9462.

McKhann, G. M., M. A. Grega, L. M. Borowicz, Jr., M. M. Bailey, S. J. Barry, S. L. Zeger, et al. (2005). Is there cognitive decline 1 year after CABG? Comparison with surgical and non-surgical controls. *Neurology* 65(7):991–99.

Mogi, M., & M. Horiuchi. (2011). Neurovascular Coupling in Cognitive Impairment Associated With Diabetes Mellitus. *Circ J* 75(5):1042–1048.

Muller, M., Y. van der Graaf, A. Algra, J. Hendrikse, W. P. Mali, & M. I. Geerlings. (2011). Carotid atherosclerosis and progression of brain atrophy: The SMART-MR Study. *Annals of Neurology* 70(2):237–244.

Napoli, C., & W. Palinski. (2005). Neurodegenerative diseases: insights into pathogenic mechanisms from atherosclerosis. *Neurobiology of Aging* 26(3):293–302.

Newman, A. B., A. L. Fitzpatrick, O. Lopez, S. Jackson, C. Lyketsos, W. Jagust, et al. (2005). Dementia and Alzheimer's disease incidence in relationship to cardiovascular disease in the Cardiovascular Health Study cohort. *Journal of the American Geriatrics Society* 53(7):1101–1107.

Newman, M. F., J. L. Kirchner, B. Phillips-Bute, V. Gaver, H. Grocott, R. H. Jones, et al. (2001). Longitudinal assessment of neurocognitive function after coronary-artery bypass surgery. *The New England Journal of Medicine* 344(6):395–402.

Nielsen, J. R., L. Gram, L. P. Rasmussen, E. M. Damsgaard, M. Dalsgaard, C. Richardt, et al. (1983). Intellectual and social function of patients surviving cardiac arrest outside the hospital. *Acta Medica Scandinavica* 213(1):37–39.

Oku, K., K. Kuboyama, P. Safar, W. Obrist, F. Sterz, Y. Leonov, et al. (1994). Cerebral and systemic arteriovenous oxygen monitoring after cardiac arrest. Inadequate cerebral oxygen delivery. *Resuscitation* 27(2):141–152.

Ott, A., M. M. Breteler, M. C. de Bruyne, F. van Harskamp, D. E. Grobbee, & A. Hofman. 1997. Atrial fibrillation and dementia in a population-based study. The Rotterdam Study. *Stroke* 28(2):316–321.

Pahnke, J., L. C. Walker, K. Scheffler, & M. Krohn. (2009). Alzheimer's disease and blood-brain barrier function-Why have anti-beta-amyloid therapies failed to prevent dementia progression? *Neurosci Biobehav Rev* 33(7):1099–1108.

Palmer, A. M. (2011). The Role of the Blood Brain Barrier in Neurodegenerative Disorders and their Treatment. *J Alzheimers Dis* 24(4):643–656.

Park, H., A. Hildreth, R. Thomson, & J. O'Connell. (2007). Non-valvular atrial fibrillation and cognitive decline: a longitudinal cohort study. *Age and Ageing* 36(2):157–163.

Park, H. L., A. J. Hildreth, R. G. Thomson, & J. O'Connell. (2005). Non-valvular atrial fibrillation and cognitive function—baseline results of a longitudinal cohort study. *Age and Ageing* 34(4):392–395.

Pasha, S., & K. Gupta. (2010). Various drug delivery approaches to the central nervous system. *Expert Opin Drug Deliv* 7(1):113–135.

Patel, R. L., M. R. Turtle, D. J. Chambers, S. Newman, & G. E. Venn. (1993). Hyperperfusion and cerebral dysfunction. Effect of differing acid-base management during cardiopulmonary bypass. *European Journal of Cardiothoracic Surgery* 7(9):457–463; discussion 464.

Paulson, O. B., S. Strandgaard, & L. Edvinsson. (1990). Cerebral autoregulation. *Cerebrovascular and Brain Metabolism Reviews* 2(2):161–192.

Petersen, P., J. Kastrup, R. Videbaek, & G. Boysen. (1989). Cerebral blood flow before and after cardioversion of atrial fibrillation. *Journal of Cerebral Blood Flow & Metabolism* 9(3):422–425.

Picchi, A., X. Gao, S. Belmadani, B. J. Potter, M. Focardi, W. M. Chilian, et al. (2006). Tumor necrosis factor-alpha induces endothelial dysfunction in the prediabetic metabolic syndrome. *Circ Res* 99(1):69–77.

Pluta, R. (2000). The role of apolipoprotein E in the deposition of beta-amyloid peptide during ischemia-reperfusion brain injury. A model of early Alzheimer's disease. *Annals of the New York Academy of Sciences* 903:324–334.

Putzke, J. D., M. A. Williams, B. K. Rayburn, J. K. Kirklin, & T. J. Boll. (1998). The relationship between cardiac function and neuropsychological status among heart transplant candidates. *Journal of Cardiac Failure* 4(4):295–303.

Qiu, C., B. Winblad, A. Marengoni, I. Klarin, J. Fastbom, & L. Fratiglioni. (2006). Heart failure and risk of dementia and Alzheimer disease: a population-based cohort study. *Archives of Internal Medicine* 166 (9):1003–1008.

Ramlawi, B., J. L. Rudolph, S. Mieno, K. Khabbaz, N. R. Sodha, M. Boodhwani, et al. (2006). Serologic markers of brain injury and cognitive function after cardiopulmonary bypass. *Annals of Surgery* 244(4):593–601.

Ravaglia, G., P. Forti, F. Maioli, M. Martelli, L. Servadei, N. Brunetti, et al. (2006). Conversion of mild cognitive impairment to dementia: predictive role of mild cognitive impairment subtypes and vascular risk factors. *Dementia and Geriatric Cognitive Disorders* 21(1):51–58.

Ridker, P. M., N. Rifai, L. Rose, J. E. Buring, & N. R. Cook. (2002). Comparison of C-reactive protein and low-density lipoprotein cholesterol levels in the prediction of first cardiovascular events. *The New England Journal of Medicine* 347(20):1557–1565.

Ross, G. W., H. Petrovitch, L. R. White, K. H. Masaki, C. Y. Li, J. D. Curb, et al. (1999). Characterization of risk factors for vascular dementia: the Honolulu-Asia Aging Study. *Neurology* 53(2):337–343.

Samuels, M. A. (2006). Can cognition survive heart surgery? *Circulation* 113 (24):2784–6.

Savageau, J. A., B. A. Stanton, C. D. Jenkins, & R. W. Frater. (1982). Neuropsychological dysfunction following elective cardiac operation. II. A six-month reassessment. *The Journal of Thoracic and Cardiovascular Surgery* 84(4):595–600.

Sendelbach, S., R. Lindquist, S. Watanuki, & K. Savik. (2006). Correlates of neurocognitive function of patients after off-pump coronary artery bypass surgery. *American Journal of Critical Care* 15(3):290–298.

Sierra, C., A. Coca, & E. L. Schiffrin. (2011). Vascular mechanisms in the pathogenesis of stroke. *Current Hypertension Reports* 13(3):200–207.

Slooter, A. J., M. Cruts, A. Hofman, P. J. Koudstaal, D. van der Kuip, M. A. de Ridder, et al. (2004). The impact of APOE on myocardial infarction, stroke, and dementia: the Rotterdam Study. *Neurology* 62(7):1196–1198.

Stanley, T. O., G. B. Mackensen, H. P. Grocott, W. D. White, J. A. Blumenthal, D. T. Laskowitz, et al. (2002). The impact of postoperative atrial fibrillation on neurocognitive outcome after coronary artery bypass graft surgery. *Anesthesia and Analgesia* 94(2):290–295.

Stewart, P. A., K. Hayakawa, M. A. Akers, & H. V. Vinters. (1992). A morphometric study of the blood-brain barrier in Alzheimer's disease. *Lab Invest* 67(6):734–742.

Tabas, I. (2011). Pulling down the plug on atherosclerosis: Finding the culprit in your heart. *Nature Medicine* 17(7):791–793.

Tarkowski, E., L. Rosengren, C. Blomstrand, C. Wikkelso, C. Jensen, S. Ekholm, et al. (1995). Early intrathecal production of interleukin-6 predicts the size of brain lesion in stroke. *Stroke* 26(8):1393–1398.

Tarkowski, E., M. Tullberg, P. Fredman, & C. Wikkelso. (2003). Correlation between intrathecal sulfatide and TNF-alpha levels in patients with vascular dementia. *Dementia and Geriatric Cognitive Disorders* 15(4):207–211.

Thomas, A. J., J. T. O'Brien, R. Barber, W. McMeekin, & R. Perry. (2003). A neuropathological study of periventricular white matter hyperintensities in major depression. *Journal of Affective Disorders* 76(1–3):49–54.

Tresch, D. D., M. F. Folstein, P. V. Rabins, & W. R. Hazzard. (1985). Prevalence and significance of cardiovascular disease and hypertension in elderly patients with dementia and depression. *Journal of the American Geriatric Society* 33(8):530–537.

Tzeng, Y. C., C. K. Willie, G. Atkinson, S. J. Lucas, A. Wong, & P. N. Ainslie. (2010). Cerebrovascular regulation during transient hypotension and hypertension in humans. *Hypertension* 56(2):268–273.

Udaka, F., H. Sawada, & M. Kameyama. (2002). White matter lesions and dementia: MRI-pathological correlation. *Ann N Y Acad Sci* 977:411–415.

van der Cammen, T. J., C. J. Verschoor, C. P. van Loon, F. van Harskamp, I. de Koning, W. J. Schudel, et al. (1998). Risk of left ventricular dysfunction in patients with probable Alzheimer's disease with APOE*4 allele. *Journal of the American Geriatrics Society* 46(8):962–967.

van Dijk, D., M. Spoor, R. Hijman, H. M. Nathoe, C. Borst, E. W. Jansen, et al. (2007). Cognitive and cardiac outcomes 5 years after off-pump vs on-pump coronary artery bypass graft surgery. *The Journal of the American Medical Association* 297(7):701–708.

van Dijk, E. J., N. D. Prins, S. E. Vermeer, H. A. Vrooman, A. Hofman, P. J. Koudstaal al. (2005). C-reactive protein and cerebral small-vessel disease: the Rotterdam Scan Study. *Circulation* 112(6):900–905.

Vasan, R. S., L. M. Sullivan, R. Roubenoff, C. A. Dinarello, T. Harris, E. J. Benjamin, et al. (2003). Inflammatory markers and risk of heart failure in elderly subjects without prior myocardial infarction: the Framingham Heart Study. *Circulation* 107(11):1486–1491.

Vukic, V., D. Callaghan, D. Walker, L. F. Lue, Q. Y. Liu, P. O. Couraud, et al. (2009). Expression of inflammatory genes induced by beta-amyloid peptides in human brain endothelial cells and in Alzheimer's brain is mediated by the JNK-AP1 signaling pathway. *Neurobiol Dis* 34(1):95–106.

Wann, B. P., T. M. Bah, M. Boucher, J. Courtemanche, N. Le Marec, G. Rousseau, et al. (2007). Vulnerability for apoptosis in the limbic system after myocardial infarction in rats: a possible model for human postinfarct major depression. *Journal of Psychiatry & Neuroscience* 32(1):11–16.

Watanabe, T., S. Koba, M. Kawamura, M. Itokawa, T. Idei, Y. Nakagawa, et al. (2004). Small dense low-density lipoprotein and carotid atherosclerosis in relation to vascular dementia. *Metabolism* 53(4):476–482.

Wilson, P. W., J. M. Hoeg, R. B. D'Agostino, H. Silbershatz, A. M. Belanger, H. Poehlmann, et al. (1997). Cumulative effects of high cholesterol levels, high blood pressure, and cigarette smoking on carotid stenosis. *The New England Journal of Medicine* 337(8):516–522.

Wisniewski, H. M., & D. Maslinska. (1996). Beta-protein immunoreactivity in the human brain after cardiac arrest. *Folia Neuropathologica* 34(2):65–71.

Wityk, R. J., M. A. Goldsborough, A. Hillis, N. Beauchamp, P. B. Barker, L. M. Borowicz, Jr., et al. (2001). Diffusion- and perfusion-weighted brain magnetic resonance imaging in patients with neurologic complications after cardiac surgery. *Archives of Neurology* 58(4):571–576.

Wolf, P. A., R. D. Abbott, & W. B. Kannel. (1987). Atrial fibrillation: a major contributor to stroke in the elderly. The Framingham Study. *Archives of Internal Medicine* 147(9):1561–1564.

Xie, Z., Y. Dong, U. Maeda, P. Alfille, D. J. Culley, G. Crosby, et al. (2006). The common inhalation anesthetic isoflurane induces apoptosis and increases amyloid beta protein levels. *Anesthesiology* 104(5):988–994.

Yaffe, K., K. Lindquist, B. W. Penninx, E. M. Simonsick, M. Pahor, S. Kritchevsky, et al. (2003). Inflammatory markers and cognition in well-functioning African-American and white elders. *Neurology* 61(1):76–80.

Yang, X., S. Askarova, & J. C. Lee. (2010). Membrane biophysics and mechanics in Alzheimer's disease. *Mol Neurobiol* 41(2-3):138–148.

Yasojima, K., C. Schwab, E. G. McGeer, & P. L. McGeer. (2000). Human neurons generate C-reactive protein and amyloid P: upregulation in Alzheimer's disease. *Brain Research* 887(1):80–89.

Yusuf, S., S. Hawken, S. Ounpuu, T. Dans, A. Avezum, F. Lanas, et al. (2004). Effect of potentially modifiable risk factors associated with myocardial infarction in 52 countries (the INTERHEART study): case-control study. *Lancet* 364(9438):937–952.

Zhiyou, C., Y. Yong, S. Shanquan, Z. Jun, H. Liangguo, Y. Ling, et al. (2009). Upregulation of BACE1 and beta-amyloid protein mediated by chronic cerebral hypoperfusion contributes to cognitive impairment and pathogenesis of Alzheimer's disease. *Neurochem Res* 34(7):1226–1235.

Zuccala, G., C. Cattel, E. Manes-Gravina, M. G. Di Niro, A. Cocchi, & R. Bernabei. (1997). Left ventricular dysfunction: a clue to cognitive impairment in older patients with heart failure. *Journal of Neurology, Neurosurgery, and Psychiatry* 63(4):509–512.

Zuccala, G., G. Onder, C. Pedone, L. Carosella, M. Pahor, R. Bernabei, et al. (2001). Hypotension and cognitive impairment: Selective association in patients with heart failure. *Neurology* 57(11):1986–1992.

Zuliani, G., M. Cavalieri, M. Galvani, A. Passaro, M. R. Munari, C. Bosi, et al. (2008). Markers of endothelial dysfunction in older subjects with late onset Alzheimer's disease or vascular dementia. *J Neurol Sci* 272(1-2):164–170.

4

Obesity and Cognitive Health: Implications of an Altered Adiposity Milieu Over the Life-Course

RACHEL A. WHITMER, PHD AND DEBORAH R. GUSTAFSON, MS, PHD

Public Health Significance

Obesity is a significant public health problem worldwide that, while increasing, is pandemic (Ramos, Xu et al., 2003). The exact processes and mechanisms linking obesity to the onset of clinically relevant cognitive impairment and dementia are complex and somewhat undiscovered. Although obesity has established effects on cardiovascular and metabolic health, only recently has its potential influence on cognitive health been evaluated. If obesity has even a modest effect on cognition, then it is important to quantify because obesity is a potentially modifiable risk factor.

Obesity and Cognition Within the Context of Changes in Population Heath Trends

Overweight and obesity are defined by the World Health Organization (WHO) and Centers for Disease Control and Prevention (CDC) as a body mass index (BMI) of 25 kg/m^2 to 29.9 kg/m^2 and 30 kg/m^2 or greater, respectively. Morbid obesity is a BMI of 40 kg/m^2 or greater. As aforementioned, overweight and obesity are increasing and pandemic in most of the world (Ford, Giles et al., 2002). The CDC estimates that in the United States, the prevalence of overweight and obesity is almost 70%. In Europe estimates are highest in the United Kingdom, with 62% of adults estimated as overweight and obese, according to the Department of Health (www.dh.gov.uk). Globally, and taking into consideration both high- and low-income countries that have data to report on

BMI, the prevalence of overweight and obesity is estimated to be at least 30% among adults (Visscher, Seidell et al., 2000; Flegal, 2005; http://www.who.int/en/, 2011). The highest prevalences have been observed among women age 50 years and older (Flegal, 2005); however, this is changing as men and children are becoming increasingly more overweight and obese as well (Li, Ford et al., 2007; Schokker, Visscher et al., 2007). Of the top 10 causes of death worldwide, half are related to obesity and account for 40.3% of all deaths. These include ischemic heart disease (14.2%), cerebrovascular disease (12.1%), chronic obstructive pulmonary disease (8.6%), type 2 diabetes (T2DM; 3.3%), and hypertensive heart disease (2.1%) (http://www.who.int/en/; WHO, 2008).

Concomitant with the increase in obesity is also a trend in the prevalence of abdominal obesity, a condition that is considered separately and that carries its own risk but is highly correlated with total body obesity. Results from the National Health and Nutrition Examination Survey (NHANES) show a marked increase between 1999 to 2000 and 2003 to 2004 in prevalence of abdominal obesity as evaluated by waist circumference. In men, the prevalence increased from 37% to 42%, and in women from 55.3% to 61.3%. In the period of 2003 to 2004, more than half of the U.S. adults met the criteria for abdominal obesity (Li, Ford et al., 2007). Similar trends have been observed in the United Kingdom and worldwide (NHANES, U.K. study). The changing population prevalence of abdominal obesity is not limited to adults but has also been observed in children. Thus the potential impact of increased adiposity on population health could commence at earlier ages such as that illustrated by recent increases in children with type 2 diabetes (T2DM). This is especially salient for cognitive health, as conditions associated with abdominal obesity (e.g., T2DM, hypertension) are also risk factors for dementia and cognitive impairment.

Aging and Body Composition Changes

Assessment of obesity and adiposity *prior* to old age is an important consideration when evaluating its potential relationship to cognition. Body mass index in elderly populations is an insensitive measure of adipose tissue. With aging, there is loss of muscle and bone mass, and BMI, as a weight per height measurement, declines with aging (Baumgartner & Roche, 1995). Elderly also accumulate fat in the abdominal area. Body mass index in the elderly often underestimates actual adiposity, or amount of adipose tissue—a problem that worsens with advancing age. Studies using BMI measurement in old age to predict disease outcomes may therefore be underestimating the true effect of adiposity on disease risk (Baumgartner & Roche, 1995). Therefore, a life-course approach may be needed to better understand the effects of adiposity on cognition (see Figure 4.1).

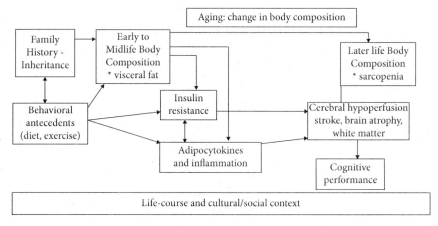

Figure 4.1 Lifecourse context of the influence of obesity on cognition.

OBESITY AND COGNITION IN EARLY LIFE TO MIDLIFE

The effects of adiposity on brain health in late life cannot be completely evaluated without considering cognitive reserve or level of intelligence earlier in life (Gustafson, 2008). However, measurement of cognitive reserve or intelligence is infrequent or unavailable in many epidemiologic studies of dementia; level of education is often used as a surrogate marker. Intelligence correlates with positive health behaviors, such as eating properly and maintaining a healthy body weight (Gottfredson, 2004). Lower childhood IQ score is related to later adiposity, smoking behavior, high blood pressure, cardiovascular disease, and mortality (Chandola, Deary et al., 2006). Childhood IQ has been related to the subsequent development of obesity and related adverse sequelae in the National Child Development Survey, a longitudinal study in the United Kingdom, and the Aberdeen Children of the 1950s cohort in Scotland, each including almost 10,000 men and women (Chandola, Deary et al., 2006; Lawlor, Clark et al., 2006). These studies are particularly important because of their long follow-ups. In the United Kingdom., lower IQ measured at 11 years was related to obesity 31 years later, even after adjustment for numerous other factors, such as childhood height, BMI at 16 years, pubertal development, parents' BMI, birth weight, father's occupational social class, sports activity, and sweets consumption. Among those with an IQ in the lowest tertile, risk for obesity was doubled among women and 60% higher in men. In Scotland, there was a strong age- and sex-adjusted inverse relationship between IQ score at age 7 years and adult BMI measured at age 45 to 52 years (Lawlor, Clark et al., 2006). However, in both studies, if educational attainment was considered, then childhood IQ was not related to obesity risk.

Postnatal weight change, as well as adult weight and height attainment, has also been related to cognition. Although birth weight and length may be positively related to childhood IQ, data related to postnatal growth show divergence. In the British 1946 birth cohort, it was shown that weight gain after age 15 years was related to lower cognition at age 26 years but that height continued to be related to better cognition (Richards, Hardy et al., 2002). Consideration of education did not alter these findings. In a Danish study of draft board registrants (Halkjaer, Holst et al., 2003), a mean decrease in BMI after age 19 years among non-obese men was related to a higher mean intelligence score at age 19 years, and intelligence score was protective for the development of obesity. However, adjustment for education overwhelmed the latter findings (Halkjaer, Holst et al., 2003). Also in the Danish study, among juvenile-onset obesity, higher intelligence was related to a greater decrease in BMI after age 19 years, which disappeared with consideration of education, and education was protective for the persistence of obesity. Future research should focus on tackling both the questions of "Does obesity interfere with intellectual development?" and "Does level of intelligence influence the development of obesity?"

OBESITY IN MIDLIFE AND DEMENTIA RISK

Evidence from prospective studies evaluating obesity in midlife with a follow-up period until old age suggests that midlife obesity, as measured by BMI, is strongly associated with an increased risk of developing dementia and Alzheimer's disease (AD) (Kivipelto, Ngandu et al., 2005; Rosengren, Skoog et al., 2005; Whitmer, Gunderson et al., 2005) independently from common comorbidities. Whitmer and colleagues prospectively examined the role of obesity and overweight (measured via BMI and skinfold thickness) in middle age (ages 40–45 years) and risk of dementia, AD, and vascular dementia (VaD) more than two decades later (Whitmer, Gunderson et al., 2005; Whitmer, 2007). Those with a midlife BMI of 30 or greater were 75% more likely to get dementia compared to those with a normal midlife BMI (18.5–24.9). Similarly, those in the top 20% of subscapular and tricep skinfold thickness had a 60% to 70% increased risk of dementia compared to those in the bottom 20% of skinfold thickness. When examining the risk of dementia subtypes in a separate study (AD and VaD), the magnitude of the effect was even greater; those obese had a threefold increased risk of AD and a fivefold increased risk of VaD (Whitmer, 2007). Four other large cohort studies from Finland, Sweden, and the United States also examining midlife obesity (as measured by BMI and risk of dementia and AD) have reported similar results (Kivipelto, Ngandu et al., 2005). A recent meta-analysis examining BMI in both midlife and late life across 16 studies found a pooled relative risk of 1.26 for midlife overweight on any dementia and a pooled relative risk of 1.64 for midlife obesity. Estimates were even higher when considering only AD. There was no pooled relative risk of obesity in late life and increased risk of dementia (Anstey, Cherbuin et al., 2011). Taken together, these studies suggest the role of midlife obesity on dementia risk is ubiquitous across different study populations and different markers of obesity (BMI, regional skinfold thickness, waist circumference).

There is one study published from the Gothenburg Birth Cohort Studies on the 37-year natural history of BMI in relation to dementia onset in women (Gustafson, Bäckman et al., 2012). In this population of women, in whom midlife central obesity is related to dementia risk (Gustafson, Bäckman et al., 2009), there has been observed a distinct midlife to late-life BMI trajectory among women who have developed dementia versus those who have not. In this report (Gustafson, Bäckman et al., 2012), the "apparent" difference in BMI decline after age 70 years, between those who have and have not developed dementia, results from different rates of BMI increase from midlife to late life. Among women who have developed late-onset dementia, the rate of midlife BMI increase has been less. Thus observed declines in BMI begin at a lower level of BMI. A variety of hypotheses have been put forward related to this observation (Gustafson, Bäckman et al., 2012). In addition, this report highlights the importance of a life-course approach in understanding the relation between different adiposity traits of a lifetime and dementia, the neurodegenerative disorder of latest life.

OBESITY AND COGNITION IN LATE ADULTHOOD

Cross-sectional studies of obesity and cognitive function in late life have shown mixed results. Some studies have suggested that obesity is associated with poorer cognitive performance (Sørensen, Christensen, & Kreiner, 1982; Kilander, Nyman et al., 1997; Waldstein & LI, 2006). However, two of these did not adjust for comorbidities(Sørensen et al., 1982; Kilander, Nyman et al., 1997), and one included adults of both middle and old age (Waldstein & LI, 2006).

Although many studies have incorporated one global measure of cognitive function, there has not been as much work comparing the contribution of adiposity to performance across different cognitive domains. This is important because varying performance on different cognitive domains may be reflective of different mechanistic pathways through which adiposity affects cognition and may or may not reflect incipient/prodromal dementia or other diseases. The Baltimore Longitudinal Study of Aging examined the association between obesity and cognitive test performance across different domains. A higher BMI was associated with worse performance on measures of global cognitive function, memory, and language. However, there was no association between central obesity, as measured by waist to hip ratio and these measures. In addition, there was no association between higher BMI and worse executive function; in fact, trends suggested that a higher BMI was associated with better performance on cognitive texts of attention, psychomotor speed, and visuospatial skills.

Beyond cross-sectional comparisons, it is important to also evaluate the association between adiposity and cognitive *change over time*. Longitudinal analyses from the Baltimore Study of Aging have indicated that a higher BMI is associated with more rapid decline on global cognitive functioning, executive function, and memory.

Prospective findings from the Framingham Study indicated that obesity and hypertension were both risk factors for 4-year cognitive decline in middle-aged and elderly men (Elias, Sullivan et al., 2003) but not women. The authors re-analyzed the data using a longer follow-up time between obesity and assessment of cognition (Elias, Elias et al., 2005) and found the same gender effect of obesity and poorer cognitive performance in men only. A cross-sectional study of middle-aged adults found no association between BMI and cognition but did observe that those participants who were obese (BMI ≥30) had less total brain volume as measured by MRI (Ward, Carlsson et al., 2005).

OBESITY AND BODY WEIGHT IN LATE LIFE AND DEMENTIA

Unlike the studies of midlife obesity and dementia, there is no consistent story thus far on obesity and adiposity in late life and dementia risk. Most evidence to date has suggested either a null or inverse association, whereas a few studies have shown an increased risk if individuals have been followed over a longer late-life period. There are challenges in determining adiposity in late life as a risk factor because of the long prodromal phase of dementia, weight loss in the early stages of dementia, and healthy survivor bias in studies of the oldest-old. Overall, the evidence has suggested that a higher weight in late life is associated with a reduced risk of dementia over the short term, however it may increase risk over the long term.

The first study to show an association between overweight and risk of dementia was performed by Gustafson and colleagues, who evaluated individuals in the Gothenburg Birth Cohort Studies (Gustafson, Rothenberg et al., 2003). Individuals were 70 years old at baseline and followed for 18 years. For women only, being more overweight was associated with an increased risk of AD. However cross-sectional and case–control analyses or studies have suggested that low body weight is associated with increased dementia risk (Wang, 2002; Gustafson, Bäckman et al., 2009; Gustafson, Bäckman et al., 2012). This finding most likely results from the long prodromal phase of dementia as well as the effect of early phase dementia on appetite and weight loss. Studies also have shown that weight loss precedes diagnosis of dementia as well as AD (Barrett-Connor, Corey-Bloom, & Wiederholt, 1998) and that weight loss occurs prior to clinical manifestations of dementia and by the time of diagnosis(Stewart, Xue et al., 2005; Gao, Hendrie et al., 2011). One prospective study with a follow-up of 5 years showed that declining weight increased risk of AD (Buchman, Bienias et al., 2005). Weight loss may be a part of the clinical course of AD (Guérin, Schneider et al., 2005) and worsens with disease severity. Consistent with this picture are studies showing that among patients with AD, low BMI and accelerated weight loss is associated with greater disease progression and higher risk of death (Mortel, Rauch et al.,1999; Luchsinger, Tang et al., 2008). Thus, cross-sectional studies, as well as studies assessing body weight shortly before time of dementia ascertainment, have implied that low body weight increases the short term risk of AD and dementia. Future studies need to determine how much this phenomenon is reflective of prodromal dementia processes.

Abdominal Obesity and Visceral Adiposity

Centrally distributed body fat, also known as abdominal obesity, is a stronger risk factor for developing T2DM, coronary heart disease, stroke, and cancer, as well as occurrence of total mortality, than total body obesity measured using BMI (Empana JP, Ducimetiere P et al. 2004; Smith, Herbert et al., 2005). Prior work examining obesity as a risk factor for disease has demonstrated that abdominal obesity is particularly pathogenic, even among those with normal body weight. Evidence has suggested that this may also be the case for dementia (Whitmer, Gustafson et al., 2008; Gustafson, Bäckman et al., 2009) and cognitive impairment (Whitmer, Gustafson et al., 2008; Kanaya, Harris et al., 2009). Reports by both Whitmer et al. (2008) and Gustafson et al.(2009) have shown an approximate twofold higher risk of dementia associated with midlife central obesity. Midlife abdominal obesity as measured by sagittal abdominal diameter was a stronger risk factor for dementia than global obesity as measured by BMI. In addition, abdominal obesity was a strong risk factor for dementia, even among those who were not overweight by BMI (Whitmer, Gustafson et al., 2008).

Abdominal obesity is particularly dangerous, even for those who are not overweight, because measures of abdominal adipose tissue represent both sub-cutaneous (under the skin) and visceral (around the organs) adipose tissue (*see* Mechanisms section below). Interestingly, evidence suggests that a peripheral distribution of adipose tissue (adipose distributed around the hips and buttock region) is not only *not* dangerous but may actually be protective against cardiovascular disease and T2DM because of possible beneficial effects of subcutaneous adipose tissue on insulin sensitivity (Snijder, Visser, & Seidell, 2006). Thus the dangerous increases in disease risk attributed to central obesity may result from not only increased visceral adiposity but decreased subcutaneous adiposity; however, at this point, this statement is somewhat speculative.

Whereas waist circumference and sagittal abdominal diameter offer anthropometric estimations of visceral fat (Empana, Ducimetiere et al., 2004), imaging of the abdomen may offer an accurate and sensitive method to directly distinguish in vivo the amount of visceral and organ fat (Onat, Barian et al., 2004; Stanforth, Green et al., 2004).Several imaging studies that have directly measured subcutaneous versus visceral adipose tissue (VAT) have shown that viscerally obese subjects, even those who do not have a BMI in the obese category, are individuals who have more insulin resistance, metabolic dysregulation, and dyslipidemia (Lemieux, Lesage et al., 1999; Despres, 2006; Arsenault, Lachance et al., 2007). Although there have been studies evaluating anthropometric measurements of abdominal size in association with cognition, there has also been some recent work attempting to tease out the association between amount of visceral fat and cognitive function An analysis of elderly Koreans combined information on BMI with visceral adiposity (measured by MRI) and found that a BMI of 25 kg/m^2 or more was associated with impaired cognitive function and that the effects of BMI on cognition were especially marked among those with more visceral adiposity (Jeong, Son et al., 2005). These findings were adjusted for T2DM, hypertension, and dyslipidemia. Results from the J-SHIPP study have suggested that reduced amounts of subcutaneous fat measured via MRI and adiponectin were associated with a greater likelihood of mild cognitive impairment in a Japanese sample of men (Kamogawa, Tabara et al., 2010).Yaffe and colleagues explored the association between several markers of adiposity, including anthropometic measurements, total fat mass by dual-energy X-ray absorptiometry, and subcutaneous and visceral fat by abdominal computed tomography in a community dwelling elderly sample. Higher adiposity was associated with cognitive decline in men but not in women (Kanaya, 2009).

Weight Gain and Cognition

Some studies have evaluated weight gain and cognitive performance. Among women enrolled in the Women's Health Initiative Study of Cognitive Aging, there was no association between weight gain and cognitive performance over 3.5 years of follow-up. Cognitive performance was evaluated both as a composite measure, combining information across several cognitive texts, as well as by determining whether there were associations with cognitive domains. There was, however, an association between poorer cognitive performance and weight loss, perhaps indicative of early dementia (Driscoll,Wassertheil-Smoller et al., 2011). The study also evaluated changes in waist circumference and found no association with poor cognitive performance. These findings are consistent with observations from the Framingham Study. In healthy middle-aged to elderly women, it seems that weight gain does not detrimentally impact cognitive function.

Obesity and Markers of Neuronal Degeneration

Temporal atrophy, an early hallmark of dementia and cognitive decline, is a manifestation of neuronal degeneration. Temporal atrophy measured using computed tomography (CT) at age 62 years to 84 years was related to higher BMI levels measured 24 years prior. In this same sample, higher BMI was also related to temporal atrophy cross-sectionally at the time of CT (Gustafson, Lissner et al., 2004). Higher BMI has also been shown to predict a higher rate of atrophy progression measured using serial MRI (Enzinger, Fazekas et al., 2005). Central adiposity (high waist-to-hip ratio) has been cross-sectionally related to temporal atrophy using MRI (Ward, Carlsson et al., 2005). Work that combined data from both the Cardiovascular Health Cognition Study and the Alzheimer's Disease Neuroimaging Initiative evaluated the association of obesity and brain structure among patients already with mild cognitive impairment (MCI) or AD. For both the AD and MCI groups, higher BMI was associated with a greater extent of frontal, parietal, and occipital brain volume deficits (Ho, Becker et al., 2010).

High BMI may lead to atrophy, or alternatively, some level of atrophy or susceptibility to atrophy may be present among those with a higher BMI because of involvement of common brain structures related to energy metabolism and dementia. Having a smaller temporal lobe volume early on may contribute to dysregulatory events leading to *both* higher levels of BMI throughout life and/or are reflective of diminished cognitive reserve. This latter scenario has been suggested in a study of children and adolescents using MRI to measure entorhinal cortex thickness in relationship to the primary susceptibility gene for sporadic AD, apolipoprotein E (APOE) (Saunders, Strittmatter et al., 1993; Shaw, Lerch et al., 2007). Possession of any APOE ε4 allele was related to a thinner left entorhinal cortex, with a stepwise increase in entorhinal thickness in the ε3 carriers, followed by those carrying an ε2 allele.

Morbid Obesity

With the recent increases in the prevalence of obesity, there has also been an unfortunate marked increase in morbid obesity, which is defined as a BMI of 40 or greater (WHO, 2012). Although there have only been a handful of studies examining the cognitive function of the morbidly obese, the evidence thus far has suggested that morbid obesity is harmful for cognitive health. A small study of morbidly obese adolescents found that these patients had deficits in multiple aspects of cognitive function, including attention and executive function (Lokken, Austin et al., 2009). Similarly, in two additional studies, morbidly obese adult patients seeking bariatric surgery also had deficits on tests of executive function (Boeka, 2008; Lokken, Yellumahanthi et al., 2010).

A recent neuropathology autopsy study was conducted in 12 morbidly obese individuals without a history of cognitive impairment ranging in age from 21 years to 70 years. Alzheimer-type neuropathological changes were found in the brains of those over age 65 years, whereas there was no evidence of pathology in the younger subjects, suggesting a synergistic influence of old age and morbid obesity on brain health (Mrak, 2009).

Treatment for Obesity and Cognition (clinical trials of weight loss and cognition) or Intentional Weight Loss and Cognition

Although some work has evaluated weight changes and dementia risk, a recent meta-analysis of 12 studies determined if intentional weight loss was associated with improvements in cognitive function (Siervo, Wells et al., 2011). Among obese subjects only, weight loss was associated with improvements in memory and executive functioning, however there was no significant influence of weight loss on cognition for overweight subjects. This is an evolving field, but future research should address whether weight loss has similar benefits on cognition as it does on other conditions such as vascular risk factors. Bariatric surgery is a surgical intervention for morbid obesity. A recent study evaluated whether there were cognitive changes among morbidly obese patients receiving this intervention versus morbidly obese patients not having bariatric surgery. Cognition was evaluated at baseline and 3 months after surgery. Those receiving surgery had improved memory performance (Gunstad, Devlin et al., 2011), suggesting that there could be even short-term benefits to brain health associated with weight loss. Future work needs to evaluate how this may impact long-term dementia risk.

Possible Mechanisms Linking Adiposity to Cognition

With the link among obesity and increased risk of metabolic dysfunction, cardiovascular disease, and T2DM, it is easy to postulate that these comorbidities are likely culprits in affecting cognitive function. There is numerous, consistent evidence that both cardiovascular disease, diabetes, and prediabetes contribute to the development of dementia and AD (Breteler, 2000; Whitmer, 2005) and increased risk of cognitive impairment (Yaffe, Lindquist et al., 2004; Yaffe, Blackwell et al., 2007) (*see* Chapters 5 and 6 and for in-depth discussion of diabetes, the metabolic dysfunction, and vascular influences on cognition). However, several studies that have accounted for comorbid cardiovascular disease and

T2DM have found an independent association between obesity and risk of dementia, suggesting other pathways may exist between adiposity and cognitive health (see Figures 4.2 and 4.3). Potential molecular pathways between obesity and cognitive function include the systemic effects of the adipocyte (fat cell) itself and the role of genetic influences.

ADIPOSE TISSUE ACTIONS

Contrary to earlier views, adipose tissue is no longer considered an inert byproduct of obesity; rather, it is a hormonally active tissue with several inflammatory and metabolic components (Chaldakov, Hristova, & Ghenev, 2003; Greenberg AS 2006). Although adipose tissue is the largest endocrine gland in the body, only recently has the role of adipose tissue on brain function been addressed. Obese persons have increased number and increased size of adipocytes; and adipocytes secrete a large number of protein hormones or adipokines (Bruun, Kristensen & Richelsen, 2002). Cytokines are biologically active low-molecular-weight proteins that have several endocrine and metabolic functions and are known products of the immune system and inflammation (Bruun et al., 2002). Adipocytokines are cytokines derived from adipose tissue and include resistin, interleukin (IL)-1, IL-6, tumor necrosis factor (TNF)-α, plasminogen activator inhibitor-1, leptin, and adiponectin (Prins, 2002). Mechanistic studies have determined that adipocytokines cause a pro-inflammatory response that plays a direct role in development of insulin resistance and endothelial dysfunction (Aldhahi, 2003).

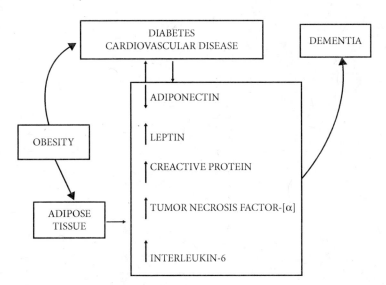

Figure 4.2 Possible adipose tissue-driven mechanisms explaining the link between obesity and cognitive impairment. (Gustafson, 2010)

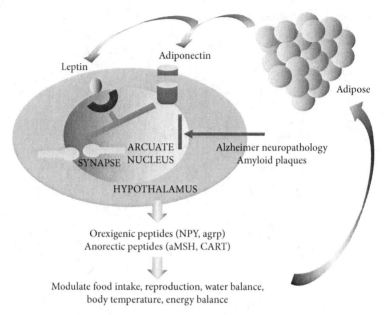

Figure 4.3 Mechanisms whereby adipose tissue hormones affect the brain and the potential modifying effects of Alzheimer's disease pathology. Leptin and adiponectin, peripheral signals from adipose tissue, interact with hypothalamic nuclei such as the arcuate nucleus. These interactions trigger the release of orexigenic and anorectic peptides from PMC neurons. These peptides exert peripheral effects, modulating food intake, reproduction, water balance, body temperature, and energy balance. In addition, leptin and adiponectin have been shown to enhance synaptic plasticity. In prodromal and clinical AD, amyloid deposited in the areas of the hypothalamus such as the arcuate nucleus potentially interfere with normal physiologic influences of leptin and adiponectin, downstream events and feedback loops. The vascular effects of adipose tissue may explain the midlife associations between overweight and obesity and dementia. The influence of AD pathology on areas of the brain involved in homeostatic regulation may explain the weight loss observed in prodromal and overt dementia.

Evidence has accumulated that supports the hypothesis that some systemically produced adipocytokines may cross the blood–brain barrier and enter the central nervous system, where adipocytokine receptors exist (Chaldakov, Hristova, & Ghenev, 2003).

FUNCTIONAL CHARACTERISTICS OF VISCERAL ADIPOSE TISSUE VERSUS SUBCUTANEOUS ADIPOSE TISSUE

Visceral adipose tissue (adipose tissue that surrounds the viscera) is functionally and morphologically different from subcutaneous adipose tissue. Visceral adipose tissue contributes to insulin resistance through being less responsive to antilipolytic effects of insulin as compared to subcutaneous adipose tissue. In comparison to subcutaneous adipose tissue cells, VAT cells have increased glucocorticoid receptors, less adiponectin secretion, and greater IL-6 and plasminogen activator inhibitor-1 levels. The portal theory (Despres, 2006) posits that it is the location of the VAT itself, which is partly drained via the portal vein, that plays a key role in free fatty acid metabolism. The processing of an increase of free fatty acids by the liver causes an increase in triglycerides, and a reduced clearance of liver insulin, leading to hyperinsulinemia and glucose intolerance. Another view is that visceral obesity indicates the inability of subcutaneous fat to clear and process surplus energy (Mauriège, Prud'homme et al., 1999). Others have proposed that visceral obesity is a marker of a neuroendocrine abnormality (Björntorp, 2000) allocating excess energy to visceral rather than subcutaneous fat. Once the visceral depot is increased, subsequent metabolic abnormalities may exaggerate existing conditions, leading to a feed-forward cascade of further metabolic dysregulation and increased risk of diabetes, cardiovascular, and other metabolic diseases (Mathieu, Larose et al., 2008).

LEPTIN

Although an exhaustive review of all adipocytokines is beyond the scope of this chapter, discussions of those that have been implicated in cognition are included. Leptin is a peptide hormone that plays a role in maintenance and regulation of body weight and is highly correlated with body fat levels (Harvey, 2003). However, research has suggested that leptin also has a role in learning and memory. Leptin crosses the blood–brain barrier, and there are leptin receptors in the neocortex and hippocampus (Benoit, Seeley, & Woods, 2004). Leptin also is transported to the brain via the cerebrospinal fluid. Leptin receptor-deficient obese mice have impaired ability on water maze tasks as well as deficiencies in long-term potentiation of neurons, suggesting a role of leptin in synaptic plasticity (Harvey, 2003; Harvey J, 2003). Leptin is secreted by the adipose cell, and one of its jobs is to increase metabolism and decrease adiposity. Although obese persons have very high levels of leptin, they also appear to be "leptin-resistant," potentially analogous to the genetically bread leptin receptor-deficient mice (Harvey, 2003).

There has been suggestion that leptin may be protective for AD neurodegeneration. Leptin is associated with decreased production and accumulation of Aβ peptide, a component of amyloid plaques found in AD (Fewlass, Pi-Sunyer et al., 2004). However, epidemiological data are mixed. A cross-sectional analysis in elderly women found that leptin is highly associated with components of the metabolic syndrome (Zamboni, Fantin et al., 2004), and those with the metabolic syndrome have shown worse cognitive decline (Yaffe, Lindquist et al., 2004). Other studies have shown that low serum leptin is associated with poorer cognitive functioning, independent of BMI in a cohort of elderly people (Holden, Tylavsky et al., 2009). However, a Swedish study reported no association with midlife blood leptin levels and dementia 32 years later (Gustafson, Bäckman et al.,2012).

ADIPONECTIN

Adiponectin is the most excessively secreted protein from adipose tissue. It is a collagen-like protein product that is known to have anti-inflammatory and anti-atherogenic properties (Pajvani & Scherer, 2003). Circulating levels of this adipocyte-derived protein are reduced in cardiovascular disease. Unlike the other adipocytokines, adiponectin does not increase with the size of the fat cell, thus it is found in lower levels among those obese. Adiponectin plays a role in regulating glucose and lipid homeostasis. A major effect of adiponectin is to enhance insulin action in the liver and reduce hepatic glucose output and triglyceride levels (Lyon & Hsueh, 2003). Mechanistic evidence from animal studies has indicated reduced levels of adiponectin causes insulin resistance, hyperlipidemia, and atherosclerosis (Aldhahi, 2003). A cross-sectional analysis of elderly men and women has shown that adiponectin and leptin together are highly associated with insulin resistance in the elderly, even after accounting for total body fat and body fat distribution (Zoico, Mazzali et al., 2004). These findings are congruent with the animal work, which has reported specific mechanistic findings of adiponectin inducing insulin resistance.

It is plausible that adipocytokines directly influence the brain or impact other processes that, in turn, affect the brain. There is stronger evidence so far to suggest that leptin may directly affect the brain and "cognition," given the distribution of receptors in the hippocampus and the findings from animal models using water maze tasks (Harvey, 2003; Harvey J, 2003).

OTHER INFLAMMATORY CYTOKINES

Visceral fat produces a greater amount of inflammatory cytokines as well. Studies have shown that obese and overweight adults and children have increased levels of several pro-inflammatory cytokines, including C-reactive protein (CRP), IL-6, and TNF-α (Greenberg & Obin, 2006). Inflammation is considered to be a consequence of obesity and the presence of increased adipocytes (Greenberg, 2006). Elevated CRP has been found in abdominally obese people, with the very highest levels among those with an excess of VAT. It is also well documented that inflammation is involved in dementia and AD-associated neurodegeneration (Singh, 1997). (*See* Chapter 11 for an in-depth discussion of inflammation and cognition.)

ACTIVATIONS OF THE RENIN-ANGIOTENSIN SYSTEM

The renin-angiotensin system (RAS) refers to a hormonal system that regulates blood pressure. Although the primary function of RAS is blood pressure regulation, RAS may also provide a link between obesity, hypertension, and vascular syndromes (such as T2DM) and health of the brain (Goossens, Blaak et al., 2003; Katzov, Bennet et al., 2004). Human brain and adipose tissue express a full RAS. Adipose RAS is involved in adipocyte growth, differentiation, and metabolism (Strazzullo, Iacone et al., 2003). The RAS is activated in response to low levels of blood pressure, when angiotensin is converted by renin to angiotensin I, which is subsequently converted to angiotensin II by ACE. Angiotensin II interacts with angiotensin receptors 1 and 2 to mediate major cardiovascular effects of the RAS, such as increasing blood pressure (Goossens, Blaak et al., 2003). In the brain, angiotensin II continues conversion to angiotensin IV, which, acting through angiotensin receptor 4 (also known as insulin-regulated aminopeptidase) (Albiston, McDowall et al., 2001; Savaskan, 2005), enhances learning and memory in animal models (Albiston, McDowall et al., 2001).

Thus, the RAS may link vascular health in the periphery, most likely in proportion to the amount of body fat present (Goossens, Blaak et al., 2003) and to dementia processes in the brain (Goossens, Blaak et al., 2003; Katzov, Bennet et al., 2004). Larger amounts of body fat increase vasoactivity and expression of vasoactive systems, which leads to increased blood levels of leptin, endothelin, adiponectin, resistin, and numerous other hormones, growth factors, and cytokines through enhanced expression of the genes encoding for these compounds in adipose tissue itself (Barton, Carmona et al., 2003).

Genetic Underpinnings of Excess Adiposity and Susceptibility to Cognitive Impairment

The role of adipose tissue, and the metabolic syndromes or milieu it represents, is underscored by Genome Wide Association Study (GWAS) results based on more than 16,000 individuals with and without AD (Harold, Abraham et al., 2009; Lambert et al., 2009; Guerreiro, Gustafson et al., 2010). These reports (Harold, Abraham et al., 2009; Lambert et al., 2009) showed not only a relationship between the major susceptibility gene for AD, *APOE*, but three other DNA variants single nucleotide polymorphisms (SNPs) within loci encoding for proteins associated with vascular and metabolic health. These include SNPs: (1) in the clusterin (*CLU*, also known as *APOJ*) gene; (2) *PICALM*; and (3) in *CR*, the gene encoding for complement component receptor 1. These genes complement the list of vascular and metabolic susceptibility genes that is maintained at www.alzgene.org (Bertram, McQueen et al., 2007) and that includes additional genes such as sortilin-related receptor (*SORL1*, which is related to the low-density lipoprotein receptor [LDLR]), angiotensin-converting enzyme (ACE), IL-8, LDLR, and cystatin 3 (CST3). The functional significance of these vascular and metabolic genes is linked to adipose tissue and its downstream effects; however, precise details are unknown.

A recent report linking the *FTO* ("fatso") gene to reduced brain volume (particularly frontal and occipital lobes) in the Alzheimer's Disease Neuroimaging Initiative (ADNI) is another example of a potential interaction between fat tissue and the brain (Ho, Stein et al., 2010). *FTO* appears to be an obesity gene and is also related to T2DM. The mechanism of action or functionality of *FTO* is not clear. However, the resulting protein appears to be a member of the non-heme dioxygenase (Fe(II)- and 2-oxoglutarate-dependent dioxygenases) superfamily. *FTO* messenger RNA is most abundant in the brain, particularly in hypothalamic nuclei governing energy balance, and levels in the arcuate nucleus are regulated by feeding and fasting (Gerken, Girard et al., 2007), thus a potential link to adipose hormones of the fat–brain axis.

Genetic Factors That May Interact with Adipose-Associated Pathways on Cognition

Genetic work on obesity and diabetes has focused on SNPs associated with leptin, adiponectin, and the peroxisome proliferators activated receptor (PPAR) (Sutton, Langefeld et al., 2005). Although a genetic background behind sporadic obesity is not clear, there are some interesting reports. Analyses from the IRAS Family Study of Hispanics have documented that adiponectin polymorphisms are associated with overall and central obesity in their population (Sutton, Langefeld et al., 2005). Other work has found that SNPs from the PPAR *ala* polymorphism are associated with cognition, insulin resistance, and diabetes (Flavell, Jamshidi et al., 2000). Preliminary work has suggested that polymorphisms in the adiponectin gene (ACDC) are associated with adipose distribution, whereas polymorphisms in the PPAR are associated with overall adiposity (Loos, Rankinen et al., 2007). One study has identified SNPs in the ADAC gene associated with visceral adiposity. Identification of individuals who have a genetic trait that causes susceptibility to overall obesity as well as visceral fat accumulation would aid in explaining the possible adipose associated effects on brain health.

Summary and Conclusions

Obesity is a growing worldwide public health problem that, if trends continue, will become pandemic (Ramos, Xu et al. 2003). Concurrent with this is a projected enormous increase in cognitive impairment. Both total body and abdominal obesity, particularly over the life-course, is associated with increased risk of developing cognitive impairment, dementia, and brain morphology indicative of neuropathology in old age. With the burgeoning epidemic of obesity and increase in excess abdominal adiposity (even among those not overweight), and the evidence that obesity increases risk of severe cognitive impairment and dementia, we may witness an unprecedented increase in of both of these conditions. Molecular and genetic mechanisms and long-term consequences of an altered adipokine milieu in humans need to be elucidated, particularly their role in neurodegenerative diseases and brain health (Gustafson, 2006; Whitmer, 2007). However, obesity is a modifiable risk factor, and research identifying these mechanisms would aid in development of measures that might prevent or delay the development of cognitive decline and dementia.

References

Albiston AL, McDowall SG, Matsacos D, Sim P, Clune E, Mustafa T, et al. (2001). Evidence that the angiotensin IV (AT(4)) receptor is the enzyme insulin-regulated aminopeptidase. *J Biol Chem*, *276*(52), 48623–48626.

Aldhahi W, & Hamdy O. (2003). Adipokines, inflammation, and the endothelium in diabetes. *Curr Diab Rep*, *3*(4), 293–298.

Anstey KJ, Cherbuin N, Budge M, & Young J. (2011). Body mass index in midlife and late-life as a risk factor for dementia: a meta-analysis of prospective studies. *Obes Rev*, *12*(5), e426–437.

Arsenault BJ, Lachance D, Lemieux I, Almeras N, Tremblay A, Bouchard C, et al. (2007). Visceral adipose tissue accumulation, cardiorespiratory fitness, and features of the metabolic syndrome. *Arch.Intern.Med.*, *167*(14), 1518–1525.

Barrett-Connor E, Edelstein S, Corey-Bloom J, & Wiederholt W. (1998). Weight loss precedes dementia in community-dwelling older adults. *J Nutr Health Aging*, *2*(2), 113–114.

Barton M, Carmona R, Ortmann J, Krieger JE, & Traupe T. (2003). Obesity-associated activation of angiotensin and endothelin in the cardiovascular system. *Int J Biochem Cell Biol*, *35*(6), 826–837.

Baumgartner RN, Heymsfield SB, & Roche AF. (1995). Human body composition and the epidemiology of chronic disease. *obes Res*, *3*(1), 73–95.

Benoit SC, Clegg DJ, Seeley RJ, & Woods SC. (2004). Insulin and leptin as adiposity signals. *Recent Prog Horm Res*, *59*, 267–285.

Bertram L, McQueen MB, Mullin K, Blacker D, & Tanzi RE. (2007). Systematic meta-analyses of Alzheimer disease genetic association studies: the AlzGene database. *Nat Genetics*, *39*(1), 17–23.

Björntorp P, & Rosmond R. (2000). Neuroendocrine abnormalities in visceral obesity. *Int J Obes Relat Metab Disord*, *24*(Suppl 2), s80–85.

Boeka AG, & Lokken KL. (2008). Neuropsychological performance of a clinical sample of extremely obese individuals. . *Arch Clin Neuropsychol*, *23*(4), 467–474.

Breteler NM. (2000). Vascular risk factors for Alzheimer's disease: an epidemiologic perspective. *Neurobiol Aging*, *21*(2), 153–160.

Bruun JM, Pedersen SB, Kristensen K, & Richelsen B. (2002). Effects of pro-inflammatory cytokines and chemokines on leptin production in human adipose tissue in vitro. *Mol Cell Endocrinol*, *190*(1-2), 91–99.

Buchman AS, Wilson RS, Bienias JL, Shah RC, Evans DA, & Bennett DA. (2005). Change in body mass index and risk of incident Alzheimer disease. *Neurology 65*(6), 892–897.

Chaldakov GN, Stankulov IS, Hristova M, & Ghenev PI. (2003). Adipobiology of disease: adipokines and adipokine-targeted pharmacology. *Curr Pharm Des*, *9*(12), 1023–1031.

Chandola T, Deary IJ, Blane D, & Batty GD. (2006). Childhood IQ in relation to obesity and weight gain in adult life: the National Child Development (1958) Study. *Int J Obes*, *30*(9), 1422–1432.

Despres JP. (2006). Is visceral obesity the cause of the metabolic syndrome? *Ann.Med.*, *38*(1), 52–63.

Driscoll I, Espeland MA, Wassertheil-Smoller S, Gaussoin SA, Ding J, Granek IA, et al. (2011). Weight change and cognitive function: findings from the Women's Health Initiative Study of Cognitive Aging. *Obesity (Silver Spring)*, *19*(8), 1595–1600.

Elias, M., Elias, P., Sullivan, L., Wolf, P., & D'Agostino, R. (2005). Obesity, diabetes and cognitive deficit: The Framingham Heart Study. *Neurobiol Aging*, *26*(Suppl. 1), 11–16.

Elias MF, Elias PK, Sullivan LM, Wolf PA, & D'Agostino RB. (2003). Lower cognitive function in the presence of obesity and hypertension: the Framingham heart study. *Int J Obes Relat Metab Disord*, *27*(2), 260–268.

Empana JP, Ducimetiere P, Charles MA, & Jouven X. (2004). Sagittal abdominal diameter and risk of sudden death in asymptomatic middle-aged men: the Paris Prospective Study I. *Circulation*, *110*(18), 2781–2785.

Enzinger C, Fazekas F, Matthews PM, Ropele S, Schmidt H, Smith S, et al. (2005). Risk factors for progression of brain atrophy in aging: six-year follow-up of normal subjects. *Neurology*, *64*(10), 1704–1711.

Fewlass DC, Noboa K, Pi-Sunyer FX, Johnston JM, Yan SD, & Tezapsidis N. (2004). Obesity-related leptin regulates Alzheimer's Abeta. *FASEB J*, *18*(15), 1870–1878.

Flavell DM, Pineda Torra I, Jamshidi Y, Evans D, Diamond JR, Elkeles RS, et al. (2000). Variation in the PPARalpha gene is associated with altered function in vitro and plasma lipid concentrations in Type II diabetic subjects. *Diabetologia 43*(5), 673–680.

Flegal KM. (2005). Epidemiologic aspects of overweight and obesity in the United States. *Physiol Behav*, *86*(5), 599–602.

Ford ES, Giles WH, & Dietz WH. (2002). Prevalence of the metabolic syndrome among US adults: Findings from the third National Health and Nutrition Examination Survey. *JAMA*, *287*, 356–359.

Gao S, Nguyen JT, Hendrie HC, Unverzagt FW, Hake A, Smith-Gamble V, et al. (2011). Accelerated weight loss and incident dementia in an elderly African-American cohort. *J Am Geriatr Soc*, *59*(1), 18–25.

Gerken T, Girard C A, Tung Y C, Webby CJ, Saudek V, Hewitson K S, et al. (2007). The obesity-associated FTO gene encodes a 2-oxoglutarate-dependent nucleic acid demethylase. *Science*, *318*(5855), 1469–1472.

Goossens GH, Blaak E E, & van Baak MA. (2003). Possible involvement of the adipose tissue renin-angiotensin system in the pathophysiology of obesity and obesity-related disorders. *Obes Rev*, *4*(1), 43–55.

Gottfredson LS. (2004). Intelligence: is it the epidemiologists' elusive "fundamental cause" of social class inequalities in health? *J Pers Soc Psychol*, *86*(1), 174–199.

Greenberg AS, & Obin MS. (2006). Obesity and the role of adipose tissue in inflammation and metabolism *Am J Clin Nutr*, *83*(2), 461s–465s.

Greenberg, A. S., & Obin, M. S. (2006). Obesity and the role of adipose tissue in inflammation and metabolism. *Am.J.Clin.Nutr.*, *83*(2), 461S–465S.

Guérin O, Andrieu S, Schneider SM, Milano M, Boulahssass R, Brocker P, et al. (2005). Different modes of weight loss in Alzheimer disease: a prospective study of 395 patients. *Am J Clin Nutr*, *82*(2), 435–441.

Guerreiro R J, Gustafson DR, & Hardy J. (2010). The genetic architecture of Alzheimer's disease: beyond APP, PSENs and APOE. *Neurobiol Aging*, *33*(3):437–456.

Gunstad J, Strain G, Devlin MJ, Wing R, Cohen RA, Paul RH, et al. (2011). Improved memory function 12 weeks after bariatric surgery. *Surg Obes Relat Dis*, *7*(4), 465–472.

Gustafson D. (2006). Adiposity indices and dementia. *Lancet Neurol*, 5(8), 713–720.

Gustafson D. (2008). A life course of adiposity and dementia. *Eur J Pharmacol*, 585(1), 163–175.

Gustafson D, Bäckman K, Joas E, Waern M, Östling S, Guo X, et al. (2012). A 37-year longitudinal follow-up of body mass index and dementia in women. *J Alzheimers Dis*, 28, 162–171.

Gustafson D, Lissner L, Bengtsson C, Björkelund C, & Skoog I. (2004). A 24-year follow-up of body mass index and cerebral atrophy. *Neurology*, 63, 1876–1881.

Gustafson DR. (2010). Adiposity hormones and dementia. *J Neurosci*, 299(1-2), 30–34.

Gustafson DR, Bäckman K, Waern M, Östling S, Guo XX, Zandi P, et al. (2009). Adiposity indicators and dementia over 32 years in Sweden. *Neurology*, 73, 1559–1566.

Gustafson DR, Bäckman K, Lissner L, Carlsson L, Waern M, Ostling S, Guo X, Bengtsson C, Skoog I,. (2012). Leptin and dementia over 32 years-The Prospective Population Study of Women. *Alzheimers Dement*, 8(4), 272–277.

Gustafson DR., Rothenberg E, Blennow K, Steen B, & Skoog I. (2003). An 18-year follow up of overweight and risk for Alzheimer's disease. *Arch Intern Med*, 163, 1524–1528.

Halkjaer, Holst C, & Sorensen T I. (2003). Intelligence test score and educational level in relation to BMI changes and obesity. *Obes Res*, 11(10), 1238–1245.

Harold D, Abraham R, Hollingworth P, Sims R, Gerrish A, Hamshere ML, et al. (2009). Genome-wide association study identifies variants at CLU and PICALM associated with Alzheimer's disease. *Nat Genet*, 41, 1088–1093.

Harvey J. (2003a). Leptin: a multifaceted hormone in the central nervous system. *Mol Neurobiol*, 28(3), 245–258.

Harvey J. (2003b). Novel actions of leptin in the hippocampus. *Ann Med*, 35(3), 197–206.

Harvey J, A. M. (2003). Leptin in the CNS: much more than a satiety signal. *Neuropharmacology*, 44(7), 845–854.

Ho AJ, Raji CA, Becker JT, Lopez OL, Kuller LH, Hua X, et al. (2010). Obesity is linked with lower brain volume in 700 AD and MCI patients. *Neurobiol Aging*, 31(8), 1326–1339.

Ho AJ, Stein J L, Hua X, Lee S, Hibar DP, Leow AD, et al. (2010). A commonly carried allele of the obesity-related FTO gene is associated with reduced brain volume in the healthy elderly. *Proc Natl Acad Sci U S A*, 107(18), 8404–8409.

Holden KF, Lindquist K, Tylavsky FA, Rosano C, Harris TB, & study., Y. K. H. A. (2009). Serum leptin level and cognition in the elderly: Findings from the Health ABC Study. *Neurobiol Aging*, 30(9), 1483–1489.

Jeong SK, Nam HS, Son MH, Son EJ, & Cho KH. (2005). Interactive effect of obesity indexes on cognition. *Dement Geriatr Cogn Disord*, 19(2-3), 91–96.

Kamogawa K, Kohara K, Tabara Y, Uetani E, Nagai T, Yamamoto M, et al. (2010). Abdominal fat, adipose-derived hormones and mild cognitive impairment: the J-SHIPP study. *Dement Geriatr Cogn Disord*, 30(5), 432–439.

Kanaya AM, Lindquist K, Harris TB, Launer L, Rosano C, Satterfield S, et al. (2009). Total and regional adiposity and cognitive change in older adults: The Health, Aging and Body Composition (ABC) study. *Arch Neurol*, 66(3), 329–335.

Katzov H, Bennet AM, Kehoe P, Wiman B, Gatz M, Blennow K, et al. (2004). A cladistic model of ACE sequence variation with implications for myocardial infarction, Alzheimer disease and obesity. *Human Mol Genetics*, 13, 2647–2657.

Kilander L, Nyman H, Boberg M, & Lithell H. (1997). Cognitive function, vascular risk factors and education. A cross-sectional study based on a cohort of 70-year-old men. *J Intern Med*, 242(4), 313–321.

Kivipelto M, Ngandu T, Fratiglioni L, Viitanen M, Kåreholt I, Winblad B, et al. (2005). Obesity and vascular risk factors at midlife and the risk of dementia and Alzheimer disease. *Arch Neurol*, 62(10), 1556–1560.

Lambert JC, Heath S, Even G, & Campion D. (2009). Genome-wide association study identifies variants at CLU and CR1 associated with Alzhimer's disease. *Nat Genet*, 41, 1094–1099.

Lawlor DA, Clark H, Davey Smith G, & Leon DA. (2006). Childhood intelligence, educational attainment and adult body mass index: findings from a prospective cohort and within sibling-pairs analysis. *Int J Obes (Lond)*, 30(12), 1758–1765.

Lemieux S, Lesage M, Bergeron J, Prud'homme D, & Despres JP. (1999). Comparison of two techniques for measurement of visceral adipose tissue cross-sectional areas by computed tomography. *Am.J.Hum.Biol.*, *11*(1), 61–68.

Li C, Ford ES, McGuire LC, & Mokdad AH. (2007). Increasing trends in waist circumference and abdominal obesity among US adults. *Obesity (Silver Spring)*, *15*(1), 216–224.

Lokken KL, Boeka AG, Austin HM, Gunstad J, & Harmon CM. (2009). Evidence of executive dysfunction in extremely obese adolescents: a pilot study. *Surg Obes Relat Dis*, *5*(5), 547–552.

Lokken KL, Boeka AG, Yellumahanthi K, Wesley M, & Clements RH. (2010). Cognitive performance of morbidly obese patients seeking bariatric surgery. *Am Surg*, *76*(1), 55–59.

Loos RJ, Ruchat S, Rankinen T, Tremblay A, Pérusse L, & Bouchard C. (2007). Adiponectin and adiponectin receptor gene variants in relation to resting metabolic rate, respiratory quotient, and adiposity-related phenotypes in the Quebec Family Study. *Am J Clin Nutr*, *85*(1), 26–34.

Luchsinger JA, Patel B, Tang MX, Schupf N, & Mayeux R. (2008). Body mass index, dementia, and mortality in the elderly. *J Nutr Health Aging 12*(2), 127–131.

Lyon CJ, Law RE, & Hsueh WA. (2003). Minireview: adiposity, inflammation, and atherogenesis. *Endocrinology 144*(6), 2195–2200.

Mathieu P, Pibarot P, Larose E, Poirier P, Marette A, & Després JP. (2008). Visceral obesity and the heart. *Int J Biochem Cell Biol.*, *40*(5), 821–836.

Mauriège P, Brochu M, Prud'homme D, Tremblay A, Nadeau A, Lemieux S, et al. (1999). Is visceral adiposity a significant correlate of subcutaneous adipose cell lipolysis in men? *J Clin Endocrinol Metab 84*(2), 736–742.

Mortel KF, Meyer JS, Rauch GM, Konno S, Haque A, & Rauch RA. (1999). Factors influencing survival among patients with vascular dementia and Alzheimer's disease. *J Stroke Cerebrovasc Dis*, *8*(2), 57–65.

Mrak RE. (2009). Alzheimer-type neuropathological changes in morbidly obese elderly individuals. *Clin Neuropathol*, *28*(1), 40–45.

Onat A, Avci GS, Barlan MM, Uyarel H, Uzunlar B, & Sansoy V. (2004). Measures of abdominal obesity assessed for visceral adiposity and relation to coronary risk. *Int J Obes Relat Metab Disord*, *28*(8), 1018–1025.

Pajvani UB, & Scherer PE. (2003). Adiponectin: systemic contributor to insulin sensitivity. *Curr.Diab.Rep.*, *3*(3), 207–213.

Prins JB. (2002). Adipose tissue as an endocrine organ *Best Pract Res Clin Endorinol Metab*, *16*(4), 639–651.

Ramos EJ, Xu Y, Romanova I, Middleton F, Chen C, Quinn R, et al. (2003). Is obesity an inflammatory disease? *Surgery*, *134*(2), 329–335.

Richards M, Hardy R, Kuh D, & Wadsworth M E. (2002). Birthweight, postnatal growth and cognitive function in a national UK birth cohort. *Int J Epidemiol*, *31*(2), 342–348.

Rosengren A, Skoog I, Gustafson D, & Wilhelmsen L. (2005). Body mass index, other cardiovascular risk factors, and hospitalization for dementia. *Arch Intern Med*, *165*(3), 321–326.

Saunders AM, Strittmatter WJ, Schmechel D, St George-Hyslop PH, Pericak-Vance MA, Joo SH, et al. (1993). Association of apolipoprotein E allele *4 with late-onset familial and sporadic Alzheimer's disease. *Neurology*, *43*, 1467–1472.

Savaskan E. (2005). The role of the brain renin-angiotensin system in neurodegenerative disorders. *Curr Alzheimer Res*, *2*(1), 29–35.

Schokker DF, Visscher TL, Nooyens AC, van Baak MA, & Seidell JC. (2007). Prevalence of overweight and obesity in the Netherlands. *Obes Rev*, *8*(2), 101–108.

Shaw P, Lerch JP, Pruessner JC, Taylor KN, Rose AB, Greenstein D, et al. (2007). Cortical morphology in children and adolescents with different apolipoprotein E gene polymorphisms: an observational study. *Lancet Neurol*, *6*(6), 494–500.

Siervo M, Arnold R, Wells JC, Tagliabue A, Colantuoni A, Albanese E, et al. (2011). Intentional weight loss in overweight and obese individuals and cognitive function: a systematic review and meta-analysis. *Obes Res*, *12*(11), 968–983.

Singh VK, & Guthikonda P. (1997). Circulating cytokines in Alzheimer's disease. *J Psychiatr Res* *31*(6), 657–660.

Smith DA, Ness EM, Herbert R, Schechter CB, Phillips RA, Diamond JA, et al. (2005). Abdominal diameter index: a more powerful anthropometric measure for prevalent coronary heart disease risk in adult males. *Diabetes Obes Metab*, *7*(4), 370–380.

Snijder MB, van Dam RM, Visser M, & Seidell JC. (2006). What aspects of body fat are particularly hazardous and how do we measure them? *In J Epidemiol*, *35*(1), 83–92.

Sørensen TI, Sonne-Holm S, Christensen U, & Kreiner S. (1982). Reduced intellectual performance in extreme overweight. *Hum Biol*, *54*(4), 765–775.

Stanforth PR, Jackson AS, Green JS, Gagnon J, Rankinen T, Després JP, et al. (2004). Generalized abdominal visceral fat prediction models for black and white adults aged 17–65 y: the HERITAGE Family Study. *Int J Obes Relat Metab Disord*, *28*(7), 925–932.

Stewart R, Masaki K, Xue QL, Peila R, Petrovitch H, White LR, et al. (2005). A 32-year prospective study of change in body weight and incident dementia: the Honolulu-Asia Aging Study. *Arch Neurol*, *62*(1), 55–60.

Strazzullo P, Iacone R, Iacoviello L, Russo O, Barba G, Russo P, et al. (2003). Genetic variation in the renin-angiotensin system and abdominal adiposity in men: the Olivetti Prospective Heart Study. *Ann Intern Med*, *138*(1), 17–23.

Sutton BS, Weinert S, Langefeld CD, Williams AH, Campbell JK, Saad MF, et al. (2005). Genetic analysis of adiponectin and obesity in Hispanic families: the IRAS Family Study. *Hum Genet*, *117*(2–3), 107–118.

Visscher TLS, Seidell JC, Menotti A, Blackburn H, Nissinen A, Feskens EJM, et al. (2000). Underweight and overweight in relation to mortality among men aged 40–59 and 50–69 years. The Seven Countries Study. *Am J Epidemiol*, *151*, 660–666.

Waldstein SR, & Katzel LI. (2006). Interactive relations of central versus total obesity and blood pressure to cognitive function. *2006*, *30*(1), 201–207.

Wang SY. (2002). Weight loss and metabolic changes in dementia. *J Nutr Health Aging 6*(3), 201–205.

Ward MA, Carlsson CM, Trivedi MA, Sager MA, & Johnson SC. (2005). The effect of body mass index on global brain volume in middle-aged adults: a cross sectional study. *BMC Neurol*, *5*, 23–29.

Whitmer RA. (2007). The epidemiology of adiposity and dementia *Curr Alzheimer Res*, *4*(2), 117–122.

Whitmer RA, Gunderson EP, Barrett-Connor E, Quesenberry CP Jr, & Yaffe K. (2005). Obesity in middle age and future risk of dementia: a 27 year longitudinal population based study. *BMJ*, *330*(7504), 1360.

Whitmer RA, Gunderson EP, Quesenberry CP Jr, Zhou J, & Yaffe K. (2007). Body mass index in midlife and risk of Alzheimer disease and vascular dementia. *Curr Alzheimer Res*, *4*(2), 103–109.

Whitmer RA, Gustafson DR, Barrett-Connor E, Haan MN, Gunderson EP, & Yaffe K. (2008). Central obesity and increased risk of dementia more than three decades later. *Neurology*, *71*(14), 1057–1064.

Whitmer RA, Sidney S, Selby J, Johnston SC, & Yaffe K. (2005). Midlife cardiovascular risk factors and risk of dementia in late life. *Neurology*, *64*(2), 277–281.

World Health Organization. (2008). *Top Ten Causes of Death*: World Health Organization.

World Health Organization Global Infobase. (2011, 20/01/2011). Retrieved 1 March 2012, from https://apps.who.int/infobase/

World Health Organization Global Database on Body Mass Index:BMI Classification (2012). Retrived 7 November 2012 from http://apps.who.int/bmi/index.jsp?introPage=intro_3.html

Yaffe K, Haan M, Blackwell T, Cherkasova E, Whitmer RA, & West N. (2007). Metabolic syndrome and cognitive decline in elderly Latinos: findings from the Sacramento Area Latino Study of Aging study. *J Am Geriatr Soc*, *55*(5), 758–762.

Yaffe K, Kanaya A, Lindquist K, Simonsick EM, Harris T, Shorr RI, et al. (2004). The metabolic syndrome, inflammation, and risk of cognitive decline. *JAMA*, *292*(18), 2237–2242.

Zamboni M, Zoico E, Fantin F, Panourgia MP, Di Francesco V, Tosoni P, et al. (2004). Relation between leptin and the metabolic syndrome in elderly women. *J Gerontol A Biol Sci Med Sci 59*(4), 396–400.

Zoico E, Di Francesco V, Mazzali G, Vettor R, Fantin F, Bissoli L, et al. (2004). Adipocytokines, fat distribution, and insulin resistance in elderly men and women. *J Gerontol A Biol Sci Med Sci, 59*(9), M935–939.

5

Insulin Resistance and Pathological Brain Aging

BRENNA CHOLERTON, PHD, LAURA D. BAKER, PHD, AND

SUZANNE CRAFT, PHD

Introduction

If I'd known I was going to live this long, I would have taken better
care of myself.
—Eubie Blake
It's not how old you are, but how you are old.
—Marie Dressler

Insulin, a hormone produced in the pancreas, has potent effects in the brain. Insulin resistance, which refers to a reduction in the ability of insulin to exert its action on target tissues, is associated with neuropathological processes that underlie both Alzheimer's disease (AD) and vascular dementia (VaD). In addition, several established risk factors implicated in hastening the cognitive aging process, including diabetes, obesity, hyperlipidemia, and metabolic syndrome, are closely linked to underlying insulin dysfunction. In Western cultures, such insulin resistance-associated conditions are reaching epidemic proportions. Given the rise in such chronic conditions, in combination with a rapidly aging population, the prevalence of AD and other cognitive disorders is likely to continue to rise exponentially. Fortunately, insulin resistance-associated conditions are often amenable to intervention, and promising new therapeutic models are currently under investigation. Such treatments could potentially lead to substantial reductions in the deleterious impact of insulin resistance on the aging brain.

Insulin and the Brain

The peripheral effects of insulin, a hormone secreted by pancreatic β-cells, have been well characterized. Recent evidence demonstrates that insulin is also active in the central nervous system (CNS). Although controversy exists as to whether insulin is synthesized in the adult brain, it is readily transported into the CNS across the blood–brain barrier (BBB) by a saturable, receptor-mediated process (Baskin, Figlewicz et al., 1987; Baura, Foster et al., 1993; Banks, Jaspan et al., 1997). Raising peripheral insulin levels acutely elevates brain and cerebrospinal fluid (CSF) insulin levels, whereas prolonged peripheral hyperinsulinemia downregulates BBB insulin receptors and reduces insulin transport into the brain (Wallum, Taborsky et al., 1987; Schwartz, Figlewicz et al., 1990). Insulin receptors are located in the synapses of both astrocytes and neurons (Abbott, Wells et al., 1999). Although insulin and insulin receptors are abundant in the brain, they are selectively distributed, with high concentrations in the olfactory bulb, cerebral cortex, hippocampus, hypothalamus, amygdala, and septum (Havrankova, Roth et al., 1978; Havrankova, Schmechel et al., 1978; Baskin, Figlewicz et al., 1987; Unger, Livingston et al., 1991).

INSULIN AND COGNITION

The localization of insulin receptors in the hippocampus and medial temporal cortex is consistent with evidence that insulin influences memory. In rats, acute intracerebroventricular insulin administration improves memory on a passive-avoidance task (Unger, Livingston et al., 1991). In humans, acute intravenous insulin administration while maintaining euglycemia reliably enhances story recall (Craft, Newcomer et al., 1996; Craft, Asthana et al., 1999; Kern, Peters et al., 2001; Craft, Asthana et al., 2003). Conversely, learning may also influence insulin receptor expression and function. For example, training rodents on a spatial memory task increased insulin receptor expression in the dentate gyrus and hippocampal CA1 field (Zhao, Chen et al., 1999). Thus, the act of learning is accompanied by changes in insulin signaling molecules in the hippocampus. Collectively, these studies suggest that insulin may contribute to normal memory functioning.

There are several mechanisms through which insulin may affect memory. One mechanism may be through effects on cerebral energy metabolism. Although insulin does not appear to influence glucose transport into brain, it may have more selective effects on cerebral glucose metabolism. Bingham et al. (2002) demonstrated an increase in cerebral glucose metabolism that was particularly pronounced in the cortex following administration of a low dose of insulin. Regional insulin effects on glucose metabolism may result from the distribution of glucose transporter isoforms (GLUTs) (Schulingkamp, Pagano et al., 2000;

Reagan, Gorovits et al., 2001). The insulin-sensitive GLUTs 4 and 8 are selectively distributed in the brain, and insulin increases brain GLUT 4 expression and translocation (Piroli, Grillo et al., 2007). In rats, GLUT 4 is expressed in the cerebellum, sensorimotor cortex, hippocampus, pituitary, and hypothalamus (Brant, Jess et al., 1993; Livingstone, Lyall et al., 1995; El Messari, Leloup et al., 1998; Apelt, Mehlhorn et al., 1999), and GLUT 8 has been observed in the hippocampus and hypothalamus (Reagan, Gorovits et al., 2001). Notably, substantial colocalization exists for insulin-containing neurons, insulin receptors, and GLUTs 4 and 8 (Apelt, Mehlhorn et al., 1999; Schulingkamp, Pagano et al., 2000). These overlapping distributions are consistent with insulin-stimulated glucose uptake in selective brain regions, including medial temporal lobe structures that support learning and memory.

Other insulin-related mechanisms that are not directly related to modulation of glucose uptake have also been implicated in normal hippocampal functioning (Zhao & Alkon, 2001). For example, insulin may influence components of the long-term potentiation (LTP) cascade, such as the cell membrane expression of NMDA receptors (Skeberdis, Lan et al., 2001), which affect the likelihood of LTP induction. Insulin also modulates levels of acetylcholine and norepinephrine, neurotransmitters that are known to influence cognitive function (Figlewicz, Szot et al., 1993; Kopf & Baratti, 1999) in the CNS. Thus, insulin affects numerous mechanisms relating to neuronal activity and cognitive function supported by such activity.

INSULIN RESISTANCE AND IMPAIRED COGNITION

In contrast to the beneficial effects of acute hyperinsulinemia described above, insulin dysfunction resulting from persistently high levels of circulating insulin may exert a negative influence on memory and other cognitive functions. For example, type 2 diabetes mellitus (T2DM) has been associated with impaired learning in both animal and human studies (Greenwood & Winocur, 2001). Further, impaired verbal memory has been observed in individuals with chronic hyperinsulinemia in the absence of hyperglycemia (Vanhanen, Koivisto et al., 1998). Additionally, impaired glucose tolerance has been associated with reduced hippocampal volume and memory impairment (Convit, Wolf et al., 2003). Taken together, these findings are consistent with the notion that acute and chronic hyperinsulinemia have opposing effects on the neural substrates of memory.

Chronic high levels of insulin can produce insulin resistance, a syndrome characterized by high peripheral insulin and diminished insulin-mediated glucose clearance (Reaven, 1983; Reaven, 2003). Over time, selective tissues become unresponsive to insulin, producing significant damaging effects in muscle, liver, adipose tissue, endothelium, and brain. Acute increases in insulin may temporarily overcome insulin resistance and facilitate memory and other cognitive functions; however, chronically elevated insulin serves to exacerbate insulin resistance and lead to a cascade of potentially negative effects in the periphery and in brain. The insulin resistance syndrome has been linked to several chronic medical conditions, including cardiovascular disease, metabolic syndrome, and diabetes, yet it has a "silent" phase, in which the pancreas is able to compensate by generating adequate levels of insulin to maintain lower glucose levels. As a result, insulin resistance may exert a negative influence on several body systems, including the CNS, for some time prior to the onset of frank diabetes. There is increasing support that such early insulin abnormalities may be associated with the initiation of AD pathology in some individuals years, or even decades, before the first clinical dementia symptoms are manifest (Xu, Qiu et al., 2009).

INSULIN ABNORMALITIES AND ALZHEIMER'S DISEASE PATHOLOGY

Converging evidence supports that insulin resistance raises the risk for developing AD neuropathology. The manner in which insulin abnormalities may contribute to the symptoms and pathogenesis of AD have been examined in a variety of experimental models. Hoyer and colleagues (2002) were the first group to suggest that desensitization of the neuronal insulin receptor plays a role in AD. They have demonstrated a reduction in insulin receptors and tyrosine kinase activity markers in AD brain (Frolich, Blum-Degen et al., 1998). This initial finding has been confirmed and extended in a larger sample of patients, which demonstrated reduced insulin and insulin-like growth factor IGF-I message with increasing AD pathology and cholinergic deficit (Rivera, Goldin et al., 2005).

Animal and in vitro studies have documented relationships between insulin and mechanisms with clear pathogenic implications for AD. In vitro, insulin modulates levels of the β-amyloid (Aβ) peptide, the aggregation of which is a fundamental neuropathological hallmark of AD. For example, insulin promotes release of intracellular Aβ in neuronal cultures, affecting both its short (Aβ40) and long (Aβ42) forms and accelerating their trafficking from the Golgi and trans-Golgi network to the plasma membrane (Gasparini, Gouras et al., 2001). Thus, low brain insulin may reduce the trafficking of Aβ from intracellular to extracellular compartments.

Interestingly, Aβ also regulates brain insulin signaling. Soluble Aβ binds to the insulin receptor and disrupts its signaling capacity and LTP induction in mouse hippocampal slice preparations (Townsend, Mehta et al., 2007). These effects could be prevented by exposing tissue to insulin prior to Aβ exposure. Synthetic soluble Aβ oligomers, known as Aβ-derived diffusible ligands, downregulate plasma membrane insulin receptors in primary hippocampal-cultured neurons, leading to synaptic spine loss. This process was also prevented by pretreatment with insulin (De Felice, Vieira et al., 2009). A related mechanism through which insulin and Aβ may interact to modulate AD pathology is via synaptotoxic effects. Loss of synapses is the earliest structural defect observed in AD. Soluble oligomeric species of Aβ are synaptotoxic, and insulin prevents binding of Aβ to synapses, thereby preserving synaptic integrity (De Felice, Vieira et al., 2009). Insulin also reduces oligomer formation, which may have additional protective effects; a functional consequence of these effects appears to be protection against Aβ-induced disruption of LTP integrity, the process of synaptic remodeling believed to underlie memory formation (Lee, Kuo et al., 2009). Collectively, these findings suggest that soluble Aβ may induce neuronal insulin resistance and synapse loss and that treatment with insulin such as that provided by intranasal insulin therapy may prevent these pathological processes.

A growing understanding of the importance of impaired Aβ clearance as opposed to increased Aβ production in late-onset AD has created intense focus on mechanisms regulating Aβ degradation. Insulin may modulate Aβ degradation by regulating expression of insulin degrading enzyme (IDE), a metalloprotease that catabolizes insulin (Zhao, Teter et al., 2004). Insuling degrading enzyme is highly expressed in brain as well as in liver, kidney, and muscle (Authier, Posner et al., 1996) and may play a critical role in Aβ clearance in brain (Kurochkin & Goto, 1994; McDermott & Gibson, 1997; Qiu, Walsh et al., 1998). Insulin degrading enzyme has also been implicated in the intracellular degradation of Aβ (Sudoh, Frosch et al., 2002) Further, decreased IDE activity, levels, and mRNA have been observed in AD brain tissue, and IDE knockout mice have reduced degradation of Aβ and insulin in brain (Perez, Morelli et al., 2000; Cook, Leverenz et al., 2003; Farris, Mansourian et al., 2003). Thus, low CNS insulin may reduce IDE levels in brain and thereby impair Aβ clearance.

Chronic peripheral hyperinsulinemia may lower brain insulin levels and interfere with peripheral Aβ clearance. Chronic peripheral hyperinsulinemia has been associated with a pattern in which brain insulin levels are initially higher then decrease as transport of insulin into the brain is downregulated (Banks, Jaspan et al., 1997). Consistent with this pattern, it has been shown that genetically obese Zucker rats have reduced insulin binding to brain capillaries (Schwartz, Figlewicz et al., 1990) and reduced hypothalamic insulin levels (Gerozissis, Orosco et al., 1993) in comparison with lean controls. Additionally, in an elegant study in which insulin resistance was induced in dogs through diet, brain uptake of labeled insulin was reduced and peripheral insulin clearance was inhibited (Kaiyala, Prigeon et al., 2000). Adults with AD show lower CSF insulin levels, higher plasma insulin levels, and reduced CSF-to plasma insulin ratios compared to healthy controls (Craft, Peskind et al., 1998). High plasma insulin levels may interfere with degradation of Aβ transported out of the brain, thereby obstructing a peripheral Aβ-clearing "sink." Concomitantly, low brain insulin levels reduce release of Aβ from intracellular compartments into extracellular compartments, where clearance is believed to occur. Thus, for some patients with

AD, high peripheral insulin levels and low brain insulin levels would result in reduced clearance of Aβ both in brain and in the periphery (Fig. 5.1).

Support for the validity of this model is provided by a recent study that induced insulin resistance in the T2576 mouse model of AD with a high-fat diet. Diet manipulation resulted in a metabolic profile of high peripheral insulin and low brain insulin and IDE levels compared with Tg2576 mice fed a normal diet (Ho, Qin et al., 2004). Diet-induced insulin resistance caused twofold increases in Aβ40 and 42, and earlier, larger Aβ deposits compared with non-insulin-resistant Tg2576 mice. Further, insulin-resistant mice had impaired learning on a water maze test. These results are consistent with a subsequent study showing that insulin regulates IDE and Aβ through a phosphatidylinositol-3-kinase-dep endent signaling mechanism (Zhao, Teter et al., 2004) in which treatment of primary hippocampal neurons with insulin produced a 25% increase in IDE expression. In another model of insulin resistance, APP/PS1 mice were given sucrose-sweetened beverages and also demonstrated increased brain Aβ deposition and reduce Morris water maze learning (Cao, Lu et al., 2007). Together these results suggest that insulin resistance can precipitate the neuropathological and

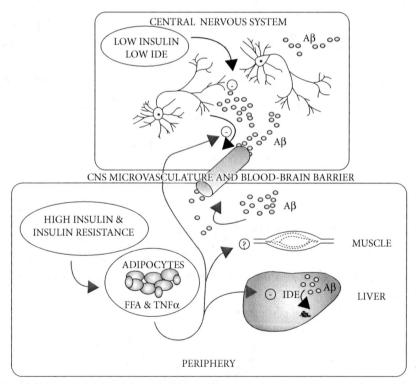

Figure 5.1 Model of peripheral hyperinsulinemia, insulin resistance, and AD pathogenesis.

behavioral features of AD and that raising brain insulin levels may reduce neuro-pathological changes related to AD.

A role for insulin has also been suggested for other AD-related mechanisms. Insulin inhibits phosphorylation of tau, the protein whose tortuous scaffolds form neurofibrillary tangles, a second neuropathological hallmark of AD. Insulin may affect tau through its regulation of glycogen synthase kinase (GSK)3β, a downstream target in the insulin signaling pathway (Hong & Lee, 1997). Schubert and colleagues (2004) abolished insulin signaling in vivo with a conditional knockout mouse model in which the insulin receptor gene was inactivated in the CNS. Phosphorylation of GSK3β and Akt was reduced and phosphorylation of tau increased 3.5-fold. Recent work has also implicated insulin receptor substrate 2, in that mice in which this gene has been knocked out have increased tangles and hyperphosphorylated tau (Schubert, Brazil et al., 2003). As reviewed earlier in this section, insulin has relevant effects on neurotransmitter levels, energy metabolism, and membrane physiology. Insulin dysregulation is also associated with oxidative stress, inflammation, and impaired neurogenesis (Craft & Watson, 2004).

Insulin Resistance-Related Conditions and Dementia

The above research provides compelling evidence concerning insulin's role in the CNS and the connection between impaired insulin action and the pathology that underlies AD. The association between dementia and insulin resistance is further substantiated by investigations of conditions related to insulin dysfunction. Insulin resistance is likely a primary underlying cause of multiple chronic diseases and thus by itself is a probable key risk factor for dementia. However, because insulin resistance is rarely identified in its earliest stages and independent of these conditions, it is seldom incorporated as a primary variable of interest in population-based models. Here, we focus on the increased dementia risk and AD/VaD neuropathology associated with insulin resistance syndromes, including diabetes, hyperlipidemia, and hypertension.

DIABETES

Diabetes is a strong predictor of cognitive decline in older adults; people with diabetes may be twice as likely to experience decline in global cognitive functions over a 5-year period than those without diabetes (Tilvis, Kahonen-Vare et al., 2004). Multiple population-based studies have reported an association between insulin resistance and cognitive impairment in elderly populations (Hassing, Grant et al., 2004; Yaffe, Blackwell et al., 2004; Strachan, 2011), and T2DM confers a significantly increased risk of dementia (both AD and VaD)

(Lu, Lin et al., 2009; Profenno, Porsteinsson et al., 2010). For example, in the prospective, community-based Rotterdam study, Ott et al. (1996) found that T2DM significantly increased the risk for all-cause dementia and AD, with greater risk apparent in people who were insulin-treated (and therefore likely to be in the more severe stages of the disease) at baseline. Similar results were reported by Leibson et al. (1997), and the Religious Orders Study reported a 65% increased risk for AD among those with T2DM (Arvanitakis, Wilson et al., 2004). Findings from the Mayo Clinic Alzheimer's Disease Patient Registry show an increased prevalence of T2DM (35% vs. 18% in non-demented control subjects) and impaired glucose tolerance (46% vs. 24%) for patients with AD (Janson, Laedtke et al., 2004). Further, AD risk is raised independently from VaD or other dementias (Ott, Stolk et al., 1999; Maher & Schubert, 2009), a finding that is not surprising given the wealth of literature that connects insulin dysfunction with AD-specific brain pathology. Interestingly, dementia risk does not appear to be associated with the age at which diabetes is diagnosed (Kloppenborg, van den Berg et al., 2008).

Coupled with animal and in vitro studies that support the influence of insulin on AD pathophysiological processes, the above epidemiological evidence provides further support for the association between diabetes and dementia. Recent neuropathological studies, however, have produced interesting and somewhat conflicting results. For example, dementia patients with treated diabetes had Aβ plaque loads that were similar to those of non-demented controls, while untreated diabetic dementia patients had plaque loads consistent with dementia patients without diabetes (Beeri, Schmeidler et al., 2008). Treated diabetics with dementia had higher levels of microvascular infarcts and anti-inflammatory markers to a degree not present in untreated diabetics (Sonnen, Larson et al., 2009). Given the preliminary nature of these results and small sample sizes, these studies must be replicated prior to making any firm conclusions as to their meaning. If supported by larger studies, however, these findings could bring into question the relative impact of both Aβ and microvascular disease in the development of clinical dementia symptoms. It is possible that treated diabetics, who are likely to be at a more advanced stage of disease, express the symptoms of dementia at lower levels of amyloid burden because of co-existing microvascular damage. Future neuropathological studies that carefully examine disease duration, treatment duration and dose, and concomitant vascular risk factors will certainly help to clarify these questions.

DYSLIPIDEMIA

Insulin is a key modulator of lipid metabolism, and insulin resistance is associated with dyslipidemia. By increasing lipolysis and free fatty acids (FFAs) in adipocytes, insulin resistance leads to an influx of FFAs into the liver. This inhibits insulin-mediated suppression of very low-density lipid (VLDL) secretion, which is crucial for preventing post-prandial hyperlipidemia and for maintaining an optimal lipid balance (Kamagate, Qu et al., 2008). Insulin resistance thus results in higher and more prolonged post-prandial VLDL and other lipids, a process that may represent yet another pathway by which insulin potentially exacerbates pathological Aβ processes in the brain. Although the mechanisms underlying the association between lipids, lipoproteins, and Aβ are not well understood, it is increasingly clear that these interactions play a vital role in Aβ production and clearance.

VASCULAR IMPAIRMENT AND HYPERTENSION

Through both direct effects and insulin resistance-related dyslipidemia and inflammation, insulin dysfunction can substantially impact the vasculature. Insulin mediates capillary recruitment, vasodilation, and regional blood flow (Cersosimo & DeFronzo, 2006; Schinzari, Tesauro et al., 2010). When not disrupted, insulin increases vasodilation and regulates vasoconstriction via modulation of nitric oxide (NO) and endothelian-1. Conversely, insulin resistance-associated declines in NO and increases in endothelin-1 activity results in vasoconstriction and reduced blood flow. This process, in turn, exacerbates both glucose and lipid dysfunction. As a result, increasing insulin resistance and progressive vascular dysfunction work together in a negative feedback loop (Cersosimo & DeFronzo, 2006). In the brain, such vasoconstriction and reduced capillary recruitment may ultimately impede neural activity and thus negatively impact cognitive function.

Approximately one in three adults have hypertension (CDC, 2011), and 50% of hypertensive patients are insulin resistant (Lima, Abbasi et al., 2009). Hypertension impairs neuron-dependent blood flow (known as functional hyperemia) via a number of insulin resistance-related processes, including oxidative stress, dysregulation of vasoactive mediators (including NO and endothelin-1), structural alteration of the blood vessels, and insufficient cerebral autoregulation (Iadecola & Davisson, 2008). Animal models evidence increased Aβ deposition with hypertension, which leads to vascular dysfunction and reduced functional hyperemia (Iadecola & Davisson, 2008).

Insulin Resistance-Related Conditions: Conclusions

It is becoming increasingly apparent that diabetes is associated with a higher dementia risk. Shared neuropathological processes underlie several conditions related to insulin resistance and both AD and VaD. Modification of central insulin resistance may thus have a positive impact on cognitive function in people with early clinical changes associated with AD pathology. More broadly, therapeutic intervention may lead to notable reductions on the community burden of dementia.

Novel Therapeutic Strategies

As described above, the harmful effects of insulin resistance on the periphery and brain are well characterized. Type 2 diabetes, cardiovascular disease, hyperlipidemia, and other chronic health conditions are related to underlying insulin resistance and have known detrimental effects on brain aging. Therapeutic interventions that address the challenges presented by insulin resistance and related conditions could significantly reduce the social and economic burden associated with late-onset dementia. Here, we examine two potential novel therapeutic strategies aimed at reducing pathological processes associated with insulin resistance and dementia: intranasal insulin (INI) and PPAR-γ agonists.

INTRANASAL INSULIN

One innovative therapeutic strategy currently under investigation is the normalization of brain insulin levels through INI administration. As reviewed in the previous sections, insulin has pleiotropic effects on pathways implicated in AD pathogenesis. As such, augmenting CNS insulin, in contrast to the majority of therapeutic approaches that focus on narrowly defined mechanisms such as acetylcholine modulation or amyloid accumulation, may have greater potential to impact the clinical symptomatology associated with AD pathology. Studies administering intravenous insulin while maintaining euglycemia have shown increased CNS insulin and improved cognition (Craft, Newcomer et al., 1996; Craft, Asthana et al., 1999; Park, Seeley et al., 2000; Craft, Asthana et al., 2003). However, chronic peripheral insulin administration is not a viable therapy because of risks associated with hypoglycemia and prolonged peripheral hyperinsulinemia. Any long-term treatment strategy for normalizing CNS insulin levels in persons with AD must avoid significantly increasing insulin in the periphery. There is increasing support that this may be achieved via intranasal pathways.

The nasal cavity is unique in that olfactory sensory neurons are directly exposed to the external environment in the upper nasal cavity, while their axons extend through the cribriform plate to the olfactory bulb. Following intranasal administration, drugs can be directly transported to the CNS, bypassing the periphery, via extracellular pathways (Born, Lange et al., 2002; Frey, 2002; Thorne, Pronk et al., 2004). Additionally, an intraneuronal pathway delivers drugs to the CNS hours or days later (Broadwell & Balin, 1985; Shipley, 1985; Baker & Spencer, 1986; Balin, Broadwell et al., 1986). Kern et al. (1999) administered 40 IU of insulin intranasally in young, healthy adults, resulting in increased

CSF insulin levels within 10 minutes of administration compared to placebo, with peak levels noted within 30 minutes. Cerebrospinal fluid insulin levels had not returned to baseline by the end of the 80-minute study. Blood glucose and insulin levels did not change, demonstrating that the effects in CSF do not result from transport from the nasal cavity to systemic circulation. This finding is consistent with a large literature that demonstrates insulin's poor transport from the nasal cavity into blood (Illum, 2002). Although elevated CSF insulin levels do not conclusively demonstrate that brain insulin levels are similarly elevated, animal studies have shown labeled INI uptake to hippocampus and cortex (Francis, Martinez et al., 2008). In a murine diabetes model, INI reduced brain atrophy and neuronal NFkB activation, while increasing synaptic markers, choline acetyltranferase levels, and activation of Akt, CREB, and GSK3β. These effects were accompanied by memory enhancement on Water Maze and radial arm tasks (Francis, Martinez et al., 2008).

Human functional and cognitive studies of INI also support insulin's transport to the CNS. Intranasal insulin treatment induced changes in auditory-evoked brain potentials (AEPs) compared to placebo (Kern, Born et al., 1999). Several studies have reported that two months of daily insulin administration (4 x 40 IU/day) significantly improves verbal memory and enhanced mood in young healthy adults (Benedict, Hallschmid et al., 2004; Stockhorst, de Fries et al., 2004; Benedict, Kern et al., 2008; Hallschmid, Benedict et al., 2008; Stockhorst, de Fries et al., submitted for publication) In a series of groundbreaking trials, acute and chronic effects of INI administration on cognitive function, CSF biomakers, and functional PET imaging were evaluated in memory-impaired older adults. Initial pilot data from these studies showed that INI improved verbal memory acutely in persons with AD or amnestic MCI without affecting plasma insulin or glucose levels and that 20 IU of insulin produced the greatest benefit (Reger, Watson et al., 2008; Reger, Watson et al., 2006) Subsequently, investigation of the chronic effects of 20 IU of INI (Reger, Watson et al. 2008) demonstrated that insulin-treated subjects had better declarative memory and selective attention performance following 21 days of treatment. In addition, caregivers rated those with greater impairment at baseline as performing significantly better functionally following treatment with insulin, whereas there was no noted improvement in the placebo group. Fasting plasma insulin and glucose levels were unchanged for both groups, whereas Aβ40/42 ratios increased for INI-treated adults compared to placebo, reflecting increased Aβ40 relative to Aβ42.

A follow-up study examined daily INI treatment for 4 months in 104 adults with AD or amnestic MCI and compared two doses (10 or 20 IU bid vs. placebo) (Craft, Baker et al., 2012). Compared with the placebo group, the lower dose of insulin improved delayed memory, and both insulin doses preserved caregiver-rated ability to carry out daily functions. General cognitive abilities (assessed using the ADAS-Cog) was also preserved by both doses of INI (Fig. 5.2).

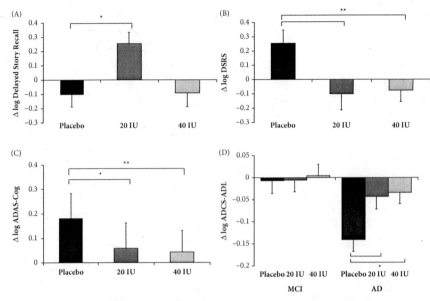

Figure 5.2 Log mean (A) delayed story recall, (B) Dementia Severity Rating Scale (DSRS), (C) Alzheimer Disease's Assessment Scale-cognitive subscale (ADAS-cog), and (D) Alzheimer's Disease Cooperative Study-activities of daily living (ADCS-ADL) scale change scores (from baseline to month 4) with standard errors of the mean (error bars) for placebo, 20-IU dose insulin, and 40-IU dose insulin groups.

In exploratory analyses, changes in CSF Aβ42 and tau/Aβ42 ratios were associated with cognitive and functional changes for insulin-treated participants. Participants in this trial also underwent FDG-PET imaging; compared with placebo-assigned participants, the lower dose insulin group showed reduced progression of hypometabolism in bilateral frontal, right temporal, bilateral occipital, and right precuneus/cuneus regions over the 4-month treatment period. The higher dose insulin group showed even greater treatment effects, indicating less hypometabolism progression in most regions and in left parietal cortex.

The above results provide compelling evidence that INI may benefit adults with amnestic MCI or AD and thus may represent a promising novel therapeutic approach to the treatment of degenerative memory disorders. Longer, larger, multisite trials will address the question of whether INI represents a viable therapeutic approach to the treatment of AD and MCI.

INSULIN-SENSITIZING AGENTS: PEROXISOME PROLIFERATORS ACTIVATED RECEPTOR-γ AGONISTS

Peroxisome proliferator activated receptor-γ agonists have been shown to improve insulin sensitivity by decreasing circulating insulin and increasing insulin-mediated glucose uptake, with minimal risk of hypoglycemia (Olefsky, 2000). In addition to improving insulin sensitivity, several investigators have reported that PPAR-γ activity may reduce both Aβ accumulation and inflammatory reactants and protect against neurotoxicity (Combs, Johnson et al., 2000; Paik, Ju et al., 2000; Delerive, Fruchart et al., 2001; Landreth, 2007). Insulin resistance leads to increased central Aβ levels; PPAR-γ agonist therapy may, by decreasing insulin resistance, help to normalize Aβ levels in brain and improve associated behavioral symptoms. In vitro, treatment with a low dose of the PPAR-γ agonist rosiglitazone increased Aβ clearance via upregulation of LRP1 (Moon, Kim et al., 2011). Another PPAR-γ agonist, pioglitazone, prevented insulin resistance and related increases in Aβ in fructose-drinking rats (Luo, Hou et al., 2011).

Activation of PPAR-γ receptors has also been shown to regulate inflammatory responses and apoptosis (Corton, Anderson et al., 2000; Escher & Wahli, 2000). Peroxisome proliferate activated receptor-γ agonists inhibit Aβ-stimulated secretion of pro-inflammatory products, arrest the evaluation of activated macrophages, and inhibit the expression of cyclooxygenase-2 (Combs, Johnson et al., 2000). Decreased oxidative stress and reduced inflammation have been demonstrated with PPAR-γ treatment in both in vitro and in vivo models (Hirsch, Breidert et al., 2003; Schmidt, Moric et al., 2003). Rosiglitazone suppressed inflammation in brain cells in vitro (Park, Park et al., 2003) and reversed the negative effects of TNF-α on insulin signaling and insulin-mediated glucose uptake (Hernandez, Teruel et al., 2004). Animal models have suggested that treatment with rosiglitazone significantly reduces inflammation in response to acute injury and also improves endothelium-dependent vasodilation and coronary arteriole function (Tao, Liu et al., 2003; Bagi, Koller et al., 2004; Cuzzocrea, Pisano et al., 2004). Treatment with pioglitazone improved cognitive performance and cerebral glucose metabolism and reduced oxidative stress in rats treated with intracerebroventricular streptozotocin (Pathan, Viswanad et al., 2006). In humans, non-diabetic patients with cardiovascular disease were treated with rosiglitazone and demonstrated notable peripheral anti-inflammatory effects (Sidhu, Cowan et al., 2003; Sidhu, Cowan et al., 2004). In obese non-diabetic patients, rosiglitazone reduced C-reactive protein (CRP), plasma monocyte chemoattractant protein-1(MCP-1), serum amyloid A, and TNF-α; reductions of CRP and MCP-1 were also noted in the obese diabetic group (Mohanty, Aljada et al., 2004). These findings suggest that PPAR-γ agonists may protect neural tissue from inflammatory damage and are thus attractive candidates for the treatment of insulin resistance and inflammation associated with early cognitive decline.

Despite a strong rationale to examine the effectiveness of PPAR-γ agonist treatment in persons with AD, results from human clinical trials have been mixed. One trial of rosigilitazone in patients with amnestic MCI and early AD resulted in improved performance on selective cognitive functions and a more favorable plasma Aβ40/42 ratio (Fig. 5.3) (Watson, Cholerton et al., 2005).

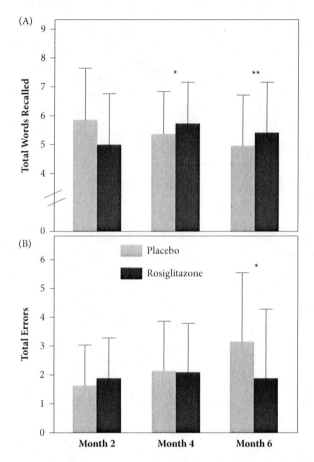

Figure 5.3 Data are depicted as group means and standard deviations and are statistically adjusted for baseline performance, age; and Dementia Rating Scale score. Figure 5.3A depicts delayed verbal memory scores from the Buscke Selective Reminding task. At month 2, groups were equivalent; however, the rosiglitazone-treated group recalled significantly more words than did the placebo-assigned group at months 4 and 6. Figure 5.3B depicts total errors for the Stroop Color-Word Interference task. At months 2 and 4, groups were equivalent; however, the rosiglitazone-treated group made significantly fewer errors than did the placebo group at month 6 (*Am J Geriatr Psychiatry* 2005; *13*: 950–958).

A larger 6-month trial failed to yield overall cognitive benefit; however, improvement was noted in subjects without an APOE ε4 allele on a task of general cognitive function at the highest dose (Risner, Saunders et al., 2006). Subsequent phase 3 clinical trials, however, failed to show any cognitive improvements in patients with mild to moderate AD, regardless of genetic status (Gold, Alderton et al., 2010; Harrington, Sawchak et al., 2011). Pioglitazone has produced similarly mixed results. Treatment with pioglitazone in patients with both T2DM and AD produced improvement on general cognitive status and declarative verbal memory following 6 months of treatment, as well as improved regional cerebral blood flow in the parietal lobe (Hanyu, Sato et al., 2009; Sato, Hanyu et al., 2011). Follow-up data demonstrated that improvements in cognitive function were associated with reduced TNF-α, supporting the anti-inflammatory actions of pioglitazone (Hanyu, Sato et al., 2010). However, another trial that was designed to primarily assess the safety of pioglitazone in non-diabetic patients with AD failed to show any improvements on secondary outcome cognitive and functional measures (Geldmacher, Fritsch et al., 2011).

The inconsistent results from clinical trials using PPAR-γ agonists have led to doubt as to whether these compounds represent effective treatments for memory disorders in older adults. In addition, safety concerns related to the effects of rosiglitazone on cardiovascular functioning and heart failure in diabetic patients have been reported. Doubts have been raised concerning reports of increased cardiovascular events with rosiglitazone treatment; however, such safety concerns may nonetheless limit willingness of physicians to prescribe rosiglitazone (Mannucci, Monami et al., 2010). Interestingly, a recent in vitro model suggested that a subclinical dose of rosiglitazone may produce more beneficial effects on Aβ clearance than higher doses (Moon, Kim et al., 2011). Follow-up animal and human studies may help to determine whether lower doses may also be accompanied by a better safety/tolerability profile. Further, the above trials all included patients with clinically diagnosed AD; however, it is possible that treating insulin resistance prior to the onset of clinically significant dementia (e.g., MCI) may produce more favorable cognitive results. Although a few of these trials included amnestic MCI patients, to date, none have examined the effects of these medications on people with MCI alone. Finally, larger clinical trials utilizing pioglitazone, which seems to have a more favorable safety profile, may help to illuminate whether PPAR-γ agonist treatment improves cognitive decline associated with AD pathological processes.

Summary

With an aging population and concurrent rise in chronic health conditions comes a rapid escalation in the incidence of dementia. Although notable strides have been made with regard to discerning the pathophysiological processes associated with AD and other dementias, pharmacological treatment trials have generally produced minimal or disappointing results. Many of the processes that underlie the neuropathological features of dementia may be related to risk factors that are responsive to the treatment of insulin resistance. As a result, novel therapeutic agents that target insulin resistance and brain insulin levels represent promising strategies to reduce the escalating burden of dementia.

References

Abbott, M. A., Wells, D. G., & Fallon, J. R. (1999). The insulin receptor tyrosine kinase substrate p58/53 and the insulin receptor are components of CNS synapses. *J Neurosci*, *19*(17), 7300–7308.

Apelt, J., Mehlhorn, G., & Schliebs, R. (1999). Insulin-sensitive GLUT4 glucose transporters are colocalized with GLUT3-expressing cells and demonstrate a chemically distinct neuron-specific localization in rat brain. *J Neurosci Res*, *57*(5), 693–705.

Arvanitakis, Z., Wilson, R. S., Bienias, J. L., Evans, D. A., & Bennett, D. A. (2004). Diabetes mellitus and risk of Alzheimer disease and decline in cognitive function. *Arch Neurol*, *61*(5), 661–666.

Authier, F., Posner, B. I., & Bergeron, J. J. (1996). Insulin-degrading enzyme. *Clin Invest Med*, *19*(3), 149–160.

Bagi, Z., Koller, A., & Kaley, G. (2004). PPAR{gamma} activation, by reducing oxidative stress, increases NO bioavailability in coronary arterioles of mice with Type 2 diabetes. *Am J Physiol Heart Circ Physiol*, *286*(2), H742-H748.

Baker, H., & Spencer, R. F. (1986). Transneuronal transport of peroxidase-conjugated wheat germ agglutinin (WGA-HRP) from the olfactory epithelium to the brain of the adult rat. *Exp Brain Res*, *63*(3), 461–473.

Balin, B. J., Broadwell, R. D., Salcman, M., & el-Kalliny, M. (1986). Avenues for entry of peripherally administered protein to the central nervous system in mouse, rat, and squirrel monkey. *J Comp Neurol*, *251*(2), 260–280.

Banks, W. A., Jaspan, J. B., Huang, W., & Kastin, A. J. (1997). Transport of insulin across the blood-brain barrier: saturability at euglycemic doses of insulin. *Peptides*, *18*(9), 1423–1429.

Banks, W. A., Jaspan, J. B., & Kastin, A. J. (1997). Selective, physiological transport of insulin across the blood-brain barrier: novel demonstration by species-specific radioimmunoassays. *Peptides*, *18*(8), 1257–1262.

Baskin, D. G., Figlewicz, D. P., Woods, S. C., Porte, D., Jr., & Dorsa, D. M. (1987). Insulin in the brain. *Annu Rev Physiol*, *49*, 335–347.

Baura, G. D., Foster, D. M., Porte, D., Jr., Kahn, S. E., Bergman, R. N., Cobelli, C., et al. (1993). Saturable transport of insulin from plasma into the central nervous system of dogs in vivo. A mechanism for regulated insulin delivery to the brain. *J Clin Invest*, *92*(4), 1824–1830.

Beeri, M. S., Schmeidler, J., Silverman, J. M., Gandy, S., Wysocki, M., Hannigan, C. M., et al. (2008). Insulin in combination with other diabetes medication is associated with less Alzheimer neuropathology. *Neurology*, *71*(10), 750–757.

Benedict, C., Hallschmid, M., Hatke, A., Schultes, B., Fehm, H. L., Born, J., et al. (2004). Intranasal insulin improves memory in humans. *Psychoneuroendocrinology*, *29*(10), 1326–1334.

Benedict, C., Kern, W., Schultes, B., Born, J., & Hallschmid, M. (2008). Differential sensitivity of men and women to anorexigenic and memory-improving effects of intranasal insulin. *J Clin Endocrinol Metab*, *93*(4), 1339–1344.

Bingham, E. M., Hopkins, D., Smith, D., Pernet, A., Hallett, W., Reed, L., et al. (2002). The role of insulin in human brain glucose metabolism: an 18fluoro-deoxyglucose positron emission tomography study. *Diabetes*, *51*(12), 3384–3390.

Born, J., Lange, T., Kern, W., McGregor, G. P., Bickel, U., & Fehm, H. L. (2002). Sniffing neuropeptides: a transnasal approach to the human brain. *Nat Neurosci*, *5*(6), 514–516.

Brant, A. M., Jess, T. J., Milligan, G., Brown, C. M., & Gould, G. W. (1993). Immunological analysis of glucose transporters expressed in different regions of the rat brain and central nervous system. *Biochem Biophys Res Commun*, *192*(3), 1297–1302.

Broadwell, R. D., & Balin, B. J. (1985). Endocytic and exocytic pathways of the neuronal secretory process and trans-synaptic transfer of wheat germ agglutinin-horseradish peroxidase in vivo. *J Comp Neurol*, *242*(4), 632–650.

Cao, D., Lu, H., Lewis, T. L., & Li, L. (2007). Intake of sucrose-sweetened water induces insulin resistance and exacerbates memory deficits and amyloidosis in a transgenic mouse model of Alzheimer disease. *J Biol Chem*, *282*(50), 36275–36282.

CDC (2011). Health, United States, 2010: With Special Feature on Death and Dying. Hyattsville, MD, National Center for Health Statistics.

Cersosimo, E., & DeFronzo, R. A. (2006). Insulin resistance and endothelial dysfunction: the road map to cardiovascular diseases. *Diabetes Metab Res Rev, 22*(6), 423–436.

Combs, C. K., Johnson, D. E., Karlo, J. C., Cannady, S. B., & Landreth, G. E. (2000). Inflammatory mechanisms in Alzheimer's disease: inhibition of beta-amyloid-stimulated proinflammatory responses and neurotoxicity by PPARgamma agonists. *J Neurosci, 20*(2), 558–567.

Convit, A., Wolf, O. T., Tarshish, C., & de Leon, M. J. (2003). Reduced glucose tolerance is associated with poor memory performance and hippocampal atrophy among normal elderly. *Proc Natl Acad Sci U S A, 100*(4), 2019–2022.

Cook, D. G., Leverenz, J. B., McMillan, P. J., Kulstad, J. J., Ericksen, S., Roth, R. A., et al. (2003). Reduced hippocampal insulin-degrading enzyme in late-onset Alzheimer's disease is associated with the apolipoprotein E-epsilon4 allele. *Am J Pathol, 162*(1), 313–319.

Corton, J. C., Anderson, S. P., & Stauber, A. (2000). Central role of peroxisome proliferator-activated receptors in the actions of peroxisome proliferators. *Annu Rev Pharmacol Toxicol, 40*, 491–518.

Craft, S., Asthana, S., Cook, D. G., Baker, L. D., Cherrier, M., Purganan, K., et al. (2003). Insulin dose-response effects on memory and plasma amyloid precursor protein in Alzheimer's disease: interactions with apolipoprotein E genotype. *Psychoneuroendocrinology, 28*(6), 809–822.

Craft, S., Asthana, S., Newcomer, J. W., Wilkinson, C. W., Matos, I. T., Baker, L. D., et al. (1999). Enhancement of memory in Alzheimer disease with insulin and somatostatin, but not glucose. *Arch Gen Psychiatry, 56*(12), 1135–1140.

Craft, S., Baker, L. D., Montine, T. J., Minoshima, S., Watson, G. S., Claxton, A., et al. (2012). Intranasal Insulin Therapy for Alzheimer Disease and Amnestic Mild Cognitive Impairment: A Pilot Clinical Trial. *Arch Neurol., 69*(1), 29–38.

Craft, S., Newcomer, J., Kanne, S., Dagogo-Jack, S., Cryer, P., Sheline, Y., et al. (1996). Memory improvement following induced hyperinsulinemia in Alzheimer's disease. *Neurobiol Aging, 17*(1), 123–130.

Craft, S., Peskind, E., Schwartz, M. W., Schellenberg, G. D., Raskind, M., & Porte, D., Jr. (1998). Cerebrospinal fluid and plasma insulin levels in Alzheimer's disease: relationship to severity of dementia and apolipoprotein E genotype. *Neurology, 50*(1), 164–168.

Craft, S., & Watson, G. S. (2004). Insulin and neurodegenerative disease: shared and specific mechanisms. *Lancet Neurol, 3*(3), 169–178.

Cuzzocrea, S., Pisano, B., Dugo, L., Ianaro, A., Maffia, P., Patel, N. S., et al. (2004). Rosiglitazone, a ligand of the peroxisome proliferator-activated receptor-gamma, reduces acute inflammation. *Eur J Pharmacol, 483*(1), 79–93.

De Felice, F. G., Vieira, M. N., Bomfim, T. R., Decker, H., Velasco, P. T., Lambert, M. P., et al. (2009). Protection of synapses against Alzheimer's-linked toxins: insulin signaling prevents the pathogenic binding of Abeta oligomers. *Proc Natl Acad Sci U S A, 106*(6), 1971–1976.

Delerive, P., Fruchart, J. C., & Staels, B. (2001). Peroxisome proliferator-activated receptors in inflammation control. *J Endocrinol, 169*(3), 453–459.

El Messari, S., Leloup, C., Quignon, M., Brisorgueil, M. J., Penicaud, L., & Arluison, M. (1998). Immunocytochemical localization of the insulin-responsive glucose transporter 4 (Glut4) in the rat central nervous system. *J Comp Neurol, 399*(4), 492–512.

Escher, P., & Wahli, W. (2000). Peroxisome proliferator-activated receptors: insight into multiple cellular functions. *Mutat Res, 448*(2), 121–138.

Farris, W., Mansourian, S., Chang, Y., Lindsley, L., Eckman, E. A., Frosch, M. P., et al. (2003). Insulin-degrading enzyme regulates the levels of insulin, amyloid beta-protein, and the beta-amyloid precursor protein intracellular domain in vivo. *Proc Natl Acad Sci U S A, 100*(7), 4162–4167.

Figlewicz, D. P., Szot, P., Israel, P. A., Payne, C., & Dorsa, D. M. (1993). Insulin reduces norepinephrine transporter mRNA in vivo in rat locus coeruleus. *Brain Res, 602*(1), 161–164.

Francis, G. J., Martinez, J. A., Liu, W. Q., Xu, K., Ayer, A., Fine, J., et al. (2008). Intranasal insulin prevents cognitive decline, cerebral atrophy and white matter changes in murine type I diabetic encephalopathy. *Brain, 131*(Pt 12), 3311–3334.

Frey, W. H., 2nd. (2002). Intranasal delivery: bypassing the blood-brain barrier to deliver therapeutic agents to the brain and spinal cord. *Drug Deliv Technol*, 2(5), 46–49.

Frolich, L., Blum-Degen, D., Bernstein, H. G., Engelsberger, S., Humrich, J., Laufer, S., et al.
(1998). Brain insulin and insulin receptors in aging and sporadic Alzheimer's disease. *J
Neural Transm*, 105(4–5), 423–438.

Gasparini, L., Gouras, G. K., Wang, R., Gross, R. S., Beal, M. F., Greengard, P., et al. (2001).
Stimulation of beta-amyloid precursor protein trafficking by insulin reduces intraneuronal beta-amyloid and requires mitogen-activated protein kinase signaling. *J Neurosci*,
21(8), 2561–2570.

Geldmacher, D. S., Fritsch, T., McClendon, M. J., & Landreth, G. (2011). A randomized pilot
clinical trial of the safety of pioglitazone in treatment of patients with Alzheimer disease.
Arch Neurol, 68(1), 45–50.

Gerozissis, K., Orosco, M., Rouch, C., & Nicolaidis, S. (1993). Basal and hyperinsulinemia-induced
immunoreactive hypothalamic insulin changes in lean and genetically obese Zucker rats
revealed by microdialysis. *Brain Res*, 611(2), 258–263.

Gold, M., Alderton, C., Zvartau-Hind, M., Egginton, S., Saunders, A. M., Irizarry, M., et al.
(2010). Rosiglitazone monotherapy in mild-to-moderate Alzheimer's disease: results
from a randomized, double-blind, placebo-controlled phase III study. *Dement Geriatr Cogn
Disord*, 30(2), 131–146.

Greenwood, C. E., & Winocur, G. (2001). Glucose treatment reduces memory deficits in young
adult rats fed high-fat diets. *Neurobiol Learn Mem*, 75(2), 179–189.

Hallschmid, M., Benedict, C., Schultes, B., Born, J., & Kern, W. (2008). Obese men respond to
cognitive but not to catabolic brain insulin signaling. *Int J Obes (Lond)*, 32(2), 275–282.

Hanyu, H., Sato, T., Kiuchi, A., Sakurai, H., & Iwamoto, T. (2009). Pioglitazone improved cognition in a pilot study on patients with Alzheimer's disease and mild cognitive impairment
with diabetes mellitus. *J Am Geriatr Soc*, 57(1), 177–179.

Hanyu, H., Sato, T., Sakurai, H., & Iwamoto, T. (2010). The role of tumor necrosis factor-alpha
in cognitive improvement after peroxisome proliferator-activator receptor gamma agonist
pioglitazone treatment in Alzheimer's disease. *J Am Geriatr Soc*, 58(5), 1000–1001.

Harrington, C., Sawchak, S., Chiang, C., Davies, J., Donovan, C., Saunders, A. M., et al. (2011).
Rosiglitazone does not improve cognition or global function when used as adjunctive
therapy to AChE inhibitors in mild-to-moderate Alzheimer's disease: two phase 3 studies.
Curr Alzheimer Res, 8(5), 592–606.

Hassing, L. B., Grant, M. D., Hofer, S. M., Pedersen, N. L., Nilsson, S. E., Berg, S., et al. (2004).
Type 2 diabetes mellitus contributes to cognitive decline in old age: a longitudinal
population-based study. *J Int Neuropsychol Soc*, 10(4), 599–607.

Havrankova, J., Roth, J., & Brownstein, M. (1978). Insulin receptors are widely distributed in
the central nervous system of the rat. *Nature*, 272(5656), 827–829.

Havrankova, J., Schmechel, D., Roth, J., & Brownstein, M. (1978). Identification of insulin in
rat brain. *Proc Natl Acad Sci U S A*, 75(11), 5737–5741.

Hernandez, R., Teruel, T., De Alvaro, C., & Lorenzo, M. (2004). Rosiglitazone ameliorates insulin resistance in brown adipocytes of Wistar rats by impairing TNF-alpha induction of p38
and p42/p44 mitogen-activated protein kinases. *Diabetologia*, 47(9), 1615–1624.

Hirsch, E. C., Breidert, T., Rousselet, E., Hunot, S., Hartmann, A., & Michel, P. P. (2003). The role
of glial reaction and inflammation in Parkinson's disease. *Ann N Y Acad Sci*, 991, 214–228.

Ho, L., Qin, W., Pompl, P. N., Xiang, Z., Wang, J., Zhao, Z., et al. (2004). Diet-induced insulin
resistance promotes amyloidosis in a transgenic mouse model of Alzheimer's disease.
Faseb J, 18(7), 902–904.

Hong, M., & Lee, V. (1997). Insulin and insulin-like growth factor-1 regulate tau phosphorylation in cultured human neurons. *Journal of Biological Chemistry*, 272(8), 19547–19553.

Hoyer, S. (2002). The aging brain. Changes in the neuronal insulin/insulin receptor signal
transduction cascade trigger late-onset sporadic Alzheimer disease (SAD). A mini-review.
J Neural Transm, 109(7–8), 991–1002.

Iadecola, C., & Davisson, R. L. (2008). Hypertension and cerebrovascular dysfunction. *Cell
Metab*, 7(6), 476–484.

Illum, L. (2002). Nasal drug delivery: new developments and strategies. *Drug Discov Today*, 7(23), 1184–1189.

Janson, J., Laedtke, T., Parisi, J. E., O'Brien, P., Petersen, R. C., & Butler, P. C. (2004). Increased risk of type 2 diabetes in Alzheimer disease. *Diabetes*, 53(2), 474–481.

Kaiyala, K. J., Prigeon, R. L., Kahn, S. E., Woods, S. C., & Schwartz, M. W. (2000). Obesity induced by a high-fat diet is associated with reduced brain insulin transport in dogs. *Diabetes*, 49(9), 1525–1533.

Kamagate, A., Qu, S., Perdomo, G., Su, D., Kim, D. H., Slusher, S., et al. (2008). FoxO1 mediates insulin-dependent regulation of hepatic VLDL production in mice. *J Clin Invest*, 118(6), 2347–2364.

Kern, W., Born, J., Schreiber, H., & Fehm, H. L. (1999). Central nervous system effects of intranasally administered insulin during euglycemia in men. *Diabetes*, 48(3), 557–563.

Kern, W., Peters, A., Fruehwald-Schultes, B., Deininger, E., Born, J., & Fehm, H. L. (2001). Improving influence of insulin on cognitive functions in humans. *Neuroendocrinology*, 74(4), 270–280.

Kloppenborg, R. P., van den Berg, E., Kappelle, L. J., & Biessels, G. J. (2008). Diabetes and other vascular risk factors for dementia: which factor matters most? A systematic review. *Eur J Pharmacol*, 585(1), 97–108.

Kopf, S. R., & Baratti, C. M. (1999). Effects of posttraining administration of insulin on retention of a habituation response in mice: participation of a central cholinergic mechanism. *Neurobiol Learn Mem*, 71(1), 50–61.

Kurochkin, I. V., & Goto, S. (1994). Alzheimer's beta-amyloid peptide specifically interacts with and is degraded by insulin degrading enzyme. *FEBS Lett*, 345(1), 33–37.

Landreth, G. (2007). Therapeutic use of agonists of the nuclear receptor PPARgamma in Alzheimer's disease. *Curr Alzheimer Res*, 4(2), 159–164.

Lee, C. C., Kuo, Y. M., Huang, C. C., & Hsu, K. S. (2009). Insulin rescues amyloid beta-induced impairment of hippocampal long-term potentiation. *Neurobiol Aging*, 30(3), 377–387.

Leibson, C. L., Rocca, W. A., Hanson, V. A., Cha, R., Kokmen, E., O'Brien, P. C., et al. (1997). The risk of dementia among persons with diabetes mellitus: a population-based cohort study. *Ann N Y Acad Sci*, 826, 422–427.

Lima, N. K., Abbasi, F., Lamendola, C., & Reaven, G. M. (2009). Prevalence of insulin resistance and related risk factors for cardiovascular disease in patients with essential hypertension. *Am J Hypertens*, 22(1), 106–111.

Livingstone, C., Lyall, H., & Gould, G. W. (1995). Hypothalamic GLUT 4 expression: a glucose- and insulin-sensing mechanism? *Mol Cell Endocrinol*, 107(1), 67–70.

Lu, F. P., Lin, K. P., & Kuo, H. K. (2009). Diabetes and the risk of multi-system aging phenotypes: a systematic review and meta-analysis. *PLoS One*, 4(1), e4144.

Luo, D., Hou, X., Hou, L., Wang, M., Xu, S., Dong, C., et al. (2011). Effect of pioglitazone on altered expression of Abeta metabolism-associated molecules in the brain of fructose-drinking rats, a rodent model of insulin resistance. *Eur J Pharmacol*, 664(1–3), 14–19.

Maher, P. A., & Schubert, D. R. (2009). Metabolic links between diabetes and Alzheimer's disease. *Expert Rev Neurother*, 9(5), 617–630.

Mannucci, E., Monami, M., Di Bari, M., Lamanna, C., Gori, F., Gensini, G. F., et al. (2010). Cardiac safety profile of rosiglitazone: a comprehensive meta-analysis of randomized clinical trials. *Int J Cardiol*, 143(2), 135–140.

McDermott, J. R., & Gibson, A. M. (1997). Degradation of Alzheimer's beta-amyloid protein by human and rat brain peptidases: involvement of insulin-degrading enzyme. *Neurochemical Research*, 22(1), 49–56.

Mohanty, P., Aljada, A., Ghanim, H., Hofmeyer, D., Tripathy, D., Syed, T., et al. (2004). Evidence for a potent antiinflammatory effect of rosiglitazone. *J Clin Endocrinol Metab*, 89(6), 2728–2735.

Moon, J. H., Kim, H. J., Yang, A. H., Kim, H. M., Lee, B. W., Kang, E. S., et al. (2011). The effect of rosiglitazone on LRP1 expression and amyloid beta uptake in human brain microvascular endothelial cells: a possible role of a low-dose thiazolidinedione for dementia treatment. *Int J Neuropsychopharmacol*, Nov 1, 1–8 [Epub ahead of print].

Olefsky, J. M. (2000). Treatment of insulin resistance with peroxisome proliferator-activated receptor gamma agonists. *J Clin Invest, 106*(4), 467–472.

Ott, A., Stolk, R. P., Hofman, A., van Harskamp, F., Grobbee, D. E., & Breteler, M. M. (1996). Association of diabetes mellitus and dementia: the Rotterdam Study. *Diabetologia, 39*(11), 1392–1397.

Ott, A., Stolk, R. P., van Harskamp, F., Pols, H. A., Hofman, A., & Breteler, M. M. (1999). Diabetes mellitus and the risk of dementia: The Rotterdam Study. *Neurology, 53*(9), 1937–1942.

Paik, J. H., Ju, J. H., Lee, J. Y., Boudreau, M. D., & Hwang, D. H. (2000). Two opposing effects of non-steroidal anti-inflammatory drugs on the expression of the inducible cyclooxygenase. Mediation through different signaling pathways. *J Biol Chem, 275*(36), 28173–28179.

Park, C. R., Seeley, R. J., Craft, S., & Woods, S. C. (2000). Intracerebroventricular insulin enhances memory in a passive-avoidance task. *Physiology and Behavior, 68*, 509–514.

Park, E. J., Park, S. Y., Joe, E. H., & Jou, I. (2003). 15d-PGJ2 and rosiglitazone suppress Janus kinase-STAT inflammatory signaling through induction of suppressor of cytokine signaling 1 (SOCS1) and SOCS3 in glia. *J Biol Chem, 278*(17), 14747–14752.

Pathan, A. R., Viswanad, B., Sonkusare, S. K., & Ramarao, P. (2006). Chronic administration of pioglitazone attenuates intracerebroventricular streptozotocin induced-memory impairment in rats. *Life Sci, 79*(23), 2209–2216.

Perez, A., Morelli, L., Cresto, J. C., & Castano, E. M. (2000). Degradation of soluble amyloid B-peptides 1–40, 1–42, and the Dutch variant 1–40Q by insulin degrading enzyme from Alzheimer disease and control brains. *Neurochemical Research, 25*(2), 247–255.

Piroli, G. G., Grillo, C. A., Reznikov, L. R., Adams, S., McEwen, B. S., Charron, M. J., et al. (2007). Corticosterone impairs insulin-stimulated translocation of GLUT4 in the rat hippocampus. *Neuroendocrinology, 85*(2), 71–80.

Profenno, L. A., Porsteinsson, A. P., & Faraone, S. V. (2010). Meta-analysis of Alzheimer's disease risk with obesity, diabetes, and related disorders. *Biol Psychiatry, 67*(6), 505–512.

Qiu, W., Walsh, D., Ye, Z., Vekrellis, K., Zhang, J., Podlisny, M., et al. (1998). Insulin-degrading enzyme regulates extracellular levels of amyloid beta-protein by degradation. *Journal of Biological Chemistry, 273*(49), 32730–32738.

Reagan, L. P., Gorovits, N., Hoskin, E. K., Alves, S. E., Katz, E. B., Grillo, C. A., et al. (2001). Localization and regulation of GLUTx1 glucose transporter in the hippocampus of streptozotocin diabetic rats. *Proc Natl Acad Sci U S A, 98*(5), 2820–2825.

Reaven, G. M. (1983). Insulin resistance in noninsulin-dependent diabetes mellitus. Does it exist and can it be measured? *Am J Med, 74*(1A), 3–17.

Reaven, G. M. (2003). The insulin resistance syndrome. *Curr Atheroscler Rep, 5*(5), 364–371.

Reger, M. A., Watson, G. S., Frey II, W. H., Baker, L. D., Cholerton, B., Keeling, M. L., et al. (2006). Effects of intranasal insulin on cognition in memory-impaired older adults: Modulation by APOE genotype. *Neurobiol Aging, 27*(3), 451–458.

Reger, M. A., Watson, G. S., Green, P. S., Baker, L. D., Cholerton, B., Fishel, M. A., et al. (2008). Intranasal insulin administration dose-dependently modulates verbal memory and plasma amyloid-beta in memory-impaired older adults. *Journal of Alzheimers Disease, 13*(3), 323–331.

Reger, M. A., Watson, G. S., Green, P. S., Wilkinson, C. W., Baker, L. D., Cholerton, B., et al. (2008). Intranasal insulin improves cognition and modulates beta-amyloid in early AD. *Neurology, 70*(6), 440–448.

Risner, M. E., Saunders, A. M., Altman, J. F., Ormandy, G. C., Craft, S., Foley, I. M., et al. (2006). Efficacy of rosiglitazone in a genetically defined population with mild-to-moderate Alzheimer's disease. *Pharmacogenomics J, 6*(4), 246–254.

Rivera, E., Goldin, A., Fulmer, N., Tavares, R., Wands, J., & de la Monte, S. (2005). Insulin and insulin-like growth factor expression and function deteriorate with progression of Alzheimer's disease: Link to brain reductions in acetylcholine. *J Alzheimer's Disease, 8*, 247–268.

Sato, T., Hanyu, H., Hirao, K., Kanetaka, H., Sakurai, H., & Iwamoto, T. (2011). Efficacy of PPAR-gamma agonist pioglitazone in mild Alzheimer disease. *Neurobiol Aging, 32*(9), 1626–1633.

Schinzari, F., Tesauro, M., Rovella, V., Galli, A., Mores, N., Porzio, O., et al. (2010). Generalized impairment of vasodilator reactivity during hyperinsulinemia in patients with obesity-related metabolic syndrome. *Am J Physiol Endocrinol Metab, 299*(6), E947–952.

Schmidt, S., Moric, E., Schmidt, M., Sastre, M., Feinstein, D. L., & Heneka, M. T. (2003). Anti-inflammatory and antiproliferative actions of PPAR-{gamma} agonists on T lymphocytes derived from MS patients. *J Leukoc Biol, 75*(3), 478–485.

Schubert, M., Brazil, D. P., Burks, D. J., Kushner, J. A., Ye, J., Flint, C. L., et al. (2003). Insulin receptor substrate-2 deficiency impairs brain growth and promotes tau phosphorylation. *J Neurosci, 23*(18), 7084–7092.

Schubert, M., Gautam, D., Surjo, D., Ueki, K., Baudler, S., Schubert, D., et al. (2004). Role for neuronal insulin resistance in neurodegenerative diseases. *Proc Natl Acad Sci U S A, 101*(9), 3100–3105.

Schulingkamp, R. J., Pagano, T. C., Hung, D., & Raffa, R. B. (2000). Insulin receptors and insulin action in the brain: review and clinical implications. *Neurosci Biobehav Rev, 24*(8), 855–872.

Schwartz, M. W., Figlewicz, D. F., Kahn, S. E., Baskin, D. G., Greenwood, M. R., & Porte, D., Jr. (1990). Insulin binding to brain capillaries is reduced in genetically obese, hyperinsulinemic Zucker rats. *Peptides, 11*(3), 467–472.

Shipley, M. T. (1985). Transport of molecules from nose to brain: transneuronal anterograde and retrograde labeling in the rat olfactory system by wheat germ agglutinin-horseradish peroxidase applied to the nasal epithelium. *Brain Res Bull, 15*(2), 129–142.

Sidhu, J. S., Cowan, D., & Kaski, J. C. (2003). The effects of rosiglitazone, a peroxisome proliferator-activated receptor-gamma agonist, on markers of endothelial cell activation, C-reactive protein, and fibrinogen levels in non-diabetic coronary artery disease patients. *J Am Coll Cardiol, 42*(10), 1757–1763.

Sidhu, J. S., Cowan, D., & Kaski, J. C. (2004). Effects of rosiglitazone on endothelial function in men with coronary artery disease without diabetes mellitus. *Am J Cardiol, 94*(2), 151–156.

Skeberdis, V. A., Lan, J., Zheng, X., Zukin, R. S., & Bennett, M. V. (2001). Insulin promotes rapid delivery of N-methyl-D- aspartate receptors to the cell surface by exocytosis. *Proc Natl Acad Sci U S A, 98*(6), 3561–3566.

Sonnen, J. A., Larson, E. B., Brickell, K., Crane, P. K., Woltjer, R., Montine, T. J., et al. (2009). Different patterns of cerebral injury in dementia with or without diabetes. *Archives of Neurology, 66*(3), 315–322.

Stockhorst, U., de Fries, D., Schottenfeld-Naor, Y., Huebinger, A., Steingrueber, H. J., & Scherbaum, W. A. (Submitted for publication). Intranasally administered insulin and its CNS effects in healthy humans: unconditioned and conditioned responses.

Stockhorst, U., de Fries, D., Steingrueber, H. J., & Scherbaum, W. A. (2004). Insulin and the CNS: effects on food intake, memory, and endocrine parameters and the role of intranasal insulin administration in humans. *Physiol Behav, 83*(1), 47–54.

Strachan, M. W. (2011). R D Lawrence Lecture 2010. The brain as a target organ in Type 2 diabetes: exploring the links with cognitive impairment and dementia. *Diabet Med, 28*(2), 141–147.

Sudoh, S., Frosch, M. P., & Wolf, B. A. (2002). Differential effects of proteases involved in intracellular degradation of amyloid b-protein between detergent-soluble and -insoluble pools in CHO-695 cells. *Biochemistry, 41*(4), 1091–1099.

Tao, L., Liu, H. R., Gao, E., Teng, Z. P., Lopez, B. L., Christopher, T. A., et al. (2003). Antioxidative, antinitrative, and vasculoprotective effects of a peroxisome proliferator-activated receptor-gamma agonist in hypercholesterolemia. *Circulation, 108*(22), 2805–2811.

Thorne, R. G., Pronk, G. J., Padmanabhan, V., & Frey, W. H., 2nd. (2004). Delivery of insulin-like growth factor-I to the rat brain and spinal cord along olfactory and trigeminal pathways following intranasal administration. *Neuroscience, 127*(2), 481–496.

Tilvis, R. S., Kahonen-Vare, M. H., Jolkkonen, J., Valvanne, J., Pitkala, K. H., & Strandberg, T. E. (2004). Predictors of cognitive decline and mortality of aged people over a 10-year period. *J Gerontol A Biol Sci Med Sci, 59*(3), 268–274.

Townsend, M., Mehta, T., & Selkoe, D. J. (2007). Soluble Abeta inhibits specific signal transduction cascades common to the insulin receptor pathway. *J Biol Chem, 282*(46), 33305–33312.

Unger, J. W., Livingston, J. N., & Moss, A. M. (1991). Insulin receptors in the central nervous system: localization, signalling mechanisms and functional aspects. *Prog Neurobiol, 36*(5), 343–362.

Vanhanen, M., Koivisto, K., Kuusisto, J., Mykkanen, L., Helkala, E. L., Hanninen, T., et al. (1998). Cognitive function in an elderly population with persistent impaired glucose tolerance. *Diabetes Care, 21*(3), 398–402.

Wallum, B. J., Taborsky, G. J., Jr., Porte, D., Jr., Figlewicz, D. P., Jacobson, L., Beard, J. C., et al. (1987). Cerebrospinal fluid insulin levels increase during intravenous insulin infusions in man. *J Clin Endocrinol Metab, 64*(1), 190–194.

Watson, G. S., Cholerton, B. A., Reger, M. A., Baker, L. D., Plymate, S. R., Asthana, S., et al. (2005). Preserved cognition in patients with early Alzheimer disease and amnestic mild cognitive impairment during treatment with rosiglitazone: a preliminary study. *Am J Geriatr Psychiatry, 13*(11), 950–958.

Xu, W., Qiu, C., Gatz, M., Pedersen, N. L., Johansson, B., & Fratiglioni, L. (2009). Mid- and late-life diabetes in relation to the risk of dementia: a population-based twin study. *Diabetes, 58*(1), 71–77.

Yaffe, K., Blackwell, T., Kanaya, A. M., Davidowitz, N., Barrett-Connor, E., & Krueger, K. (2004). Diabetes, impaired fasting glucose, and development of cognitive impairment in older women. *Neurology, 63*(4), 658–663.

Zhao, W., Chen, H., Xu, H., Moore, E., Meiri, N., Quon, M. J., et al. (1999). Brain insulin receptors and spatial memory. Correlated changes in gene expression, tyrosine phosphorylation, and signaling molecules in the hippocampus of water maze trained rats. *J Biol Chem, 274*(49), 34893–34902.

Zhao, W. Q., & Alkon, D. L. (2001). Role of insulin and insulin receptor in learning and memory. *Mol Cell Endocrinol, 177*(1–2), 125–134.

6

Metabolic Syndrome, Other Composite Vascular Risk Scores, and Cognitive Impairment

JOSÉ ALEJANDRO LUCHSINGER, MD, MPH

Introduction

Here we provide a brief review of definitions, burden, and causes of cognitive impairment that is pertinent to the subject of this review. The most extreme form of cognitive impairment and the most commonly studied and diagnosed in clinical practice is dementia, defined as cognitive impairment accompanied by functional impairment severe enough to cause loss of independence (*Diagnostic and statistical manual of mental disorders, 4th edition: DSM IV*, 1997). Another common diagnostic category used in clinical practice is mild cognitive impairment (MCI; Petersen, 2004). Mild cognitive impairment is defined as cognitive impairment not accompanied by loss of independence, evidenced by complaints and by abnormal cognitive tests in the absence of significant functional impairment. Mild cognitive impairment may be an intermediate level of cognitive impairment between normal cognition and dementia. Mild cognitive impairment and dementia are the most commonly used cognitive categories in research and clinical practice. However, cognition may also be ascertained, particularly in research, by performance in cognitive tests. These cognitive tests may test global cognition (e.g., the widely used Folstein Mini Mental Status Exam; Folstein, Folstein et al., 1975) or may test particular cognitive domains. Arguably, the two most important cognitive domains in clinical practice and research are memory and executive function. Memory is defined as the ability to recollect information (Small & Mayeux, 1999). Executive function could be defined as the ability to plan, execute, and finish complex tasks or behaviors (Royall, Lauterbach et al., 2002). Collecting information on particular cognitive domains is useful because performance on cognitive tests may be proxies or markers for particular causes of cognitive impairment. Traditionally, cognitive impairment caused by cerebrovascular disease, called vascular cognitive impairment (VCI) has been thought to be manifested as impairment in executive functions caused by disruption of frontal-subcortical pathways (Hachinski, Iadecola et al., 2006). However, cerebrovascular disease can also cause memory problems resulting from retrieval deficits or by causing "strategic" strokes in areas that disrupt memory, such as the thalamus. Memory impairment, particularly consolidation deficits, is thought to be a proxy of Late-Onset Alzheimer's disease (LOAD) (Small & Mayeux, 1999).

Estimates of the relative importance of LOAD and VCI are controversial because their diagnosis is usually based on clinical information that assumes underlying pathology. Recent pathology studies show that the neuropathology of dementia is more heterogeneous than traditionally accepted (Savva, Wharton et al., 2009). It has been traditionally accepted that the majority of dementia results from LOAD, whereas a minority result from VCI. Other causes of dementia such as Lewy Body disease, fronto-temporal dementia, and Parkinson's dementia are less common and are not covered in this chapter. There is growing acceptance that cerebrovascular disease is important in LOAD. It is thought that infarcts decrease the threshold of LOAD pathology needed to manifest cognitive impairment (Snowdon, Greiner et al., 1997). In other words, LOAD and VCI pathology act synergistically to cause cognitive impairment. Some have suggested that LOAD and VCI pathology co-exist so often that characterization of dementia subtypes should no longer be attempted. The importance of cerebrovascular disease for the two main types of cognitive impairment anchors the rationale for exploration of vascular risk factors as predictors or causes of cognitive impairment. This chapter focuses on the role of clusters of risk factors, rather than individual risk factors, for cognitive impairment.

Mechanisms Linking Vascular Risk Factors and Cognitive Impairment

Other chapters in this book describe in detail the associations of some specific vascular risk factors with cognitive impairment and the underlying mechanisms for these associations. Here we briefly summarize the mechanisms that may link vascular risk factors, and, therefore, their clusters, to cognitive impairment. Although the specific mechanisms through which vascular risk factors affect the risk of LOAD are largely unclear, it seems reasonable to hypothesize that two main pathways are possible. One pathway is through cerebrovascular disease. The other pathway is through the deposition of amyloid β protein—the main putative culprit of LOAD—in the brain (Petrovitch, White et al., 2000; Sparks, Martin et al., 2000). The relation between vascular risk factors and cerebrovascular disease is clear (Sacco, Benjamin et al., 1997). As mentioned previously, vascular risk factors increase the risk of cerebrovascular disease, and cerebrovascular disease seems to lower the threshold of amyloid pathology necessary to manifest dementia (Snowdon, Greiner et al., 1997).

The relation between vascular risk factors and amyloid β is less clear, but there is evidence of plausible mechanisms. For example, type 2 diabetes may increase the risk of dementia via oxidative stress or protein glycosilation (Biessels, 1999), both possibly related to LOAD. Hyperinsulinemia, an antecedent and correlate of type 2 diabetes and the main underlying mechanism of the metabolic syndrome, is an important potential mechanism relating vascular risk factors and amyloid β deposition (*see* Chapter 5). Peripheral insulin is transported to the CNS across the blood–brain barrier (Schwartz, Sipols et al., 1990; Banks, Jaspan et al., 1997), and insulin receptors have been found in the hippocampus (Park, 2001), the part of the brain first affected by AD (Small, 2002), indicating the potential for peripheral insulin to cause direct injury in AD. In addition, insulin-degrading enzyme in the brain is a regulator of extracellular Aβ levels(Vekrellis, Ye et al., 2000), which competes with insulin (Farris, Mansourian et al., 2003). Insulin also has a role in the regulation of phosphorylation of tau protein, the main component of neurofibrillary tangles (Park, 2001). Vascular risk factors may contribute to dementia in other ways. Heart disease, such as congestive heart failure or arrhythmias, can lead to cognitive impairment through cerebral hypoperfusion or embolism (Breteler, Claus et al., 1994) and is also known to be linked with the apolipoprotein E (APOE) ε4 allele, a known risk factor for AD (*see* Chapter 3; Treves, Bornstein et al., 1996; Wang & Zhou, 2003). Hypertension may also contribute to a blood–brain barrier dysfunction, which has been suggested to be involved in the etiology of AD (Skoog, 1997) or through the formation of free oxygen radicals (*see* Chapter 1; Skoog, 1997). Finally, it is important to point out that synaptic integrity and brain reserve may also determine the susceptibility of the brain to amyloid burden and cerebrovascular disease in manifesting cognitive impairment. More research is needed in how vascular risk factors may affect cognitive impairment by affecting brain susceptibility.

Rationale for the Study of Composite Measures of Vascular Risk

Although vascular risk factors are usually examined individually, researchers and clinicians have recognized that "traditional" risk factors, which include diabetes, dyslipidemia, and hypertension, usually occur together in individuals. One of the first names for this phenomenon was the "metabolic syndrome X," a term coined by Reaven and Laws (1999) also referred to as insulin resistance syndrome, and more recently as the metabolic syndrome. The metabolic syndrome (MeSy) is a constellation of interrelated risk factors of metabolic origin that appear to directly promote atherosclerotic cardiovascular disease and lead to an increased risk of type 2 diabetes mellitus (Grundy, Cleeman et al., 2005). The pathogenesis of the MeSy is multifactorial, but insulin resistance, obesity and sedentary lifestyle, and unknown genetic factors interact in its occurrence (Eckel, Grundy et al., 2005). To introduce the MeSy into clinical practice, several organizations have attempted to formulate simple criteria for its diagnosis, with the goal to reduce atherosclerotic disease risk through lifestyle changes and drug therapy (Grundy, Cleeman et al., 2005). However, because of age-related changes in risk factors, it is not clear whether the MeSy captures the increased risk of diabetes and atherosclerotic disease in the elderly (Abbott, Curb et al., 2002). In addition, different criteria for the MeSy may be required for different ethnic groups because of racial variation in development of insulin resistance in response to increased adiposity (Luchsinger, 2006). Although the MeSy is associated with other factors that increase the risk of cardiovascular disease, such as increased inflammation and thrombogenicity (Reaven, 2002), these factors are not part of the existing definitions of the syndrome. Few of the studies that we summarize below include ascertainment of inflammation. Increased inflammation can increase insulin resistance, thereby worsening components of the syndrome; thus, inflammatory markers such as high-sensitivity C-reactive protein (hsCRP) may add predictive value to MeSy (Libby & Ridker, 2004). High-sensitivity CRP seems to be a marker of vascular disease, rather than a mediator (Schunkert & Samani, 2008) and thus may identify persons with the MeSy who already have atherosclerosis and are thus more susceptible to adverse outcomes.

One study estimated the prevalence of the MeSy in middle-aged adults without diabetes or cardiovascular disease to be 26.8% in men and 16.6% in women (Wilson, D'Agostino et al., 2005).. These individuals have a twofold increase in the risk of atherosclerotic cardiovascular disease and a sixfold increase in the risk of developing diabetes (Grundy, Cleeman et al., 2005). In the elderly, the prevalence of the MeSy ranges between one-fourth and one-half of all persons, depending on the definition used (Rathmann, Haastert et al., 2006).

Over the years, several groups have developed criteria to define the metabolic syndrome (Grundy, Cleeman et al., 2005). They include the World Health Organization (WHO), the European Group for the Study of Insulin Resistance (EGIR), the National Cholesterol Education Program (NCEP), the Adult Treatment Panel III (ATPIII), the International Diabetes Foundation (IDF), and the American Association of Clinical Endocrinologists (AACE). The proposed criteria are similar but have some important differences. Those developed by WHO and EGIR include measures of insulin resistance, whereas the others do not. In addition, criteria by EGIR and AACE exclude diabetes because the metabolic syndrome is thought to be an antecedent to diabetes; the criteria developed by other groups include it in their definitions. The AACE criteria use body mass index (BMI) as a measure of adiposity, whereas the other criteria emphasize waist circumference because of the importance of abdominal obesity as a cardiovascular risk factor. In general, the criteria differ on the specific cut-points used for waist circumference and blood pressure and concentrations of triglycerides, high-density lipoprotein (HDL), and glucose. The heterogeneity in definitions of the MeSy reflects the difficulty in defining the syndrome. This difficulty likely involves measurement error, which affects the results of studies summarized below.

The American Heart Association (AHA) and the National Heart Blood and Lung Institute (NHLBI) at the National Institutes of Health published a statement to harmonize existing criteria for the metabolic syndrome and formulated new ones (Grundy, Cleeman et al., 2005) According to their definition, which reflects minor modifications from that of the ATPIII and NCEP, the metabolic syndrome has to meet three of the following five criteria: (1) elevated waist circumference, defined as 102 centimeters or greater for men and 88 centimeters or greater for women; (2) triglycerides concentrations 150 mg/dL or greater, or drug treatment for elevated triglycerides; (3) HDL concentrations less than 40 mg/dL for men and less than 50 mg/dL for women, or drug treatment for low HDL; (4) systolic blood pressure 130 mmHg or greater and diastolic blood pressure 85 mmHg or greater, or drug treatment for hypertension; (5) fasting glucose concentrations 100 mg/dL or greater, or drug treatment for elevated glucose. Most of the studies described in this review use this definition or some modification to ascertain the MeSy. The definition has some limitations. It does not take into account racial and ethnic differences in susceptibility to increased adiposity. For example, Asians require smaller increases in abdominal fat and waist circumference to develop insulin resistance compared to Europeans (Reaven & Laws, 1999). Further, it does not include a direct measure of insulin resistance but, rather, assumes that the measurement of waist circumference and of fasting glucose concentrations will capture this parameter. Direct measures of insulin resistance, such as fasting insulin concentrations, may be all the information that is needed to predict risk of diabetes and cardiovascular disease (Tuan, Abbasi et al., 2003). In addition, the risk factors that comprise the metabolic syndrome may have a linear association with atherosclerotic cardiovascular disease—that is, the higher the level of risk factor (blood pressure, lipids, glucose, waist circumference), the higher the risk—and their dichotomization (use of cutoffs) probably leads to misclassification of individuals as having or not having a criterion and does not take into account the graded risk related to different levels of the risk factor. Finally, most of the evidence for the existing definitions of the metabolic syndrome comes from middle-aged populations, and work is needed to determine its clinical significance in other age groups, particularly the elderly, who are most susceptible to cognitive impairment.

The relevance of the metabolic syndrome to cognitive impairment is that its components, type 2 diabetes (Luchsinger, Reitz et al., 2005), hyperinsulinemia (Luchsinger, Tang et al., 2004), obesity (Whitmer, Gunderson et al., 2005), dyslipidemia (Reitz, Tang et al., 2010), and hypertension (Kivipelto, Laakso et al., 2002), are increasingly recognized as risk factors for dementia and cognitive impairment. Thus, one would expect the metabolic syndrome to be related to these conditions.

The metabolic syndrome is based largely on the presumption that its components are caused by insulin resistance. However, this definition does not take into account important CV risk factors, such as smoking, that are not caused by insulin resistance and are related to behavior. Other risk scores have been developed to take into account the coexistence of risk factors, regardless of whether they are related pathophysiologically. Valuable tools for targeting preventive measures to those at risk for the disease are "risk scores"(Hall, Jung et al., 2003). They have been frequently used in population-based settings, particularly to predict the risks of vascular disorders such as stroke, cardiovascular events, diabetes, and mortality from vascular causes (Pocock, McCormack et al., 2001; Assmann, Cullen et al., 2002; Hall, Jung et al., 2003; Clayton, Lubsen et al., 2005; Fowkes, Murray et al., 2008; Yang, So et al., 2008; de Ruijter, Westendorp et al., 2009). They commonly include few known risk factors that are easily measureable to calculate the subsequent risk of an event or disease within a given time frame. Although the absolute risk of an event may differ across populations, risk ranking by use of risk scores is consistent (D'Agostino, Grundy et al., 2001; Bastuji-Garin, Deverly et al., 2002). An additional benefit of risk scores is that they can be used to transmit easily understandable information about risk factors to the general population. The most commonly used risk scores is the Framingham coronary heart disease prediction score (D'Agostino, Grundy et al., 2001). Other investigators have developed risk scores using methods similar to the Framingham score to predict cognitive impairment, and the studies are summarized in this review.

Summary of the Literature

METABOLIC SYNDROME AND COGNITIVE IMPAIRMENT

As previously described, cognitive impairment can be ascertained as performance in global or domain-specific cognitive tests or as diagnoses such as MCI and dementia. We divide the review of the literature in studies examining the relation between the MeSy and cognitive performance and studies relating the MeSy with cognitive impairment diagnoses. Table 6.1 summarizes the studies relating the MeSy with cognitive performance. All studies used the ATP III

Table 6.1 **Summary of Studies Relating the Metabolic Syndrome With Cognitive Performance (Ordered by Year)**

Author (year)	Study design and sample	Exposure and outcome	Findings
(Yaffe, Kanaya et al., 2004)	Longitudinal study; 2632 black and white elders with a mean age of 74 years.	Metabolic syndrome by National Cholesterol Education Program (NCEP) Guidelines, inflammation measured with interleukin-6 and C-reactive protein. Cognitive imp airment defined as 5-point decline in the modified mini-mental state examination (3MS)	Prevalence of the metabolic syndrome was 38.6%. Persons with the MeSy were more likely to have cognitive impairment (RR = 1.21; 95% CI = 1.02–1.41). This association was limited to those with the metabolic syndrome and high inflammation.
(Dik, Jonker et al., 2007)	Cross-sectional study; 1183 participant in the Longitudinal Aging Study Amsterdam ages 65 years to 88 years.	MeSy by NCEP guidelines. Inflammation assessed by CRP and α-1 antichymotripsin (ACT). Cognition assessed with the mini-mental status exam, a verbal learning test (memory), fluid intelligence (Ravens Matrices) and information processing speed (coding task).	Prevalence of MeSy was 36.3%. MeSy was related to lower performance in all tests with the exception of delayed recall, but this association was limited to persons with high inflammation.
(Komulainen, Lakka et al., 2007)	Longitudinal study; 101 women ages 60 years to 70 years from Kuopio, Finland.	MeSY defined by NCEP guidelines. Outcomes were memory and cognitive speed.	MeSY prevalence was 13% at baseline and increased to 49% at follow-up. MeSy at baseline associated with increased risk of poor memory at follow-up (4.27; 95% CI 1.02–17.90) Increasing components increased risk of poor memory. Low HDL related to worse memory.

(continued)

Table 6.1 **(Continued)**

Author (year)	Study design and sample	Exposure and outcome	Findings
(Roriz-Cruz, Rosset et al., 2007)	Cross-sectional study; 422 community dwelling persons ages 60 years and older in Brazil without stroke	MeSy defined by modified ATP III criteria Outcome: Frontal subcortical geriatric syndrome, which included three or more of the following: cognitive impairment, late-onset depression, neuromotor dysfunction, urgency incontinence.	MeSy associated with higher risk of FSCS (OR = 5.9; CI = 1.5–23.4).
(van den Berg, Biessels et al., 2007)	Longitudinal study; 599 persons ages 85 years and older from the Leiden Study in the Netherlands	MeSy defined by ATP III Criteria. Global cognition measured with MMSE, Attention with Stroop test, speed with Letter digit processing test, memory with 12 word learning test.	MeSy not associated with cognition in cross-sectional analyses. MeSy associated with decelerated cognitive decline
(Yaffe, Haan et al., 2007)	Longitudinal study; 1624 Latinos ages 60 years and older in the Sacramento Latino Study of Aging	MeSy defined by ATP III. Cognition measured with 3 MS, delayed word recall test. 3-year changes.	44% had MeSy. MeSy related to decline in MS and recall test, but latter attenuated after adjustment. The association with 3 MS stronger in persons with inflammation.
(Gatto, Henderson et al., 2008)	Cross-sectional study; 853 adult men and women without diabetes and cognitive impairment with a mean age of 60 years, in two trials in the United States.	MeSy defined by NCEP guidelines; outcome six areas of cognitive function.	MeSy associated with lower verbal learning non significant ($p = 0.09$). Increasing components associated with lower global cognition, lower verbal learning, and lower semantic memory. Hypertension-only component associated with lower scores.

Study	Description	Findings
(van den Berg, Dekker et al., 2008)	Cross-sectional study; 64 persons with type 2 diabetes, 83 with MeSy without diabetes, 100 controls ages 50 years to 75 years from the Hoorn Study in the Netherlands. Cross-sectional analysis	MeSy defined by ATP III criteria. Abstract reasoning, memory, information processing, attention and executive function, and language and visuoconstruction, assessed with a comprehensive neuropsychological battery and ascertained as z scores	The MeSy group and diabetes group behaved similarly. Both showed worse performance in information processing speed and attention and executive functioning. None of the components of the metabolic syndrome was related to cognitive performance individually.
(Liu, Zhou et al., 2009)	Cross-sectional study; 3216 participants ages 60 years and older in China	MeSy defined by ATP II criteria. Outcomes MMSE and ADL.	Prevalence of MeSy was 22.8%. MeSy was associated with a cognitive impairment (OR = 2.55; 95 % CI; 2.07–3.13).
(Akbaraly, Kivimaki et al., 2010,)	Cross-sectional study; 4150 participants from the Whitehall Study in the United Kingdom mean age 60.5 years	MeSy defined by ATP III; cognition assessed with tests of memory, reasoning, vocabulary, phonemic fluency, semantic fluency, and global cognition.	Only persistent MeSy (present in at least two of three follow-ups) was related to lower cognitive performance in memory, reasoning, vocabulary, and verbal and semantic fluency. Adjustment for Occupational position significantly attenuated the associations.
(Cavalieri, Ropele et al., 2010)	Cross-sectional study; 819 participants without stroke or dementia from the Austrian Stroke Prevention Study with a mean age of 65 years	MeSy defined by ATP III criteria. Inflammation measured with C-reactive protein. Outcomes included the MMSE and tests of memory, psychomotor skills, and executive functions.	MeSy prevalence was 28.3%. Persons with MeSy performed worse in memory and executive function, but there were no differences in MRI findings, including WMLs, lacunes, infarcts, and brain percentage.

(continued)

Table 6.1 (Continued)

Author (year)	Study design and sample	Exposure and outcome	Findings
(Lee, Eom, et al., 2010)	Longitudinal study; 596 participants ages 60 years and older from South Korea	MeSy defined by the ATP III. Head circumference measured as a proxy of early life exposures. Cognitive impairment defined as MMSE < 24.	MeSy associated with increased cognitive impairment at follow-up independent of head circumference.
(Lee, Jang et al., 2010)	Cross-sectional study; 2944 participants older than age 60 years from South Korea	MeSy defined by ATP III criteria. Cognition measured with MMSE < 18	MeSy prevalence was 53.8%. MeSy was not associated with cognitive impairment. High triglycerides and low HDL associated with cognitive impairment in the presence of the APOE-ε4 allele.
(Muller, van Raamt et al., 2010)	Cross-sectional study; 823 participants with atherosclerotic disease from the SMART study in the Netherlands aged 58 ± 10 years old.	MeSY defined by ATP III criteria. Cognition assessed with tests of memory, executive, and visuospatial function. Cognitive impairment defined as performance in the lowest 10% percentile.	MeSy prevalence was 36%. MeSy related to increased risk of memory (OR = 2.0; 95% CI 1.1–3.3) and visuospatial dysfunction (OR = 2.3; 95% CI = 1.4–2.7).
(Raffaitin, Feart et al., 2011)	Longitudinal study; 4323 women and 2764 men ages 65 years and older from the Three City Study in France.	MeSY defined by ATP III. Cognition measured by MMSE, a test of verbal fluency, and a test of visual working memory. Decline defined as worst quintile in difference between two measurements at 2- or 4-year follow-up	MeSy prevalence was 15.8%. MeSy was related to a decline in global cognition (HR = 1.22; 95% CI 1.08–1.37), and visual memory (1.13, 95% CI = 1.01–1.26).

or NCEP definition, and three studies included a measure of systemic inflammation. Most studies were in Europe, followed by Asia, the United States, and Latin America. Out of 15 studies, 9 were cross-sectional and 6 were longitudinal. Four studies included persons younger than aged 60 years, 10 studies were in samples of persons age 60 years and older, and 1 study included persons only 85 years and older. Four studies reported on only global cognitive function, and 12 reported on several cognitive domains. Only two studies reported no association between the MeSy and cognitive impairment. One of those, by Lee et al. (2009), was a cross-sectional study in South Korea that defined cognitive impairment by a global measure, the MMSE, using a relatively low MMSE score as a cutoff (score < 18) that may have detected only severe cognitive impairment, which could explain the negative finding. However, this study reported that two components of the metabolic syndrome, high triglycerides and low HDL, were related to a higher risk of cognitive impairment in persons with the APOE ε4 allele. The other negative study, by Van den Berg (2007), was a study of persons age 85 years and older from the Netherlands that reported no association with cognition in several cognitive domains, and an inverse association with cognitive decline.

Among the studies that reported a positive association with MeSy and cognitive impairment, the relationship with particular cognitive domains was inconsistent. Among the 11 studies that reported on several cognitive domains and were positive, only 4 reported associations of the MeSy with impairment in all cognitive domains. Three reported associations with cognitive impairment excluding memory, and two reported associations with memory but not with other cognitive domains. The studies that measured inflammation with CRP or other measures reported an association only among those with high inflammation.

Table 6.2 summarizes studies relating the association of the MeSy with incident MCI or dementia. Out of the seven studies in the table, all studies were longitudinal. Four studies had dementia as an outcome, two studies had both MCI and dementia, and one study examined dementia alone. One study included measures of inflammation. One study was in middle-aged participants and the rest were in elderly subjects. Three studies were in Europe, and four were in the United States. One of the studies in the United States was among Japanese-Americans. Two studies reported no association between the MeSy and MCI or dementia. However, the MCI study reported an association between the MeSy and non-amnestic MCI, but not amnestic MCI, among those with high inflammation. The other negative study examining AD as the outcome found that while the MeSy was not associated with AD, both diabetes and high insulin levels, both important correlates of the metabolic syndrome, were related to a higher risk of LOAD. Among the studies that reported positive associations, one reported that the association was limited only to younger elderly (75 years or younger), two

Table 6.2 **Summary of Studies Relating the Presence of the Metabolic Syndrome With Risk of Mild Cognitive Impairment or Dementia (Ordered by Year)**

Author (year)	Study design and sample sign	Exposure and outcome	Findings
(Kalmijn, Foley et al., 2000)	Longitudinal study; 3734 Japanese American Men aged 52.7 years from the Honolulu Asia Aging Study	MeSy ascertained as the addition of z-scores from seven risk factors (random postload glucose, diastolic and systolic blood pressures, body mass index, subscapular skinfold thickness, random triglycerides, and total cholesterol). Outcome was incident dementia.	The risk of dementia increased 5% per one SD increase in z-scores of risk factors, particularly for vascular dementia but not Alzheimer's disease
(Muller, Tang et al., 2007)	Longitudinal study; 2476 men and women ages 65 years and older in Northern New York City.	MeSy defined by NCEP and by the European Group for the study of Insulin Resistance. Cognitive outcome: dementia	MeSy not associated with dementia or dementia subtypes in cross-sectional or longitudinal analyses but diabetes and insulin levels were.
(Raffaitin, Gin et al., 2009)	Longitudinal study; 7087 community dwelling persons ages 65 years and older from the three city study in France	MeSy defined by ATP III. Outcome as incident dementia.	MeSy prevalence was 15.8%. MeSy related to VD (2.42; 95% CI = 1.24–4.73) but not AD (0.81; 0.5–1.31).
(Yaffe, Weston et al., 2009)	Longitudinal study; 4895 women with a mean age of 66.2 years from a study of osteoporosis.	MeSy defined by ATP III guidelines; composite outcome was the presence of dementia, MCI, or a short blessed test score greater than 6.	Prevalence of MeSy was 10.2%. Risk of cognitive impairment increased after 4 years of observation (OR = 1.66; 95% CI 1.14–2.41).

Study	Study Description	Methods	Results
(Solfrizzi, Scafato et al., 2009)	Longitudinal study; 2097 participants ages 65years to 84 years from the Italian Longitudinal Study of Aging	MeSy defined by ATP II criteria. Outcomes were MCI and progression from MCI to dementia	MCI patients with MeSy had higher risk of progression to dementia (HR =4.4; 95% CI = 1.3–14.8) However, MeSY was not associated with MCI among those without cognitive impairment (1.07; 95% CI = 0.67,1.7)
(Roberts, Geda et al., 2010)	Longitudinal study; 1969 participants ages 70 years to 89 years from Olmstead, MN.	MeSy Defined by ATP III criteria, international diabetes federation, and American Heart Association. Cognition was defined as amnestic and non-amnestic MCI.	MeSY was not associated with either na-MCI or a-MCI. High C-reactive protein (CRP; highest tertile vs lowest tertile) was associated with na-MCI [odds ratio (OR) = 1.85; 95% confidence interval (CI) =1.05, 3.24] but not with a-MCI, after adjusting for sex, age, and years of education. The combination of MeSY and high CRP (compared to no MetS and lowest CRP tertile) was associated with na-MCI (OR = 2.31; 95% CI = 1.07, 5.00) but not with a-MCI (OR = 0.96; 95% CI = 0.59, 1.54). The combined presence of MeSY and high levels of inflammation is associated with na-MCI in this elderly cohort, and suggests etiologic differences in MCI subtypes.
(Forti, Pisacane et al., 2010)	Longitudinal study; 749 subjects ages 65 years and older without cognitive impairment aged in a study of aging in Italy	MeSy was defined by NCEP criteria; outcome was incident dementia	MeSY prevalence was 28.5%. MeSy was not related to incident dementia in persons younger than age 75 years and was associated with lower risk in persons age 75 years and older.

studies reported associations with vascular dementia, but not AD, and one study reported that the MeSy was related to the progression from MCI to dementia but was not associated with incident MCI.

The studies summarized in Tables 6.1 and 6.2 provide a heterogeneous mix of results, but some patterns can be discerned. The number of studies reporting some association between the MeSy and cognitive impairment outnumber those reporting no association. Among some studies that were negative, there were associations between components of the metabolic syndrome (e.g., diabetes, dyslipidemia) or high inflammation with cognitive impairment. The few studies that examined the association of the MeSy with cognitive impairment among the oldest old found no association, whereas those in younger age groups found associations. Given that the MeSy and its components are known cerebrovascular risk factors, one would expect to find a stronger association of the MeSy with executive-frontal cognitive abilities, non-amnestic MCI, and vascular dementia. In general, most studies follow this pattern, but there were some studies that found an association of the MeSy with memory impairment but not executive frontal impairment.

The limitations of the MeSy described previously should be taken into account when putting this summary of the literature in context. Longitudinal studies have shown that cholesterol levels and measures of adiposity, two of the main components of the MeSy, decrease with age (Weijenberg, Feskens et al., 1996; Stevens, Cai et al., 1998), and it has been suggested that lower cholesterol levels and lower BMI in the elderly represent surrogate markers of frailty or subclinical disease (Reitz, Tang et al., 2004; Schupf, Costa et al., 2005). Blood pressure decreases in the years preceding onset of LOAD and continues to decline during the course of the disorder (Skoog, 2003). The cause of this decline may be that brain structures affected in this disease course are involved in BP regulation. Alternatively, higher blood pressure levels may be needed to maintain an adequate cerebral perfusion (Skoog, 2003). Thus, it seems that the components of the MeSy do not capture in the elderly what they intend to capture in middle age because of survival bias and metabolic changes with aging. On the contrary, diabetes and insulin resistance increase with aging (Ferrannini & Balkau, 2002). Decreases in some of the parameters that define the MeSy may explain some of the negative findings in elderly populations, particularly in the oldest old. Another limitation of the MeSy is that it does not take ethnicity into account. The definition of obesity in particular should vary by ethnic group because some ethnic groups are more susceptible to the effects of adiposity (e.g., insulin resistance) than others (Luchsinger, 2006). For example, Asians are known to develop insulin resistance with lower levels of abdominal adiposity compared to Whites (McKeigue, 1999). Hispanics of Mexican origin are also known to be more susceptible to the effects of adiposity than Whites (McKeigue, 1999; Luchsinger, 2001). Geographic and corresponding ethnic variability in the literature may explain some of the inconsistencies in findings. Finally, and related to the previous points, the components of the MeSy are likely related to adverse outcomes in a continuous way, and the somewhat arbitrary, cutoff-defined ascertainment of the MeSy may not capture these continuous associations.

OTHER COMPOSITE VASCULAR MEASURES

Compared to the MeSy, the literature examining other aggregate measures of vascular risk with cognitive impairment are fewer. Table 6.3 summarizes five representative studies. Two studies are from related elderly cohorts from New York City, one recruited in 1992 to 1994, and the other recruited in 1999 to 2001, and examine LOAD as an outcome. One study is from a middle-aged cohort in Finland and examines late-onset dementia as the outcome. One study is from the landmark Framingham offspring study and examined neuropsychological performance and brain imaging measures as outcomes. One study is from the Kaiser-Permanente middle-aged cohort in California. All the studies used a similar approach in constructing the score, but two studies used a simple count of risk factors, whereas three weighed the presence of the risk factors. In general, all studies found that the higher the risk factor burden, the higher the risk of cognitive impairment. The two studies from New York City found strong associations with both LOAD and vascular dementia. The studies from Finland and California did not discriminate between LOAD and vascular dementia, and the study from Framingham found and association with lower performance in tests of executive frontal function but not memory. These results strongly support the role of increasing cardiovascular risk factor burden on cognitive impairment but do not resolve the issue of whether the association is mostly for VCI compared with LOAD.

There are several issues that must be taken into account when interpreting these findings. Some of the limitations of the MeSy apply to vascular scores as well. One issue is the influence of age on both the risk of dementia and on the ascertainment of the risk factors for dementia. Some of the risk factors or measures may be more robust through the lifespan. For example, a longitudinal study in New York City reported the seemingly paradoxical finding that low cholesterol predicts dementia (Reitz, Tang et al., 2004). It seemed likely that this finding resulted from aging-related changes (cholesterol decreases with frailty and aging). A second study from a related cohort identified elevated HDL as an inverse risk factor for dementia that was independent of the inverse association with cholesterol, suggesting that HDL is a lipid measure independent of aging-related changes and thus was included in a vascular score (Reitz, Tang, et al., 2010). The same study also found that elevated waist-to-hip ratio (WHR) was a robust predictor of dementia risk (Luchsinger, Cheng et al., 2012) even in the elderly, whereas there was no association or an inverse association between

Table 6.3 **Summary of Studies Relating the Association Between Clusters of Cardiovascular Risk Factors and Cognitive Outcomes (Ordered by Year)**

Author (year)	Study design and sample	Exposure and outcome	Findings
(Seshadri, Wolf et al., 2004)	Longitudinal study; 1841 subjects from the Framingham Offspring study with a mean age of 62 years without baseline stroke or dementia	The exposure was the Framingham stroke Risk profile. Outcomes included total cerebral brain volume ratio (from MRI), neuropsychological tests.	The Framingham Stroke Risk Score was inversely associated with brain volume and with performance in tests of attention, executive function, and visuospatial function but not tests of verbal memory or naming.
(Whitmer, Sidney et al., 2005)	Retrospective cohort study; 8,845 participants from a managed care organization in the United States	Composite risk score of smoking, hypertension, high cholesterol, and diabetes; outcome was late-life incident dementia.	Compared with participants having no risk factors, the risk for dementia increased from 1.27 for having one risk factor to 2.37 for having all four risk factors
(Luchsinger, Reitz et al., 2005)	Longitudinal study; 1138 individuals from Northern New York City with a mean age of 76.2 years recruited between 1992 and 1994	A aggregate of four risk factors (diabetes, hypertension, heart disease, and current smoking) was constructed. The presence of each risk factor without weights (score = 1 for the presence of each risk factor) was constructed. Outcome was incident AD.	The adjusted hazards ratio of probable AD for the presence of three or more risk factors was 3.4 (95% CI: 1.8, 6.3; p for trend < 0.0001). Diabetes was strongest individual risk factor, but clusters of the other risk factors were also strong predictors.
(Kivipelto, Ngandu et al., 2006)	Longitudinal study; 1409 middle-aged population from Finland	Risk score created with the variables high age, low education, hypertension, hypercholesterolemia and obesity. Risk score was weighed by OR for each risk factor.	Higher risk score in middle age predicted higher dementia risk in older age. The best cut-off found (risk score 9 points or more) had a sensitivity of 0.77 and a specificity of 0.63, with a negative predictive value of 0.98.
(Reitz, Tang et al., 2010)	Longitudinal study; 1051 participants from Northern New York City recruited between 1999 and 2001 ages 65 years and older	Risk score was constructed with age, sex, education, ethnicity, APOE-ε4, diabetes, hypertension, smoking, HDL, and waist-to-hip ratio. The coefficients relating each individual variable to LOAD were used as weights for each variable in the score. Outcome was incident AD.	The risk of LOAD increased 20-fold for individuals in the highest score quintile.

low body mass index and increased dementia risk. It seems important to determine how the risk score performs independently of age when only modifiable risk factors are included (i.e., diabetes, smoking, dyslipidemia, waist-hip-ratio, hypertension). Also these models performed well: the associations were slightly attenuated but showed a clear increase of LOAD risk with increasing risk score and the strongest risk in the highest category.

All risk scores have limitations in the estimation of absolute risks and generalizability to different populations and clinical settings. A community-developed score may not be useful in a referral setting such as a memory disorders clinic. However, a community-based score may represent the risk in populations attending primary care clinics or even senior centers where screening is available. This is the principle behind scores such as the Framingham cardiovascular risk score (Wilson, D'Agostino et al., 1998). The Framingham risk score was developed in a community-based sample but is widely used in clinical settings in the United States to calculate cardiovascular risk and make decisions about therapies, such as lipid-lowering therapy.

The c-statistic or area under the receiver operating characteristic (ROC) curve is often used to assess the accuracy of a risk score. C-statistics reported for the Framingham cardiovascular risk score, the most studied and well-known risk score for prediction of cardiovascular disease, ranges between 0.75 and 0.8 (Lloyd-Jones). The study by Kivipelto reported a C-statistic of 0.77 (Kivipelto, Ngandu et al., 2006). In the study by Reitz et al., the c-statistics for the original model, including demographics, APOE, and vascular risk factors, was 0.79. An important question is whether aggregate measures of vascular risk factor add predictive ability to age (Barnes & Yaffe, 2004). Reitz et al. found that when only demographic variables are included in the predictive score, the c-statistic is 0.72, indicating that vascular risk factors increase the predicitivity of the model. However, it is important to point out that the c-statistic is better for evaluating discriminatory or diagnostic models compared to the evaluation of predictive models, such as the ones summarized here (Cook, 2008). The C-statistic is insensitive to the predictive contribution of variables with effect estimate sizes such as those that we report for vascular risk factors. Thus, the contribution of the addition of the vascular risk factors to the model is likely an underestimation. A future direction should be to use calibration methods (Cook, 2008) to evaluate how the addition of modifiable risk factors to the demographic variables improves the estimates of probability of dementia and clinical risk stratification.

Summary and Conclusions

The literature examining the association of aggregates of vascular risk factors in relation to cognitive impairment demonstrate that the effect of multiple risk factors may be greater than the effect of individual risk factors. In addition, this literature provides strong support for the role of vascular risk factors in cognition, one of the most important functional domains in aging. Thus, prevention, modification, and treatment of vascular risk factors and their clusters may improve cognition in our aging societies and seem to justify the conduct of clinical trials targeting treatment of clusters of risk factors examining cognition as a primary outcome.

More studies are needed to refine the measurement of clusters of risk factors that affect cognition in particular and understand how these clusters change throughout the lifespan. Finally, it is important to understand whether these clusters operate primarily through cerebrovascular mechanisms or whether nonvascular mechanisms are also important. If nonvascular mechanisms are also important, specific therapies that do not target traditional vascular risk factors may be used, such as agents targeting advanced products of glycosilation.

References

Abbott, R. D., Curb, J. D., Rodriguez, B. L., Masaki, K. H., Yano, K., Schatz, I. J., et al. (2002). Age-related changes in risk factor effects on the incidence of coronary heart disease. *Ann Epidemiol*, *12*(3), 173–181.

Akbaraly, T. N., Kivimaki, M., Shipley, M. J., Tabak, A. G., Jokela, M., Virtanen, M., et al. (2010) Metabolic syndrome over 10 years and cognitive functioning in late midlife: the Whitehall II study. *Diabetes Care*, *33*(1), 84–89.

Assmann, G., Cullen, P., & Schulte, H. (2002). Simple scoring scheme for calculating the risk of acute coronary events based on the 10-year follow-up of the prospective cardiovascular Munster (PROCAM) study. *Circulation*, *105*(3), 310–315.

Banks, W. A., Jaspan, J. B., & Kastin, A. J. (1997). Selective, physiological transport of insulin across the blood-brain barrier: novel demonstration by species-specific radioimmunoassays. *Peptides*, *18*(8), 1257–1262.

Barnes, D. E., & Yaffe, K. Accuracy of summary risk score for prediction of Alzheimer disease: better than demographics alone? *Arch Neurol*, *68*(2), 268; author reply 268–270.

Bastuji-Garin, S., Deverly, A., Moyse, D., Castaigne, A., Mancia, G., de Leeuw, P. W., et al. (2002). The Framingham prediction rule is not valid in a European population of treated hypertensive patients. *J Hypertens*, *20*(10), 1973–1980.

Biessels, G. J. (1999). Cerebral complications of diabetes: clinical findings and pathogenetic mechanisms. *Neth J Med*, *54*(2), 35–45.

Breteler, M. M., Claus, J. J., Grobbee, D. E., & Hofman, A. (1994). Cardiovascular disease and distribution of cognitive function in elderly people: the Rotterdam Study. *Bmj*, *308*(6944), 1604–1608.

Cavalieri, M., Ropele, S., Petrovic, K., Pluta-Fuerst, A., Homayoon, N., Enzinger, C., et al. (2010) Metabolic syndrome, brain magnetic resonance imaging, and cognition. *Diabetes Care*, *33*(12), 2489–2495.

Clayton, T. C., Lubsen, J., Pocock, S. J., Voko, Z., Kirwan, B. A., Fox, K. A., et al. (2005). Risk score for predicting death, myocardial infarction, and stroke in patients with stable angina, based on a large randomised trial cohort of patients. *Bmj*, *331*(7521), 869.

Cook, N. R. (2008). Statistical evaluation of prognostic versus diagnostic models: beyond the ROC curve. *Clin Chem*, *54*(1), 17–23.

D'Agostino, R. B., Sr., Grundy, S., Sullivan, L. M., & Wilson, P. (2001). Validation of the Framingham coronary heart disease prediction scores: results of a multiple ethnic groups investigation. *Jama, 286*(2), 180–187.

de Ruijter, W., Westendorp, R. G., Assendelft, W. J., den Elzen, W. P., de Craen, A. J., le Cessie, S., et al. (2009). Use of Framingham risk score and new biomarkers to predict cardiovascular mortality in older people: population based observational cohort study. *Bmj, 338*, a3083.

Diagnostic and statistical manual of mental disorders, 4th edition.:DSM IV. (1997). Washington, D.C.: American Psychiatric Association.

Dik, M. G., Jonker, C., Comijs, H. C., Deeg, D. J., Kok, A., Yaffe, K., et al. (2007). Contribution of metabolic syndrome components to cognition in older individuals. *Diabetes Care, 30*(10), 2655–2660.

Eckel, R. H., Grundy, S. M., & Zimmet, P. Z. (2005). The metabolic syndrome. *Lancet, 365*(9468), 1415–1428.

Farris, W., Mansourian, S., Chang, Y., Lindsley, L., Eckman, E. A., Frosch, M. P., et al. (2003). Insulin-degrading enzyme regulates the levels of insulin, amyloid beta-protein, and the beta-amyloid precursor protein intracellular domain in vivo. *Proc Natl Acad Sci U S A, 100*(7), 4162–4167.

Ferrannini, E., & Balkau, B. (2002). Insulin: in search of a syndrome. *Diabetic Medicine., 19*(9), 724–729.

Folstein, M. F., Folstein, S. E., & McHugh, P. R. (1975). "Mini-mental state". A practical method for grading the cognitive state of patients for the clinician. *J Psychiatr Res, 12*(3), 189–198.

Forti, P., Pisacane, N., Rietti, E., Lucicesare, A., Olivelli, V., Mariani, E., et al. (2010) Metabolic syndrome and risk of dementia in older adults. *J Am Geriatr Soc, 58*(3), 487–492.

Fowkes, F. G., Murray, G. D., Butcher, I., Heald, C. L., Lee, R. J., Chambless, L. E., et al. (2008). Ankle brachial index combined with Framingham Risk Score to predict cardiovascular events and mortality: a meta-analysis. *Jama, 300*(2), 197–208.

Gatto, N. M., Henderson, V. W., St John, J. A., McCleary, C., Hodis, H. N., & Mack, W. J. (2008). Metabolic syndrome and cognitive function in healthy middle-aged and older adults without diabetes. *Neuropsychol Dev Cogn B Aging Neuropsychol Cogn, 15*(5), 627–641.

Grundy, S. M., Cleeman, J. I., Daniels, S. R., Donato, K. A., Eckel, R. H., Franklin, B. A., et al. (2005). Diagnosis and Management of the Metabolic Syndrome: An American Heart Association/National Heart, Lung, and Blood Institute Scientific Statement. *Circulation, 112*(17), 2735–2752.

Hachinski, V., Iadecola, C., Petersen, R. C., Breteler, M. M., Nyenhuis, D. L., Black, S. E., et al. (2006). National Institute of Neurological Disorders and Stroke-Canadian Stroke Network vascular cognitive impairment harmonization standards. *Stroke, 37*(9), 2220–2241.

Hall, L. M., Jung, R. T., & Leese, G. P. (2003). Controlled trial of effect of documented cardiovascular risk scores on prescribing. *Bmj, 326*(7383), 251–252.

Kalmijn, S., Foley, D., White, L., Burchfiel, C. M., Curb, J. D., Petrovitch, H., et al. (2000). Metabolic cardiovascular syndrome and risk of dementia in Japanese- American elderly men. The Honolulu-Asia aging study. *Arterioscler Thromb Vasc Biol, 20*(10), 2255–2260.

Kivipelto, M., Laakso, M. P., Tuomilehto, J., Nissinen, A., & Soininen, H. (2002). Hypertension and hypercholesterolaemia as risk factors for Alzheimer's disease: potential for pharmacological intervention. *CNS Drugs, 16*(7), 435–444.

Kivipelto, M., Ngandu, T., Laatikainen, T., Winblad, B., Soininen, H., & Tuomilehto, J. (2006). Risk score for the prediction of dementia risk in 20 years among middle aged people: a longitudinal, population-based study. *Lancet Neurol, 5*(9), 735–741.

Komulainen, P., Lakka, T. A., Kivipelto, M., Hassinen, M., Helkala, E. L., Haapala, I., et al. (2007). Metabolic syndrome and cognitive function: a population-based follow-up study in elderly women. *Dement Geriatr Cogn Disord, 23*(1), 29–34.

Lee, K. S., Jang, Y., Chung, Y. K., Chung, J. H., Oh, B. H., & Hong, C. H. (2009) Relationship between the diagnostic components of metabolic syndrome (MS) and cognition by ApoE genotype in the elderly. *Arch Gerontol Geriatr, 50*(1), 69–72.

Lee, K.S., Eom, J.S., Cheong, H.K., Oh, B.H, &Hong, C.H. (2010). Effects of head circumference and metabolic syndrome on cognitive decline. *Gerontology, 56*(1), 32–38.

Libby, P., & Ridker, P. M. (2004). Inflammation and atherosclerosis: role of C-Reactive protein in risk assessment. *The American Journal of Medicine, 116*(6, Supplement 1), 9–16.

Liu, C. Y., Zhou, H. D., Xu, Z. Q., Zhang, W. W., Li, X. Y., & Zhao, J. (2009). Metabolic syndrome and cognitive impairment amongst elderly people in Chinese population: a cross-sectional study. *Eur J Neurol, 16*(9), 1022–1027.

Lloyd-Jones, D. M. Cardiovascular Risk Prediction: Basic Concepts, Current Status, and Future Directions. *Circulation, 121*(15), 1768–1777.

Luchsinger, J. A. (2001). Diabetes. In M. Aguirre-Molina, C. W. Molina & R. E. Zambrana (Eds.), *Health issues in the Latino community* (pp. 277–300). San Francisco: Jossey-Bass.

Luchsinger, J. A. (2006). A work in progress: the metabolic syndrome. *Sci Aging Knowledge Environ, 2006*(10), pe19.

Luchsinger, J. A., Cheng, D., Tang, M. X., Schupf, N., & Mayeux, R. (2012) Central Obesity in the Elderly is Related to Late-onset Alzheimer Disease. *Alzheimer Dis Assoc Disord.*

Luchsinger, J. A., Reitz, C., Honig, L. S., Tang, M. X., Shea, S., & Mayeux, R. (2005). Aggregation of vascular risk factors and risk of incident Alzheimer disease. *Neurology, 65*(4), 545–551.

Luchsinger, J. A., Tang, M. X., Shea, S., & Mayeux, R. (2004). Hyperinsulinemia and risk of Alzheimer disease. *Neurology, 63*(7), 1187–1192.

McKeigue, P. M. (1999). Ethnic Variation in Insulin Resistance and Risk of Type 2 Diabetes. In G. M. Reaven & A. Laws (Eds.), *Insulin Resistance: the metabolic syndrome X* (pp. 19–34). Totowa, NJ: Humana Press.

Mitchell, T. W., Nissanov, J., Han, L. Y., Mufson, E. J., Schneider, J. A., Cochran, E. J., et al. (2000). Novel method to quantify neuropil threads in brains from elders with or without cognitive impairment. *J Histochem Cytochem, 48*(12), 1627–1638.

Muller, M., Tang, M. X., Schupf, N., Manly, J. J., Mayeux, R., & Luchsinger, J. A. (2007). Metabolic syndrome and dementia risk in a multiethnic elderly cohort. *Dement Geriatr Cogn Disord, 24*(3), 185–192.

Muller, M., van Raamt, F., Visseren, F. L., Kalmijn, S., Geerlings, M. I., Mali, W. P., et al. (2010) Metabolic syndrome and cognition in patients with manifest atherosclerotic disease: the SMART study. *Neuroepidemiology, 34*(2), 83–89.

Park, C. R. (2001). Cognitive effects of insulin in the central nervous system. *Neurosci Biobehav Rev, 25*(4), 311–323.

Petersen, R. C. (2004). Mild cognitive impairment as a diagnostic entity. *J Intern Med, 256*(3), 183–194.

Petrovitch, H., White, L. R., Izmirilian, G., Ross, G. W., Havlik, R. J., Markesbery, W., et al. (2000). Midlife blood pressure and neuritic plaques, neurofibrillary tangles, and brain weight at death: the HAAS. Honolulu-Asia aging Study. *Neurobiol Aging, 21*(1), 57–62.

Pocock, S. J., McCormack, V., Gueyffier, F., Boutitie, F., Fagard, R. H., & Boissel, J. P. (2001). A score for predicting risk of death from cardiovascular disease in adults with raised blood pressure, based on individual patient data from randomised controlled trials. *Bmj, 323*(7304), 75–81.

Raffaitin, C., Feart, C., Le Goff, M., Amieva, H., Helmer, C., Akbaraly, T. N., et al. (2011) Metabolic syndrome and cognitive decline in French elders: the Three-City Study. *Neurology, 76*(6), 518–525.

Raffaitin, C., Gin, H., Empana, J. P., Helmer, C., Berr, C., Tzourio, C., et al. (2009). Metabolic syndrome and risk for incident Alzheimer's disease or vascular dementia: the Three-City Study. *Diabetes Care, 32*(1), 169–174.

Rathmann, W., Haastert, B., Icks, A., Giani, G., Holle, R., Koenig, W., et al. (2006). Prevalence of the metabolic syndrome in the elderly population according to IDF, WHO, and NCEP definitions and associations with C-reactive protein: the KORA Survey 2000. *Diabetes Care, 29*(2), 461.

Reaven, G. M. (2002). Multiple CHD risk factors in type 2 diabetes: beyond hyperglycaemia. *Diabetes Obes Metab, 4 Suppl* 1, S13–18.

Reaven, G. M., & Laws, A. (1999). *Insulin resistance: the metabolic syndrome X.* Totowa, New Jersey: Humana Press.

Reitz, C., Tang, M. X., Luchsinger, J., & Mayeux, R. (2004). Relation of plasma lipids to Alzheimer disease and vascular dementia. *Arch Neurol, 61*(5), 705–714.

Reitz, C., Tang, M. X., Schupf, N., Manly, J. J., Mayeux, R., & Luchsinger, J. (2010) Higher HDL in the elderly is associated with lower risk of late onset Alzheimer's disease. *Arch Neurol, 67*(12):1491–1497.

Reitz, C., Tang, M. X., Schupf, N., Manly, J. J., Mayeux, R., & Luchsinger, J. A. A summary risk score for the prediction of Alzheimer disease in elderly persons. *Arch Neurol, 67*(7), 835–841.

Reitz, C., Tang, M. X., Schupf, N., Manly, J. J., Mayeux, R., & Luchsinger, J. A. (2010). Association of higher levels of high-density lipoprotein cholesterol in elderly individuals and lower risk of late-onset Alzheimer disease. *Arch Neurol, 67*(12), 1491–1497.

Roberts, R. O., Geda, Y. E., Knopman, D. S., Cha, R. H., Boeve, B. F., Ivnik, R. J., et al. (2010)Metabolic syndrome, inflammation, and nonamnestic mild cognitive impairment in older persons: a population-based study. *Alzheimer Dis Assoc Disord, 24*(1), 11–18.

Roriz-Cruz, M., Rosset, I., Wada, T., Sakagami, T., Ishine, M., De Sa Roriz-Filho, J., et al. (2007). Cognitive impairment and frontal-subcortical geriatric syndrome are associated with metabolic syndrome in a stroke-free population. *Neurobiol Aging, 28*(11), 1723–1736.

Royall, D. R., Lauterbach, E. C., Cummings, J. L., Reeve, A., Rummans, T. A., Kaufer, D. I., et al. (2002). Executive control function: a review of its promise and challenges for clinical research. A report from the Committee on Research of the American Neuropsychiatric Association. *J Neuropsychiatry Clin Neurosci, 14*(4), 377–405.

Sacco, R. L., Benjamin, E. J., Broderick, J. P., Dyken, M., Easton, J. D., Feinberg, W. M., et al. (1997). American Heart Association Prevention Conference. IV. Prevention and Rehabilitation of Stroke. Risk factors. *Stroke., 28*(7), 1507–1517.

Savva, G. M., Wharton, S. B., Ince, P. G., Forster, G., Matthews, F. E., & Brayne, C. (2009). Age, neuropathology, and dementia. *N Engl J Med, 360*(22), 2302–2309.

Schunkert, H., & Samani, N. J. (2008). Elevated C-reactive protein in atherosclerosis – chicken or egg? *N Engl J Med, 359*(18), 1953–1955.

Schupf, N., Costa, R., Luchsinger, J., Tang, M. X., Lee, J. H., & Mayeux, R. (2005). Relationship between plasma lipids and all-cause mortality in nondemented elderly. *J Am Geriatr Soc, 53*(2), 219–226.

Schwartz, M. W., Sipols, A., Kahn, S. E., Lattemann, D. F., Taborsky, G. J., Jr., Bergman, R. N., et al. (1990). Kinetics and specificity of insulin uptake from plasma into cerebrospinal fluid. *Am J Physiol, 259*(3 Pt 1), E378–383.

Seshadri, S., Wolf, P. A., Beiser, A., Elias, M. F., Au, R., Kase, C. S., et al. (2004). Stroke risk profile, brain volume, and cognitive function: The Framingham Offspring Study. *Neurology, 63*(9), 1591–1599.

Skoog, I. (1997). The relationship between blood pressure and dementia: a review. *Biomed Pharmacother, 51*(9), 367–375.

Skoog, I. (2003). Highs and lows of blood pressure:a cause of Alzheimer's disease? *Lancet Neurol, 2*(6), 334.

Small, S. A. (2002). The longitudinal axis of the hippocampal formation: its anatomy, circuitry, and role in cognitive function. *Rev Neurosci, 13*(2), 183–194.

Small, S. A., & Mayeux, R. (1999). A clinical approach to memory decline. *J Pract Psychiatry Behav Health, 5*, 87–94.

Snowdon, D. A., Greiner, L. H., Mortimer, J. A., Riley, K. P., Greiner, P. A., & Markesbery, W. R. (1997). Brain infarction and the clinical expression of Alzheimer disease. The Nun Study. *Jama, 277*(10), 813–817.

Solfrizzi, V., Scafato, E., Capurso, C., D'Introno, A., Colacicco, A. M., Frisardi, V., et al. (2009). Metabolic syndrome, mild cognitive impairment, and progression to dementia. The Italian Longitudinal Study on Aging. *Neurobiol Aging.*

Sparks, D. L., Martin, T. A., Gross, D. R., & Hunsaker, J. C., 3rd. (2000). Link between heart disease, cholesterol, and Alzheimer's disease: a review. *Microsc Res Tech, 50*(4), 287–290.

Stevens, J., Cai, J., Pamuk, E. R., Williamson, D. F., Thun, M. J., & Wood, J. L. (1998). The effect of age on the association between body-mass index and mortality. *N Engl J Med*, 1–7.

Treves, T. A., Bornstein, N. M., Chapman, J., Klimovitzki, S., Verchovsky, R., Asherov, A., et al. (1996). APOE-epsilon 4 in patients with Alzheimer disease and vascular dementia. *Alzheimer Dis Assoc Disord, 10*(4), 189–191.

Tuan, C.-Y., Abbasi, F., Lamendola, C., McLaughlin, T., & Reaven, G. (2003). Usefulness of plasma glucose and insulin concentrations in identifying patients with insulin resistance. *The American Journal of Cardiology, 92*(5), 606–610.

van den Berg, E., Biessels, G. J., de Craen, A. J., Gussekloo, J., & Westendorp, R. G. (2007). The metabolic syndrome is associated with decelerated cognitive decline in the oldest old. *Neurology, 69*(10), 979–985.

van den Berg, E., Dekker, J. M., Nijpels, G., Kessels, R. P., Kappelle, L. J., de Haan, E. H., et al. (2008). Cognitive functioning in elderly persons with type 2 diabetes and metabolic syndrome: the Hoorn study. *Dement Geriatr Cogn Disord, 26*(3), 261–269.

Vekrellis, K., Ye, Z., Qiu, W. Q., Walsh, D., Hartley, D., Chesneau, V., et al. (2000). Neurons regulate extracellular levels of amyloid beta-protein via proteolysis by insulin-degrading enzyme. *J Neurosci, 20*(5), 1657–1665.

Wang, C. H., & Zhou, X. (2003). [Meta-analysis for relationship between apoE gene polymorphism and coronary heart disease]. *Zhonghua Yu Fang Yi Xue Za Zhi, 37*(5), 368–370.

Weijenberg, M. P., Feskens, E. J., & Kromhout, D. (1996). Age-related changes in total and high-density-lipoprotein cholesterol in elderly Dutch men. *Am J Public Health, 86*(6), 798–803.

Whitmer, R. A., Gunderson, E. P., Barrett-Connor, E., Quesenberry, C. P., Jr, & Yaffe, K. (2005). Obesity in middle age and future risk of dementia: a 27 year longitudinal population based study. *BMJ*, bmj.38446.466238.E466230.

Whitmer, R. A., Sidney, S., Selby, J., Johnston, S. C., & Yaffe, K. (2005). Midlife cardiovascular risk factors and risk of dementia in late life. *Neurology, 64*(2), 277–281.

Wilson, P. W., D'Agostino, R. B., Levy, D., Belanger, A. M., Silbershatz, H., & Kannel, W. B. (1998). Prediction of coronary heart disease using risk factor categories. *Circulation, 97*(18), 1837–1847.

Wilson, P. W. F., D'Agostino, R. B., Parise, H., Sullivan, L., & Meigs, J. B. (2005). Metabolic Syndrome as a Precursor of Cardiovascular Disease and Type 2 Diabetes Mellitus. *Circulation, 112*(20), 3066–3072.

Yaffe, K., Haan, M., Blackwell, T., Cherkasova, E., Whitmer, R. A., & West, N. (2007). Metabolic syndrome and cognitive decline in elderly Latinos: findings from the Sacramento Area Latino Study of Aging study. *J Am Geriatr Soc, 55*(5), 758–762.

Yaffe, K., Kanaya, A., Lindquist, K., Simonsick, E. M., Harris, T., Shorr, R. I., et al. (2004). The metabolic syndrome, inflammation, and risk of cognitive decline. *JAMA, 292*(18), 2237–2242.

Yaffe, K., Weston, A. L., Blackwell, T., & Krueger, K. A. (2009). The metabolic syndrome and development of cognitive impairment among older women. *Arch Neurol, 66*(3), 324–328.

Yang, X., So, W. Y., Tong, P. C., Ma, R. C., Kong, A. P., Lam, C. W., et al. (2008). Development and validation of an all-cause mortality risk score in type 2 diabetes. *Arch Intern Med, 168*(5), 451–457.

7

Chronic Kidney Disease and Cognitive Aging

MANJULA KURELLA TAMURA, MD, MPH

Introduction

Although cognitive impairment has long been recognized among patients with end-stage renal disease (ESRD) receiving chronic dialysis, recent evidence has suggested a link between less advanced stages of chronic kidney disease (CKD) and accelerated cognitive aging. These associations are noteworthy because CKD is common among older adults and potentially modifiable. This chapter will describe the link between age-associated declines in kidney and cognitive function, explore several possible mechanisms, and examine the implications for clinical care and subsequent research.

Definition and Prevalence of Chronic Kidney Disease According to Age

The National Kidney Foundation (2002) defines CKD as a glomerular filtration rate (GFR) less than 60 mL/min/1.73 m^2 or other evidence of kidney damage (e.g., albuminuria or proteinuria) for 3 months or more. Using this definition, 20% of adults in the United States ages 60 years to 69 years and 45% of adults older than age 70 years are estimated to have CKD (Coresh et al., 2007). The majority of older individuals with CKD have mild to moderate reductions in GFR—that is, GFR 30 mL/min/1.73 m^2 to 59 mL/min/1.73 m^2. At the other extreme, each year approximately 50,000 U.S. adults older than age 65 years develop ESRD and start chronic dialysis or receive a kidney transplant (Collins et al., 2007), an incidence rate more than double that observed among middle-age adults.

Similarly to cognitive function, it is widely accepted that kidney function declines with age. However, the extent to which age-associated decline in kidney function is attributable to "normal aging" or results from age-associated pathological processes remains a matter of debate. For example, Lindeman and colleagues (1985) measured kidney function over 8 years to 24 years in 254 healthy men ages 22 years to 97 years in the Baltimore Longitudinal Study of Aging. They noted that the rate of kidney function decline accelerated with age but also that 36% of subjects experienced no change in kidney function over time. These findings suggest that kidney function decline with age is common but not necessarily inevitable. Adding to this complexity is uncertainty about the optimal method for assessing kidney function in older individuals. Glomerular filtration rate is widely accepted as the best overall marker of kidney function; as such, it is central to the detection and staging of CKD. Most often GFR is estimated from the serum creatinine concentration. However, creatinine concentration is influenced by factors other than GFR, including muscle mass and dietary intake. This may result in some degree of misclassification of kidney function in the elderly and other populations with reduced muscle mass. With these issues in mind, the next section examines the epidemiology of cognitive impairment among persons with CKD and ESRD.

Epidemiology of Dementia and Cognitive Impairment in End-Stage Renal Disease and Chronic Kidney Disease

END-STAGE RENAL DISEASE EPIDEMIOLOGY

Based on Medicare claims data, which is known to be insensitive for ascertaining dementia, the estimated prevalence of dementia among patients in the United States with ESRD is 7% to 12% (Rakowski et al., 2006; Collins et al., 2007). Similarly to the general population, a dementia diagnosis is more common among the elderly, women, and non-White patients (Kurella et al., 2006; Rakowski et al., 2006). A diagnosis of dementia is less common in the Japanese and European ESRD populations as compared to the U.S. ESRD population (Kurella et al., 2006). Dementia incidence, based on claims data, is approximately 1% to 2% among ESRD patients younger than age 65 years and roughly doubles with each decade of age, reaching 6% to 8% for patients older than age 85 years (Collins et al., 2007).

Prevalence estimates based on neuropsychological testing are substantially higher. The prevalence of dementia among patients with ESRD is approximately threefold higher than the age-matched general population, ranging from 16% to 38% depending on the study sample and the definition of impairment (Sehgal et al., 1997; Kurella et al., 2004; Murray et al., 2006; Cook et al., 2008; Brady et al., 2009; Kurella Tamura et al., 2009; Leinau et al., 2009). The high prevalence of cognitive impairment in this population is not confined to the elderly—15% to 25% of ESRD patients ages 45 years to 64 years also have evidence of cognitive impairment (Kurella Tamura et al., 2010). Very few published studies have evaluated the longitudinal course of cognitive impairment or the incidence of dementia among ESRD patients. Fukunishi et al. (2002) studied 508 patients with ESRD on hemodialysis in Japan who had a mean age of 66 years. The diagnosis of dementia was based on psychiatric interview using Diagnostic and Statistical Manual (DSM) IV criteria. The annual incidence of dementia was 2.5%, an incidence rate seven times higher than that of the general Japanese population (Fukunishi et al., 2002).

CHRONIC KIDNEY DISEASE EPIDEMIOLOGY

Among adults with CKD, the prevalence of cognitive impairment and incidence of cognitive decline and dementia are also high. For example, in a sample of 23,000 Black and White U.S. adults with a mean age of 65 years, cognitive impairment (ascertained by a brief cognitive screen) was present in 12% of adults with an estimated GFR (eGFR) less than 60 mL/min/1.73 m^2 (Kurella Tamura et al., 2008). After adjustment for demographic characteristics and several cardiovascular risk factors, each 10 mL/min/1.73 m^2 decrease in eGFR below 60 mL/min/1.73 m^2 was associated with an 11% increased prevalence of impairment. Seliger et al. (2004) demonstrated an increased risk for incident dementia among older adults with CKD in the Cardiovascular Health Study. Chronic kidney disease, defined according to sex-specific serum creatinine cut-points, was associated with a 37% increased risk for clinically defined dementia over a median 6 years of follow-up. Several other prospective studies have demonstrated an independent relationship between CKD and risk for cognitive decline, primarily in older adults, and other studies have suggested that severity of CKD may also be related to risk for cognitive decline (Kurella et al., 2005; Buchman et al., 2009; Etgen et al., 2009; Khatri et al., 2009; Yaffe et al., 2010) (Table 7.1).

However, not all studies suggest CKD is independently associated with cognitive decline (Table 7.1). For example, in the MrOS study involving 5520 men with a mean age of 74 years, lower eGFR was associated with cross-sectional cognitive function scores but was not independently associated with cognitive decline (Slinin et al., 2008). Among 1345 adults in the Rancho Bernardo study with a mean age of 75 years, low eGFR was not independently associated with cognitive decline. Differences in the target population (especially in the prevalence of advanced CKD) or differences in the study design and cognitive outcome may underlie these divergent observations. Several alternative possibilities also deserve consideration.

The first is whether misclassification of individuals with low muscle mass from creatinine-based GFR estimates may have attenuated the association

Table 7.1 Prospective Studies Evaluating Association Between Chronic Kidney Disease (CKD) and Cognitive Decline or Dementia

Study population	Years of follow-up	CKD biomarker	CKD prevalence	Outcome	Findings
3349 adults with mean age of 75 in the Cardiovascular Health Study (Seliger et al. 2004)	6	Serum creatinine ≥1.5 mg/dL in men, and ≥1.3 mg/dL in women.	10%	Dementia, adjudicated by expert panel on the basis of neuropsychiatric battery	CKD associated with 37% higher risk for dementia
3034 adults with mean age of 74 in the Health Aging and Body Composition Study (Kurella et al. 2005)	2–4	Creatinine eGFR <60.	22%	Decline in 3MS score to <80 or decline >5 points at follow-up	32–143% increased risk for cognitive decline among adults with eGFR 45-59 and <45, respectively,
2172 adults with mean age of 72 in the Northern Manhattan Study (Khatri et al. 2009)	3	Creatinine eGFR <60.	13%	Decline in modified Telephone Interview of Cognitive Status	Increased rate of decline for adults with eGFR <60 (vs. eGFR >90)
5520 men with mean age of 74 in the Osteoporotic Fractures in Men Study (Slinin et al. 2008)	5	Creatinine eGFR <60.	17%	Decline in 3MS score to <80 or >5 points at follow-up; or decline in Trails B score more than 1 standard deviation below sample mean	No significant association of CKD with decline in 3MS or Trails B

Population	Ref	Kidney measure	Prevalence	Cognitive outcome	Findings
886 adults with mean age of 81 in the Rush Memory and Aging Project (Buchman et al. 2009)	3	Creatinine eGFR <60.	50%	Cognitive decline using a battery of 19 tests summarized into global decline and 5 domains	Lower eGFR significantly associated with accelerated decline across multiple domains
3679 adults with mean age of 68 in the INVADE study (Etgen et al. 2009)	2	Creatinine clearance <60.	18%	6-Item Cognitive Impairment Test score >7	114% increased risk for cognitive impairment among adults with creatinine clearance <45
2140 adults with mean age of 74 in the Cardiovascular Health Study (Sarnak et al. 2008)	4	Cystatin-C ≥1.16 mg/L.	25%	3MS score < 80 on 2 consecutive visits	2-fold higher frequency of developing cognitive impairment among adults with cystatin-C ≥1.16 mg/L
3030 adults with mean age of 73 in the Health Aging and Body Composition Study (Yaffe et al. 2008)	7	Cystatin-C ≥1.25 mg/L.	15%	Decline of more than 1 standard deviation during follow-up on the 3MS or Digit Symbol Substitution	54-92% increased risk for cognitive decline among adults with elevated cystatin-C
1345 adults with mean age of 75 in the Rancho Bernardo Study (Jassal et al. 2010)	7	ACR ≥30mg/g and eGFR <60.	ACR ≥30mg/g: 16%, eGFR <60: 42% among women and 27% among men.	Annual change in MMSE, Trails B, and category fluency scores	ACR of ≥30 mg/g was associated with accelerated cognitive decline in men but not women. No association between eGFR<60 and cognitive decline in men or women

(continued)

Table 7.1 (Continued)

Study population	Years of follow-up	CKD biomarker	CKD prevalence	Outcome	Findings
28,384 adults with a mean age of 66 in the ONTARGET and TRANSCEND studies (Barzilay et al. 2011)	5	ACR ≥30 mg/g	16%	Decline in MMSE of 3 points	ACR 30-299 mg/g was associated with 23% higher risk of cognitive decline, and ACR ≥300 mg/g was associated with 25% higher risk of cognitive decline. In addition, worsening albuminuria associated with 30-77% increased risk for cognitive decline.
4095 adults with mean age of 55 in the Prevention of Renal and Vascular End Stage Disease Study (Joosten et al. 2011)	6–8	ACR ≥30 mg/g, eGFR <60	ACR ≥30 mg/g: 15%, eGFR <60: 9%	Change in the Ruff Figural Fluency Test	ACR ≥30 mg/g associated with more rapid cognitive decline among ages 35–48 but not older ages. No association between eGFR and cognitive decline.

Note: eGFR – estimated glomerular filtration rate (in ml/min/1.73m2), ACR – albumin to creatinine ratio, MMSE – Mini Mental State Exam, 3MS – Modified Mini Mental State Exam, INVADE – Intervention Project on Cerebrovascular Diseases and Dementia in the Community of Ebersberg, ONTARGET – Ongoing Telmisartan Alone and in Combination With Ramipril Global End Point Trial, TRANSCEND – Telmisartan Randomized Assessment Study in ACE Intolerant Subjects With Cardiovascular Disease.

between CKD and cognitive decline in some studies. Cystatin-C is an alternate marker of kidney filtration function that is purported to be less influenced by muscle mass than serum creatinine. In two large cohort studies of older adults, elevated cystatin-C levels independently predicted cognitive decline and dementia (Sarnak et al., 2008; Yaffe et al., 2008). Importantly, cystatin-C was noted to predict cognitive decline even among individuals with normal eGFR based on measurement of creatinine. Thus, it is suggested to be a better marker of early, or preclinical, CKD, particularly in older patients with low muscle mass.

An additional or alternative possibility is that GFR is merely a confounder for albuminuria. Albuminuria is a marker of glomerular permeability that has traditionally been considered an early marker of CKD, whereas low eGFR was considered a late marker. However, this assumption is now being challenged for several reasons. First, it is now clear that in diseases like diabetes, low eGFR is often not preceded by albuminuria, and conversely, albuminuria does not always progress to low eGFR. Second, other studies demonstrate that albuminuria predicts mortality and progression to ESRD *independently* of low GFR (Hemmelgarn et al., 2010), suggesting it is not necessarily an early marker of CKD but a complementary marker to low GFR. Many have speculated that low-level albuminuria (i.e., 10-300 mg/g creatinine) reflects endothelial dysfunction as a consequence of systemic small vessel disease rather than a disease process confined to the kidney.

In the Rancho Bernardo Study, albuminuria, but not eGFR, was associated with an increased risk for cognitive decline among men (Jassal et al., 2010) but not among women. In the Prevention of Renal and Vascular End-Stage Disease (PREVEND) study, baseline level of albuminuria and the change in albuminuria over time were independently correlated with cognitive decline. Conversely, there was no association of eGFR with cognitive decline after controlling for albuminuria (Joosten et al., 2011). Similarly, in the ONTARGET and TRANSCEND clinical trials, new or worsening albuminuria over time was associated with a 30% to 77% increased risk for cognitive decline independent of eGFR (Barzilay et al., 2011). In addition, the risk for cognitive decline associated with albuminuria was modified by treatment with an angiotensin converting enzyme (ACE) inhibitor, angiotensin receptor blocker (ARB), or both. As compared to placebo, treatment with an ACE inhibitor and/or ARB reduced the incidence of cognitive decline among subjects with macroalbuminuria (albuminuria >300 mg/g creatinine/day) but not among subjects with normoalbuminuria or microalbuminuria (albuminuria 30–299 mg/g creatinine/day). In contrast, in cross-sectional analyses from the Chronic Renal Insufficiency Cohort (CRIC) involving only participants with eGFR less than 70 mL/min/1.73 m^2, lower eGFR, but not albuminuria, was associated with poorer cognitive function (Kurella Tamura et al., 2011). This observation may be explained by a subsequent study of more than 19,000 adults suggesting that low eGFR and albuminuria were complementary markers of cognitive decline. That is, when eGFR was preserved, higher levels of albuminuria predicted cognitive decline. Conversely, when albuminuria was low or absent, lower eGFR predicted cognitive decline (Kurella Tamura et al., 2011).

In sum, epidemiological data indicate that CKD is associated with an increased risk for cognitive decline and dementia that is independent of most established dementia risk factors. These associations are identifiable at early stages of CKD and become more pronounced with increasing severity of CKD. Further, these associations have been noted for multiple, potentially complementary CKD biomarkers, including creatinine eGFR, cystatin-C, and albuminuria. Finally, in two studies, changes in albuminuria appear to parallel changes in cognitive function, perhaps indicating that a shared pathophysiological process is contributing to kidney and cognitive function decline.

Risk Factors for Cognitive Impairment in Chronic Kidney Disease and End-Stage Renal Disease

Several lines of evidence point to small vessel disease as playing a central role in the development of dementia among persons with CKD. First, the anatomic and hemodynamic properties of the vascular beds in the brain and kidney share several features. Both are high-flow, low-resistance end-organs with high resting demand (Seliger et al., 2008). Blood flow is tightly regulated in both organs across a range of perfusion pressures. Second, small vessel pathology is often associated with kidney function impairment and with cognitive impairment. Small vessel pathology is often observed in patients with non-diabetic CKD who undergo kidney biopsy (Fogo et al., 1997). In the brain, analagous vascular lesions have been described in association with lacunar infarcts and white matter hyperintensities, representing complete and incomplete infarcts, respectively (Fernando et al., 2006). These lesions, in turn, are strongly correlated with cognitive impairment in the general population (Kuller et al., 2003; Vermeer et al., 2003; Smith et al., 2008; Wright et al., 2008). Third, cross-sectional studies indicate robust associations between CKD and small vessel disease in the brain, including small vessel stroke, white matter lesions, and cerebral microbleeds (Nakatani et al., 2003; Seliger et al., 2005; Ikram et al., 2008). Similar findings between cystatin-C and albuminuria with small vessel ischemic disease lesions in the brain (Seliger et al., 2005; Weiner et al., 2008) have recently been reported. Thus, some have speculated that impairments in kidney and cognitive function may be manifestations of chronic ischemia resulting from small vessel disease in different end-organs.

Could CKD be a mediator of accelerated cognitive decline rather than merely a marker, and if so, what factors and pathways might be involved? First, CKD may be a result of small vessel ischemic disease but also a cause. Traditional cerebrovascular disease risk factors, especially hypertension, become more difficult to control as CKD progresses. Moreover, a number of metabolic derangements are present in CKD, including inflammation, oxidative stress, endothelial dysfunction, insulin resistance, altered sympathetic tone, and dysregulation of bone metabolism (Himmelfarb et al., 2010). These novel risk factors tend to increase in severity as kidney function declines and are implicated in the high rates of cardiovascular events and associated with cognitive decline in this population (Go et al., 2004). Whether these risk factors contribute to cerebrovascular disease among patients with CKD is not known.

Second, CKD may contribute to dementia independently of its hypothesized effects on small vessel ischemic disease but, rather, through nonvascular mechanisms. Anemia is perhaps the best studied of these putative nonvascular risk factors. In cross-sectional studies of patients with CKD and ESRD, anemia is associated with an increased prevalence of cognitive impairment and dementia (Kurella et al., 2006; Murray et al., 2006). In uncontrolled trials among severely anemic patients with ESRD (i.e., hematocrit < 25%), amelioration of anemia with erythropoietin was associated with improvement in cognitive function (Grimm et al., 1990; Marsh et al., 1991). No randomized trials in CKD or ESRD patients have tested whether anemia correction or erythropoietin replacement improves cognitive function. However, in one large trial of patients with CKD and anemia, subjects receiving erythropoietin had higher rates of stroke as compared to subjects receiving placebo (Pfeffer et al., 2009). Because stroke is a major risk factor for dementia, this has raised questions about whether erythropoietin therapy is likely to preserve cognitive function in patients with mild anemia.

Uremia is characterized by retention of a large number of solutes, and several may have direct neurotoxicity or contribute indirectly to the pathogenesis of dementia by altering the blood–brain barrier. Because the number of retained substances is large, in practice the removal of urea during a dialysis treatment is often used as a proxy for the "dose," or adequacy of dialysis treatments. In a randomized clinical trial conducted 30 years ago, subjects with ESRD randomized to receive larger dialytic removal of urea (i.e., larger dialysis dose) had improvements in reaction time and EEG measures ((Teschan et al., 1983), although it should be noted that modern standards for urea removal are considerably higher than in this study. In several, but not all, subsequent observational studies, cognitive function has been reported to improve shortly after initiation or intensification of dialysis (Teschan et al., 1983; Jassal et al., 2006) or after kidney transplantation, although most of these studies suffer from the lack of a control group. Several uremic solutes, including guanidine compounds, asymmetric dimethylarginine, advanced glycation end-products, phenolic compounds, and parathyroid hormone, have neurotoxicity in vitro (De Deyn et al., 2001), but confirmation of their toxicity in human studies is lacking.

Third, several factors associated with treatment of ESRD may lead to delirium, and these cumulative insults may result in accelerated cognitive aging. For example, among patients with untreated ESRD, uremic encephalopathy, a syndrome of cognitive impairment attributed to the retention of as yet unidentified uremic solutes, has been well-described {Teschan et al., 1975}. Fluid shifts during hemodialysis may lead to cerebral edema (i.e., dialysis dysequilibrium syndrome). Further, the hemodynamic stress of hemodialysis may lead to cerebral hypoperfusion. Functional MRI studies before and after hemodialysis have provided conflicting evidence of this (Prohovnik et al., 2007; Lux et al., 2010). Ultrafiltration, and possibly erythropoiesis stimulating agents, may contribute to hyperviscosity and cerebral thrombotic events. In several small clinical studies that have conducted repeated assessments during the course of a weekly hemodialysis cycle, cognitive function has been shown to decline during hemodialysis and during the long intradialytic interval between treatments (Williams et al., 2004; Murray et al., 2007). Thus, repeated clinical or subclinical delirium events may have long-term detrimental effects on cognitive function.

Finally, could there be a shared genetic predisposition to CKD and cognitive decline? Polymorphisms of the apolipoprotein E (APOE) gene have been associated with CKD and cognitive decline. However, although individuals with the APOE 4 variant are three to eight times more likely to develop Alzheimer's dementia (AD), limited data suggest individuals with this variant are *less* likely to develop ESRD (Oda et al., 1999). As described above, cystatin-C is a novel marker of kidney function that is reported to have greater correlation with measured GFR as compared with serum creatinine in older individuals. Cystatin-C colocalizes with β-amyloid in brains of patients with AD, and polymorphisms of the cystatin-C gene are associated with increased risk for dementia (Lin et al., 2003), suggesting that cystatin-C may play a role in the development of dementia independently of its association with kidney function. Prospective studies that control for kidney function are needed to clarify whether the association between cystatin-C and dementia is explained by its role as a kidney biomarker or by other factors.

A Conceptual Model of Cognitive Aging in Chronic Kidney Disease

Putting this information together, there seems to be a consensus that cerebrovascular disease, and small vessel disease in particular, is a key feature linking CKD with accelerated cognitive aging (Fig. 7.1). An unanswered question is the extent to which small vessel disease is a result of shared risk factors or a consequence of novel CKD risk factors. On the one hand, several risk factors, most

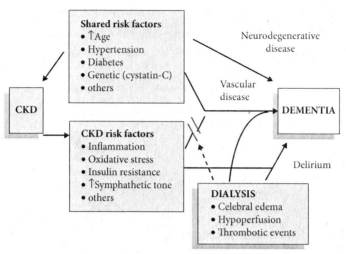

Figure 7.1 Conceptual model of pathways connecting chronic kidney disease and accelerated cognitive aging.

notably diabetes and hypertension, contribute to small vessel disease in the brain and kidney and are linked with cognitive decline and progression of CKD. On the other hand, most epidemiological studies have demonstrated independent associations between CKD and cognitive decline after controlling for the presence (although usually not the severity) of these risk factors. Further, there is widespread agreement that CKD accelerates cardiovascular disease in other end-organs (e.g., heart, lower extremity); thus it seems at least plausible that CKD might do the same in the brain.

The role of neurodegenerative disease in CKD is not well-studied, although some intriguing data linking polymorphisms of cystatin-C to dementia deserve further study. Finally, a host of factors related to dialysis therapy may affect the pace of cognitive decline in diverse ways. Specifically, although dialysis may ameliorate some aspects of uremia, it may also accelerate vascular disease and contribute to subclinical episodes of delirium. These mechanisms remain mostly speculative and have not been carefully studied in a large number of patients.

Implications

IMPLICATIONS FOR CLINICAL CARE

The high prevalence of cognitive impairment and dementia among patients with advanced CKD and ESRD has several implications for clinical care. For example, cognitive impairment may hinder adherence with the complex dietary and pharmacologic regimens prescribed to patients with CKD, increase the risk of adverse drug events, and impair informed decision making surrounding preemptive vascular access placement and ESRD treatment options. Thus, clinicians need to be aware of this high prevalence and be able to accurately identify CKD patients with cognitive impairment in their practice. Cognitive impairment may also influence the clinician's management of CKD, including timing of dialysis initiation or candidacy for kidney transplantation. Among patients with ESRD, dementia increases the risk for functional decline, hospitalization, withdrawal from dialysis, and death and increases the cost of care (Kurella Tamura et al., 2011). The clinical significance of cognitive impairment not meeting criteria for dementia has not been fully elucidated, although some evidence suggests that cognitive impairment may also be associated with longer hospitalizations and larger dialysis unit staff burden (Sehgal et al., 1997). Given this anticipated course, the diagnosis of dementia in a patient with advanced CKD or ESRD should prompt clinicians to initiate advance care planning discussions.

Whether the prevention or treatment of dementia should differ among patients with CKD is not clear. Several cholinesterase inhibitors and the N-methyl-D-aspartate receptor antagonist memantine used for treatment of dementia symptoms require dose adjustment or are contraindicated in patients with advanced CKD (Kurella Tamura et al., 2011). The ONTARGET/TRANSCEND trials support the use of ACE inhibitors or ARBs among individuals with macroalbuminuria in the setting of diabetes or vascular disease to delay cognitive decline. Combination therapy (ACE inhibitor plus ARB) did not confer benefit over monotherapy. Whether the results can be extrapolated to individuals without diabetes or vascular disease is not known. Other cardiovascular risk reduction strategies are reasonable although generally already recommended for patients with CKD and not specifically tested for the purpose of dementia prevention. There are very few data on therapies targeting novel CKD risk factors. In a randomized clinical trial of patients with advanced CKD and ESRD, homocysteine lowering with B vitamins did not delay cognitive decline (Brady et al., 2009). There is insufficient evidence to recommend increasing the intensity of dialysis to improve cognitive function. However, a randomized clinical trial to test this hypothesis has recently been completed.

Summary

In summary, CKD may be considered a model of accelerated cognitive aging acting primarily, although not exclusively, through vascular mechanisms. Additional research is needed to clarify the causal direction of these associations and mediating factors. Given the burden of cognitive impairment among patients with

CKD and the ease of assessing kidney function, future clinical trials, especially those directed at vascular mechanisms, should consider targeting this high-risk population.

References

Barzilay, J. I., Gao, P., O'Donnell, M., Mann, J. F., Anderson, C., Fagard, R., et al. (2011). Albuminuria and decline in cognitive function: The ONTARGET/TRANSCEND studies. *Arch Intern Med, 171*(2), 142–150.

Brady, C. B., Gaziano, J. M., Cxypoliski, R. A., Guarino, P. D., Kaufman, J. S., Warren, S. R., et al. (2009). Homocysteine lowering and cognition in CKD: the Veterans Affairs homocysteine study. *Am J Kidney Dis, 54*(3), 440–449.

Buchman, A. S., Tanne, D., Boyle, P. A., Shah, R. C., Leurgans, S. E., & Bennett, D. A. (2009). Kidney function is associated with the rate of cognitive decline in the elderly. *Neurology, 73*(12), 920–927.

Collins, A. J., Kasiske, B., Herzog, C., Chavers, B., Foley, R., Gilbertson, D., et al. (2007). Excerpts from the United States Renal Data System 2006 Annual Data Report. *Am J Kidney Dis, 49*(1 Suppl 1), A6-7, S1–296.

Cook, W. L., & Jassal, S. V. (2008). Functional dependencies among the elderly on hemodialysis. *Kidney Int, 73*(11), 1289–1295.

Coresh, J., Selvin, E., Stevens, L. A., Manzi, J., Kusek, J. W., Eggers, P., et al. (2007). Prevalence of chronic kidney disease in the United States. *Jama, 298*(17), 2038–2047.

De Deyn, P. P., D'Hooge, R., Van Bogaert, P. P., & Marescau, B. (2001). Endogenous guanidino compounds as uremic neurotoxins. *Kidney Int Suppl, 78*, S77–83.

Etgen, T., Sander, D., Chonchol, M., Briesenick, C., Poppert, H., Forstl, H., et al. (2009). Chronic kidney disease is associated with incident cognitive impairment in the elderly: the INVADE study. *Nephrol Dial Transplant, 24*(10), 3144–3150.

Fernando, M. S., Simpson, J. E., Matthews, F., Brayne, C., Lewis, C. E., Barber, R., et al. (2006). White matter lesions in an unselected cohort of the elderly: molecular pathology suggests origin from chronic hypoperfusion injury. *Stroke, 37*(6), 1391–1398.

Fogo, A., Breyer, J. A., Smith, M. C., Cleveland, W. H., Agodoa, L., Kirk, K. A., et al. (1997). Accuracy of the diagnosis of hypertensive nephrosclerosis in African Americans: a report from the African American Study of Kidney Disease (AASK) Trial. AASK Pilot Study Investigators. *Kidney Int, 51*(1), 244–252.

Fukunishi, I., Kitaoka, T., Shirai, T., Kino, K., Kanematsu, E., & Sato, Y. (2002). Psychiatric disorders among patients undergoing hemodialysis therapy. *Nephron, 91*(2), 344–347.

Go, A. S., Chertow, G. M., Fan, D., McCulloch, C. E., & Hsu, C. Y. (2004). Chronic kidney disease and the risks of death, cardiovascular events, and hospitalization. *N Engl J Med, 351*(13), 1296–1305.

Grimm, G., Stockenhuber, F., Schneeweiss, B., Madl, C., Zeitlhofer, J., & Schneider, B. (1990). Improvement of brain function in hemodialysis patients treated with erythropoietin. *Kidney Int, 38*(3), 480–486.

Hemmelgarn, B. R., Manns, B. J., Lloyd, A., James, M. T., Klarenbach, S., Quinn, R. R., et al. (2010). Relation between kidney function, proteinuria, and adverse outcomes. *Jama, 303*(5), 423–429.

Himmelfarb, J., & Ikizler, T. A. (2010). Hemodialysis. *N Engl J Med, 363*(19), 1833–1845.

Ikram, M. A., Vernooij, M. W., Hofman, A., Niessen, W. J., van der Lugt, A., & Breteler, M. M. (2008). Kidney function is related to cerebral small vessel disease. *Stroke, 39*(1), 55–61.

Jassal, S. K., Kritz-Silverstein, D., & Barrett-Connor, E. (2010). A prospective study of albuminuria and cognitive function in older adults: the Rancho Bernardo study. *Am J Epidemiol, 171*(3), 277–286.

Jassal, S. V., Devins, G. M., Chan, C. T., Bozanovic, R., & Rourke, S. (2006). Improvements in cognition in patients converting from thrice weekly hemodialysis to nocturnal hemodialysis: A longitudinal pilot study. *Kidney Int*, *70*(5), 956–962..

Joosten, H., Izaks, G., Slaets, J., De Jong, P. E., Visser, S. T., Bilo, H. J. G., et al. (2011). Association of cognitive function with albuminuria and eGFR in the general population. *Clin J Am Soc Nephrol*, *6*(6), 1400–1409.

National Kidney Foundation. K/DOQI clinical practice guidelines for chronic kidney disease: evaluation, classification, and stratification. Kidney Disease Outcome Quality Initiative. (2002). *Am J Kidney Dis*, *39*(2 Suppl 2), S1–246.

Khatri, M., Nickolas, T., Moon, Y. P., Paik, M. C., Rundek, T., Elkind, M. S., et al. (2009). CKD associates with cognitive decline. *J Am Soc Nephrol*, *20*(11), 2427–2432.

Kuller, L. H., Lopez, O. L., Newman, A., Beauchamp, N. J., Burke, G., Dulberg, C., et al. (2003). Risk factors for dementia in the cardiovascular health cognition study. *Neuroepidemiology*, *22*(1), 13–22.

Kurella, M., Chertow, G. M., Fried, L. F., Cummings, S. R., Harris, T., Simonsick, E., et al. (2005). Chronic kidney disease and cognitive impairment in the elderly: the health, aging, and body composition study. *J Am Soc Nephrol*, *16*(7), 2127–2133.

Kurella, M., Chertow, G. M., Luan, J., & Yaffe, K. (2004). Cognitive impairment in chronic kidney disease. *J Am Geriatr Soc*, *52*(11), 1863–1869.

Kurella, M., Mapes, D. L., Port, F. K., & Chertow, G. M. (2006). Correlates and outcomes of dementia among dialysis patients: the Dialysis Outcomes and Practice Patterns Study. *Nephrol Dial Transplant*, *21*(9),2543–2548.

Kurella Tamura, M., Larive, B., Unruh, M., Stokes, J., Beck, G., & Chertow, G. (2009). Prevalence and Correlates of Cognitive Impairment in the Frequent Hemodialysis Network (FHN) Trials. *American Society of Nephrology meeting, (abstract)*.

Kurella Tamura, M., Larive, B., Unruh, M. L., Stokes, J. B., Nissenson, A., Mehta, R. L., et al. (2010). Prevalence and correlates of cognitive impairment in hemodialysis patients: the Frequent Hemodialysis Network trials. *Clin J Am Soc Nephrol*, *5*(8), 1429–1438.

Kurella Tamura, M., Wadley, V., Yaffe, K., McClure, L. A., Howard, G., Go, R., et al. (2008). Kidney function and cognitive impairment in US adults: the Reasons for Geographic and Racial Differences in Stroke (REGARDS) Study. *Am J Kidney Dis*, *52*(2), 227–234.

Kurella Tamura, M., Xie, D., Yaffe, K., Cohen, D. L., Teal, V., Kasner, S. E., et al. (2011). Vascular risk factors and cognitive impairment in chronic kidney disease: the Chronic Renal Insufficiency Cohort (CRIC) study. *Clin J Am Soc Nephrol*, *6*(2), 248–256.

Kurella Tamura, M., & Yaffe, K. (2011). Dementia and cognitive impairment in ESRD: diagnostic and therapeutic strategies. *Kidney Int*, *79*(1), 14–22.

Leinau, L., Murphy, T. E., Bradley, E., & Fried, T. (2009). Relationship between conditions addressed by hemodialysis guidelines and non-ESRD-specific conditions affecting quality of life. *Clin J Am Soc Nephrol*, *4*(3), 572–578.

Lin, C., Wang, S. T., Wu, C. W., Chuo, L. J., & Kuo, Y. M. (2003). The association of a cystatin C gene polymorphism with late-onset Alzheimer's disease and vascular dementia. *Chin J Physiol*, *46*(3), 111–115.

Lindeman, R. D., Tobin, J., & Shock, N. W. (1985). Longitudinal studies on the rate of decline in renal function with age. *J Am Geriatr Soc*, *33*(4), 278–285.

Lux, S., Mirzazade, S., Kuzmanovic, B., Plewan, T., Eickhoff, S. B., Shah, N. J., et al. (2010). Differential activation of memory-relevant brain regions during a dialysis cycle. *Kidney Int*, *78*(8), 794–802.

Marsh, J. T., Brown, W. S., Wolcott, D., Carr, C. R., Harper, R., Schweitzer, S. V., et al. (1991). rHuEPO treatment improves brain and cognitive function of anemic dialysis patients. *Kidney Int*, *39*(1), 155–163.

Murray, A. M., Pederson, S. L., Tupper, D. E., Hochhalter, A. K., Miller, W. A., Li, Q., et al. (2007). Acute variation in cognitive function in hemodialysis patients: a cohort study with repeated measures. *Am J Kidney Dis*, *50*(2), 270–278.

Murray, A. M., Tupper, D. E., Knopman, D. S., Gilbertson, D. T., Pederson, S. L., Li, S., et al. (2006). Cognitive impairment in hemodialysis patients is common. *Neurology, 67*(2), 216–223.

Nakatani, T., Naganuma, T., Uchida, J., Masuda, C., Wada, S., Sugimura, T., et al. (2003). Silent cerebral infarction in hemodialysis patients. *Am J Nephrol, 23*(2), 86–90.

Oda, H., Yorioka, N., Ueda, C., Kushihata, S., & Yamakido, M. (1999). Apolipoprotein E polymorphism and renal disease. *Kidney Int Suppl, 71*, S25–27.

Pfeffer, M. A., Burdmann, E. A., Chen, C. Y., Cooper, M. E., de Zeeuw, D., Eckardt, K. U., et al. (2009). A trial of darbepoetin alfa in type 2 diabetes and chronic kidney disease. *N Engl J Med, 361*(21), 2019–2032.

Prohovnik, I., Post, J., Uribarri, J., Lee, H., Sandu, O., & Langhoff, E. (2007). Cerebrovascular effects of hemodialysis in chronic kidney disease. *J Cereb Blood Flow Metab, 27*(11), 1861–1869.

Rakowski, D. A., Caillard, S., Agodoa, L. Y., & Abbott, K. C. (2006). Dementia as a predictor of mortality in dialysis patients. *Clin J Am Soc Nephrol, 1*(5), 1000–1005.

Sarnak, M. J., Katz, R., Fried, L. F., Siscovick, D., Kestenbaum, B., Seliger, S., et al. (2008). Cystatin C and aging success. *Arch Intern Med, 168*(2), 147–153.

Sehgal, A. R., Grey, S. F., DeOreo, P. B., & Whitehouse, P. J. (1997a). Prevalence, recognition, and implications of mental impairment among hemodialysis patients. *Am J Kidney Dis, 30*(1), 41–49.

Seliger, S. L., & Longstreth, W. T., Jr. (2008). Lessons about brain vascular disease from another pulsating organ, the kidney. *Stroke, 39*(1), 5–6.

Seliger, S. L., Longstreth, W. T., Jr., Katz, R., Manolio, T., Fried, L. F., Shlipak, M., et al. (2005). Cystatin C and Subclinical Brain Infarction. *J Am Soc Nephro, 16*(12), 3721–37271.

Seliger, S. L., Siscovick, D. S., Stehman-Breen, C. O., Gillen, D. L., Fitzpatrick, A., Bleyer, A., et al. (2004). Moderate renal impairment and risk of dementia among older adults: the Cardiovascular Health Cognition Study. *J Am Soc Nephrol, 15*(7), 1904–1911.

Slinin, Y., Paudel, M. L., Ishani, A., Taylor, B. C., Yaffe, K., Murray, A. M., et al. (2008). Kidney function and cognitive performance and decline in older men. *J Am Geriatr Soc, 56*(11), 2082–2088.

Smith, E. E., Egorova, S., Blacker, D., Killiany, R. J., Muzikansky, A., Dickerson, B. C., et al. (2008). Magnetic resonance imaging white matter hyperintensities and brain volume in the prediction of mild cognitive impairment and dementia. *Arch Neurol, 65*(1), 94–100.

Teschan, P. E., Bourne, J. R., Reed, R. B., & Ward, J. W. (1983). Electrophysiological and neurobehavioral responses to therapy: the National Cooperative Dialysis Study. *Kidney Int Suppl*(13), S58–65.

Vermeer, S. E., Prins, N. D., den Heijer, T., Hofman, A., Koudstaal, P. J., & Breteler, M. M. (2003). Silent brain infarcts and the risk of dementia and cognitive decline. *N Engl J Med, 348*(13), 1215–1222.

Weiner, D. E., Bartolomei, K., Scott, T., Price, L. L., Griffith, J. L., Rosenberg, I., et al. (2008). Albuminuria, Cognitive Functioning, and White Matter Hyperintensities in Homebound Elders. *Am J Kidney Dis, 53*(3), 438–447.

Williams, M. A., Sklar, A. H., Burright, R. G., & Donovick, P. J. (2004). Temporal effects of dialysis on cognitive functioning in patients with ESRD. *Am J Kidney Dis, 43*(4), 705–711.

Wright, C. B., Festa, J. R., Paik, M. C., Schmiedigen, A., Brown, T. R., Yoshita, M., et al. (2008). White matter hyperintensities and subclinical infarction: associations with psychomotor speed and cognitive flexibility. *Stroke, 39*(3), 800–805.

Yaffe, K., Ackerson, L., Kurella Tamura, M., Le Blanc, P., Kusek, J. W., Sehgal, A. R., et al. (2010). Chronic kidney disease and cognitive function in older adults: findings from the chronic renal insufficiency cohort cognitive study. *J Am Geriatr Soc, 58*(2), 338–345.

Yaffe, K., Lindquist, K., Shlipak, M. G., Simonsick, E., Fried, L., Rosano, C., et al. (2008). Cystatin C as a marker of cognitive function in elders: findings from the health ABC study. *Ann Neurol, 63*(6), 798–802.

8

Sleep Disorders and Cognitive Function in Older Adults

ADAM P. SPIRA, PHD AND SONIA ANCOLI-ISRAEL, PHD

Introduction

Sleep complaints are common among older adults. Approximately half of elders have been shown to have a complaint about some aspect of their sleep or daytime sleepiness (Foley et al., 1995; Ganguli et al., 1996; Mellinger et al., 1985). A meta-analysis by Ohayon et al. (2004) found that over the lifespan, healthy individuals exhibit a decrease in sleep duration, an increase in sleep fragmentation, and a decrease in sleep efficiency (i.e., they spend a greater proportion of time in bed awake). With age, adults also take longer to fall asleep, spend more time in lighter stages of sleep, and spend less time in deeper stages and in rapid eye movement (REM) sleep (Ohayon et al., 2004). Most of these changes, however, occur before age 60 years; only sleep efficiency decreases throughout older adulthood (Ohayon et al., 2004). Thus, for healthy individuals, entering older adulthood does not necessarily mean a substantial or global loss of sleep quality (Vitiello, 2006). Beyond changes associated with normal aging, the elevated prevalence of sleep complaints among older adults is thought to arise from primary sleep disorders, circadian rhythm disruption, medical conditions, psychiatric disorders, psychosocial variables, and medication side effects (Ancoli-Israel & Cooke, 2005).

Like sleep complaints, cognitive impairment is common among older adults. Findings from the Aging, Demographics, and Memory Study indicate that approximately 14% of older adults older than age 70 years have dementia and 22% have cognitive impairment below the threshold of dementia (Plassman et al., 2007, 2008). A meta-analysis indicated that the incidence of dementia doubles almost every 5 years between ages 60 years and 80 years and then begins to slow down (Ritchie et al., 1992), although other results have suggested that exponential increases in incidence continue through the 80s (Jorm & Jolley, 1998). Recent findings from a study of women age 85 years and older found that approximately 41% had mild cognitive impairment (MCI) or dementia (Yaffe et al., 2011).

These age-related increases in both sleep complaints and cognitive impairment raise the possibility of an association between sleep disorders and cognitive decline. A causal association between sleep disturbance and cognitive decline would have significant implications for public health, given the high prevalence of sleep disorders in older adults, the burden of cognitive impairment in this population, and the fact that poor sleep often can be improved in elders. Under this scenario, prevention and treatment of sleep disorders might be a means of preventing or ameliorating cognitive decline. If, on the other hand, sleep disturbances are not causally linked to cognitive decline—as in the case that sleep disturbance and cognitive impairment both arise from a neurodegenerative process—then changes in sleep could have prognostic utility; they could assist clinicians in the identification of patients at risk for declines who require closer monitoring.

We review research findings regarding the association between common sleep disorders and cognition in older adults, including performance on neuropsychological tests, and diagnoses of dementia and MCI. When data are available, we also discuss the impact of treating sleep disorders on the cognitive health of older adults.

Sleep Quality, Insomnia, and Cognition

According to the *Diagnostic and Statistical Manual of Mental Disorders, 4th Edition, Text Revision* (DSM-IV-TR) diagnostic criteria, insomnia is characterized by problems falling or staying sleep or with sleep that is non-restorative (American Psychiatric Association; APA, 2000). In addition, this disturbance must occur for 1 month or longer, cause significant functional impairment, not occur solely in the context of another sleep disorder or mental disorder, and not result from substance use or a medical comorbidity (APA, 2000). The *International Classification of Sleep Disorders, 2nd Edition* (ICSD-2; American Academy of Sleep Medicine; AASM, 2005) general criteria for insomnia also permit a complaint of poor sleep quality and require that the disturbance must occur "...despite adequate opportunity and circumstances for sleep." (p. 2) ICSD-2 provides a list of forms of daytime consequences that amount to impairment (e.g., sleepiness, sleep-related worries; AASM, 2005).

Insomnia is highly prevalent in older adults. Lichstein et al. (2004), in a review of results from epidemiologic studies of self-reported sleep and insomnia, estimated that 25% of older adults have either insomnia or insomnia symptoms. Individual studies, however, have found higher rates. For example, a study of Italian adults ages 65 years and older found that 54% or women and 36% of men had insomnia (Maggi et al., 1998).

Compared to older adults without insomnia, those with insomnia demonstrate lower performance in tests of attention (Vignola et al., 2000; Haimov et al., 2008) and estimation of elapsed time (Haimov et al., 2008). Mixed findings have emerged regarding the association between insomnia diagnosis and memory and executive function (Haimov et al., 2006, 2008; Vignola et al., 2000). Less evidence exists for an association between insomnia diagnosis and performance on measures of general cognition, psychomotor speed, or language (Haimov et al., 2008; Vignola et al., 2000). In addition, the patterns of associations between sleep parameters and cognitive performance may differ among older adults with insomnia who use benzodiazepine medications, those with insomnia who do not use benzodiazepines, and good sleepers (Bastien et al., 2003). For example, among good sleepers, greater objectively measured latency to sleep onset was associated with lower performance on a measure of executive function, but this was not the case among older adults with insomnia who were not taking benzodiazepines or those who were taking these medications (Bastien et al., 2003).

Much of our knowledge regarding sleep and cognition in older adults is from epidemiologic studies that included one or more questions about insomnia symptoms or from questionnaires such as the Pittsburgh Sleep Quality Index (PSQI; Buysse et al., 1989), rather than formal diagnostic assessments of insomnia. In addition, a few studies have used polysomnography (PSG) or wrist actigraphy to measure sleep objectively. Actigraphy measures sleep by recording wrist movement with a device resembling a wristwatch called an actigraph and using an algorithm to differentiate sleep (inactivity) from wake (activity) (Ancoli-Israel et al., 2003). Although it cannot be used to diagnose insomnia, actigraphy is useful in studies of sleep and cognition, particularly in older adults with dementia, among whom cognitive impairment can impact the validity of self-reported sleep (Van Den Berg et al., 2008).

In a cross-sectional study of older adults, poor sleep quality (measured by the PSQI) was linked to lower performance on measures of general cognitive function and some aspects of executive function (Nebes et al., 2009), although another study, this time in older men, found no association between PSQI scores and performance in those cognitive domains (Blackwell et al., 2011). Reports of more frequent problems with falling or remaining asleep have been associated with impairment (Tworoger et al., 2006) or decline (Cricco et al., 2001; Jelicic et al., 2002) in measures of general cognitive function. Because these studies relied on only a few questionnaire items to assess sleep, these findings suggest that it may not only be clinically diagnosed insomnia that puts older adults at risk for cognitive decline but that milder cases of poor sleep may also increase this risk.

The association between sleep duration and cognition is complex (Table 8.1). Although some studies of community-dwelling older adults have found associations between reports of longer sleep duration and better objectively or

Table 8.1 **Associations Between Self-Reported Sleep Duration and Cognitive Performance in Community-Dwelling Older Adults**

Study	Sample	Significant associations	Null associations
Hart et al., 1995	insomnia patients	Longer TST associated with better immediate verbal recall	IQ, attention, psychomotor performance, visual memory, delayed recall, executive function
Alapin et al. 2000	good and poor sleepers	Longer TST associated with lower frequency of self-reported concentration difficulties	None
Ohayon & Vecchierini, 2002	population-based sample	≤5 hours TST (vs. 7–8.5 hours) associated with self-reported attention/concentration problems; 5–7 hours TST (vs. 7–8.5 hours) associated with self-reported problems with orientation to person	Delayed recall, praxis, orientation (temporal), prospective memory. No association of longer sleep with self-reported impairment in any domains.
Ohayon & Vecchierini, 2005	population-based sample	Self-reported cognitive impairment associated with self-report of short sleep (vs. intermediate 50% of sample)	No association of self-reported cognitive impairment with longer sleep.
Tworoger et al., 2006	older women in Nurses' Health Study	≤5 hours TST (vs. 7 hours) associated with lower performance or impairment in general cognition, executive function, and a composite of measures; 8 hours TST (vs. 7 hours) associated with lower executive function.	No association between sleep duration and cognitive decline. No association between longer sleep and general cognition or memory.
Schmutte et al., 2007	community-based sample	None	General cognition, attention, executive function, memory, psychomotor performance, language, or visuospatial ability

Study	Sample		
Faubel et al., 2009[*]	population-based sample	Longer sleep duration (from 7 hours to ≥11 hours) associated with lower performance and greater risk of impairment on a measure of general cognitive function.	No association between sleep <7 hours and general cognitive function
Nebes et al., 2009	good and poor sleepers	None	Executive function, psychomotor performance, memory
Loerbroks et al., 2010	population-based sample	Increases in TST from 7–8 hours to ≥9 hours associated with greater risk of impairment on measures of general cognition verbal memory	No cross-sectional associations of sleep duration and cognition. No association between decreases in sleep duration and cognition
Blackwell et al., 2011	community-based, older men	After correction for multiple comparisons, TST >8 hours associated with lower performance in attention	General cognition, executive function

[*]Included total sleep in a 24-hour period in total sleep duration (i.e., not only nocturnal sleep). TST = total sleep time.

subjectively measured cognitive performance (Hart et al., 1995; Alapin et al., 2000), others have found the opposite (Faubel et al., 2009), and some have found no association (Schmutte et al., 2007; Nebes et al., 2009). Other studies in this population have investigated potential U-shaped associations between sleep duration and cognition by comparing the performance of those with short or long sleep duration to those with sleep of a more intermediate duration. Some studies have found that compared to those with more average sleep, those reporting shorter sleep perform worse (or report performing worse) in some cognitive domains (Ohayon & Vecchierini, 2002, 2005; Tworoger et al., 2006). However, others have found that compared to more intermediate sleep duration, longer sleep is associated with lower performance (Blackwell et al., 2011; Tworoger et al., 2006). Some evidence from prospective studies suggests that increases, but not decreases, in self-reported sleep duration from an intermediate duration, are associated with a greater risk of impairment in particular cognitive domains (Loerbroks et al., 2010).

A few studies have used objective sleep measures to investigate the association between sleep duration and cognition in community-dwelling elders. Shorter actigraphically measured sleep duration has been linked to lower performance on measures of general cognitive function in at least one (Blackwell et al., 2006) but not all (Blackwell et al., 2011; Cohen-Zion et al., 2001; Yaffe et al., 2007) studies. A series of studies in a cohort of older women suggests that there is no association of actigraphic TST with set shifting, an aspect of executive function (Blackwell et al., 2006; Blackwell et al., 2011; Yaffe et al., 2007).

Difficulty remaining asleep is an increasingly common complaint with age (Lichstein et al., 2004). The term "sleep fragmentation" refers to interruptions in sleep and is commonly quantified by wake after sleep onset (WASO; the amount of time spent awake after an individual initially falls asleep). Low sleep efficiency also can, but does not necessarily, reflect fragmented sleep. Higher self-reported sleep efficiency is correlated with better performance on tests of general cognitive function and working memory, but not in other aspects of executive function among community-dwelling older adults (Nebes et al., 2009). Among older insomnia patients, self-report of lower sleep efficiency has been linked to performance on tests of sustained attention, executive function, psychomotor performance, and memory (Hart et al., 1995). Others, however, have found no association between self-reported sleep fragmentation and performance in general cognitive function (Frisoni et al., 1992).

A few studies provide data on objectively measured sleep fragmentation and cognition in community-dwelling elders. For example, greater WASO and lower sleep efficiency, as measured by actigraphy, were associated with lower performance in general cognition and executive function in a study of older women (Blackwell et al. 2006). Similar findings emerged from a study of older men (Blackwell et al., 2011). Another smaller actigraphy study, however, found no association between change in sleep fragmentation and change in general cognitive function (Cohen-Zion et al., 2001).

Researchers also have studied cognitive correlates of the interval between going to bed and falling asleep, or "sleep onset latency." Longer self-reported sleep onset latency has been linked to lower performance on tests of general cognitive function (Schmutte et al., 2007; Nebes et al., 2009) and language and visuospatial ability (Schmutte et al., 2007). In older women, longer actigraphically measured sleep onset latency was associated with impairment in general cognitive function and executive function (Blackwell et al., 2006; Yaffe et al., 2007).

In sum, studies of older adults from a range of populations indicate that insomnia diagnosis and insomnia symptoms, along with reports of relatively long and short sleep duration, are associated with lower performance or impairment in multiple cognitive domains. Studies using objective sleep measures generally support these findings. However, results are not consistent across studies, and many of the studies reviewed that reported positive associations between sleep and one or more cognitive domains reported null associations in other domains. Conflicting findings between studies could result from multiple factors, including the heterogeneity of populations sampled, differences in measures utilized, and variation in analytic methods. Although findings indicate that disturbed sleep is commonly associated with worse cognitive function in older adults, it is premature to make conclusive statements regarding associations between particular sleep parameters (e.g., sleep duration, fragmentation) and performance in specific cognitive domains, in a given population of older adults. Further, mixed findings in particular cognitive domains have emerged within individual studies. For example, in Nebes et al. (2009), good and poor sleepers differed on some, but not all, aspects of executive function. This suggests that a finer-grained categorization of cognitive domains may be necessary to most accurately account for the association between sleep disturbance and cognition.

Additional prospective studies with rigorous measures of sleep and more comprehensive and uniform assessment of cognitive domains are needed to clarify the extent to which insomnia and both objectively and subjectively estimated sleep parameters predict cognitive decline and clinically adjudicated cognitive outcomes in older adults, such as MCI and dementia. Also, to improve our understanding of the mechanisms by which insomnia and poor sleep quality impact cognition, prospective studies with neuroimaging outcomes (e.g., white matter lesions, atrophy, amyloid burden) or other neurobiological outcomes are needed. For example, preliminary research in eight younger adults with insomnia and eight controls demonstrated smaller hippocampal volumes in the insomnia patients (Riemann et al., 2007), and research in an animal models of AD has demonstrated that β-amyloid levels are increased by experimental sleep deprivation (Kang et al., 2009). Jelicic et al. (2002) found that adjusting for depressive symptoms removed the sleep-cognition association and suggested that depressive symptoms might mediate the association between insomnia symptoms and cognitive decline. Others, however, have found that adjustment for depression has no meaningful impact on findings (Nebes et al., 2009). Further research is needed to determine the extent to which depressive symptoms mediate or confound the association between insomnia symptoms and cognitive decline. Further, because it is common among older adults and can markedly affect sleep duration and continuity, sleep-disordered breathing (SDB) may account for some of the associations that have been observed between these sleep parameters and cognitive outcomes. Therefore, studies are needed that collect data on both SDB and the sleep parameters we have been discussing.

Sleep-Disordered Breathing, Cognition, and Risk of Dementia

Sleep-disordered breathing refers to disorders characterized by repeated episodes of cessation or significant reduction of respiration during sleep. In obstructive sleep apnea (OSA), these cessations (apneas) or reductions (hypopneas) result from complete or partial occlusion of the airway (AASM, 2005). Central sleep apnea refers to repeated cessation of respiratory effort during sleep that is attributed to central nervous system control, rather than obstruction, and complex sleep apnea refers to the presence of both obstructive and central apneas (Wellman & White, 2011). In this chapter, we use the term SDB to refer to the broad class of these disorders.

An overnight sleep study using PSG is the gold standard for SDB assessment, and in sleep disorder clinics these studies typically are prompted by reports of loud snoring, observed pauses in respiration during sleep, or excessive daytime sleepiness. Multiple physiological processes are recorded during PSG, and summary indices are used to quantify SDB severity, many of which involve a count of apneas and hypopneas and quantification of the amount of oxygen desaturation. In adults, apneas are defined as complete or near complete cessation of respiration for 10 seconds or longer, whereas hypopneas are defined as a significant decrease in airflow along with SaO_2 desaturation (Iber et al., 2007). The apnea-hypopnea index (AHI) refers to the mean number of apneas + hypopneas per hour of sleep and is perhaps the most commonly used SDB index. The respiratory disturbance index (RDI) is another popular summary measure, which is sometimes used interchangeably with the AHI, but is properly defined as the mean number of apneas, hypopneas, and respiratory effort-related arousals (RERAs) per hour of sleep.

According to the ICSD-2, 5 or more respiratory events per hour of sleep, plus patient complaints (e.g., daytime sleepiness, unrefreshing sleep, gasping, choking during sleep) or bed partner reports of loud snoring or witnessed apneas, are required for OSA diagnosis (AASM, 2005); in the event of 15 or more events per hour, ICSD-2 permits OSA diagnosis in the absence of patient or bed partner reports. Commonly used categories for SDB severity are an AHI of 5 to 15 for mild, 15 to 30 for moderate, and more than 30 for severe OSA.

Estimates of SDB prevalence vary by age, sex, and SDB diagnostic criteria used. However, SDB is more common in older than in middle-aged adults, and more common among men than among women. In a representative sample from Wisconsin, approximately 9% of men and 4% of women ages 30 years to 60 years were estimated to have an AHI of 15 or greater (Young et al., 1993). In a large study of more than 3,000 older men, 26.4% were found to have an RDI of 15 or greater and approximately 60% an RDI of 5 or greater (Mehra et al., 2007). The proportion of men with an RDI of 15 or greater increased with age, from 22.8% for men younger than age 72 years to 30.1% for men age 80 years or older, although the proportion of men with an RDI less than 5 did not (Mehra et al., 2007). In another population-based sample of elders, however, 62% had an AHI of 10 or greater (Ancoli-Israel et al., 1991b).

The neuropsychological correlates of SDB are well documented in primarily middle-aged and younger samples. In reviews of SDB and cognition in these mostly younger or mixed-age populations, the most consistent cognitive correlates are deficits in attention and executive function and, to a lesser extent, memory (Aloia et al., 2004; Beebe et al., 2003; Engleman et al., 2000). As displayed in Table 8.2, greater objectively measured SDB severity in older adults has been linked to lower performance, impairment, or decline in measures of global cognitive function or IQ, memory, attention, executive function, psychomotor performance, language, and visuospatial abilities. Recently, a study of older women reported that those with an AHI of 15 or greater had almost twice the odds of developing MCI or dementia approximately 5 years later, compared to those with an AHI of less than 15 (Yaffe et al., 2011). The authors presented evidence suggesting that this association is explained by hypoxia, rather than by sleep fragmentation. Despite the many positive findings, it should be noted that the literature on SDB and cognition in older adults contains numerous null findings and that no cognitive domains are consistently associated with SDB (Table 8.2).

Studies investigating the impact of treating OSA on cognitive outcomes have produced mixed findings. One review reported that treatment with continuous positive airway pressure (CPAP) was associated with improvements in global cognition, attention, executive function, and memory but found that results were not consistent across studies (Aloia et al., 2004), and another review concluded that executive dysfunction and deficits in planning and motor skills might not be responsive to CPAP (Sanchez et al., 2009).

Table 8.2 Association Between Sleep-Disordered Breathing and Cognitive Test Performance in Older Adults

Study	Sample	SDB measures	General cognition/IQ	Memory	Attention	Executive function	Psychomotor performance	Language	Visuospatial
Moldofsky et al., 1983	6 Adults aged 65+ with AD	Multiple	x	–	x	–	–	–	–
Yesavage et al., 1985	41 men (mean age = 69.5)	RDI	x	0, 0	0	x, x	x	x, 0	–
Berry et al., 1987	29 adults aged >60 years	Multiple	0, 0, 0	–	–	–	–	–	–
Berry et al., 1990	8 adults aged 60+ with SAS vs. 12 controls	SAS = AHI ≥10 and two signs/symptoms of daytime dysfunction	x, 0, 0	x, 0	–	–	–	–	–
Knight et al. 1987	27 adults aged 65+	Apnea index <5 vs. ≥5	–	0	0	–	0	0	0
Hoch et al., 1989	15 AD patients, 12 controls	AI	0	0	x	0	0, 0	–	–
Ancoli-Israel et al., 1991a	235 nursing home residents	AI, RDI	x	x	x	x, x	–	–	x
Stone et al., 1994	34 adults with insomnia aged 55+	RDI <5 vs. ≥10	0	0, 0, 0	0	0, 0	0, 0	–	–

Study	Sample	Measures						
Cohen-Zion et al., 2001	Population-based sample of 46 adults aged 65+	RDI	x	–	–	–	–	x
Aloia et al., 2003	Cohort of 12 adults >55 years with RDI >10	RDI, time in <80% blood oxygen saturation	–	x, 0	0, 0, 0	0, 0, 0	0, 0	x
Foley et al., 2003	718 Japanese American men ≥79 years	AHI	0, 0	0	0	0	–	–
Cohen-Zion et al., 2004	140 adults 65+ (50% African-American, 50% Caucasian)	RDI, ODI	x	–	–	–	–	–
O'Hara et al., 2005	36 older adults	AHI, minimum SaO$_2$	–	x*	–	–	–	–
Spira et al., 2008	448 older women	AHI, SaO$_2$ nadir, CAI	x**	–	–	0	–	–
Cole et al., 2009	90 nursing home residents with cognitive impairment	respiratory awakenings, SaO$_2$	x	–	–	–	–	–

(continued)

Table 8.2 (Continued)

Study	Sample	SDB measures	General cognition/IQ	Memory	Attention	Executive function	Psychomotor performance	Language	Visuospatial
Blackwell et al., 2011	2,909 men aged 67+	AHI, arterial oxygen saturation <80%, arousal index	0	–	x	0	–	–	–
Sforza et al., 2010	827 older adults	ODI, AHI	0	x, x, 0, 0, 0	0, 0	0, 0, 0, 0, 0	–	–	–
Kim et al., 2011	30 older adults with MCI, 30 controls	AHI, AI, HI, SaO$_2$ nadir	–	0, 0, 0, 0	–	x†	–	x†	0

Note: x = significant association with lower performance; 0 = null association; *in APOE e4 carriers only; **stronger effect in APOE e4 carriers than in entire sample; †associations significant only in participants with MCI, not in controls; – = not applicable to study. AI = apnea index; AHI = apnea hypopnea index; HI = hypopnea index; ODI = oxygen desaturation index; RDI = respiratory disturbance index; SaO$_2$ = blood oxygen saturation

In summary, findings suggest that SDB is associated with lower cognitive function in multiple domains and may contribute to the risk of cognitive impairment. However, findings have been inconsistent across studies, and mixed findings in particular cognitive domains have emerged within individual studies. Additional prospective research is needed to more clearly understand the impact of SDB on specific cognitive domains and the mechanisms linking SDB to cognitive performance, particularly in the general population of community-dwelling older people.

Circadian Rhythm Disturbances and Cognition

Patterns of sleep and wake, and many other behavioral and physiological processes, follow a circadian pattern (i.e., approximately 24-hour cycle). Normal aging is associated with a circadian phase advance; older adults tend to go to sleep earlier and awaken earlier than younger people (Czeisler et al., 1992; Duffy et al., 1998). Older adults also demonstrate a decreased circadian rhythm amplitude (Weitzman et al., 1982), which can result in sleep complaints. One explanation for changes in sleep/wake patterns in the context of normal aging includes age-related cell loss in the suprachiasmatic nucleus (SCN; Swaab et al., 1985), the circadian pacemaker in the anterior hypothalamus (Richardson, 2005). In addition, studies examining levels of light exposure in adult populations have found that the intensity and amount of light exposure are lower in older adults than in younger adults. As light is the strongest cue for strong, synchronized circadian rhythms, and the mechanism of the light is through the eyes via the retinohypothalamic tract, older adults—and especially those with cataracts—are more likely to have decreased light exposure and more desynchronized or misaligned rhythms.

Relatively few studies have investigated the association of circadian rhythms and cognition in the general population of older adults. In a study of 144 older adults, greater rest/activity rhythm fragmentation was associated with lower performance on cognitive tests (Oosterman et al., 2009). Similarly, a study of more than 1,200 older women found that those with weaker activity rhythms or delayed rhythms had a higher likelihood of developing dementia or MCI when compared to those with stronger rhythms or non-delayed phases (Tranah et al., 2011).

It has been suggested that disrupted circadian rest/activity rhythms may play a causal role in incident dementia or may be a marker of a neurodegenerative process and that trials aimed at impacting these rhythms may be needed to determine which is the case (Lim & Saper, 2011). Naylor et al. (2000) found that a social and physical activity intervention increased both slow wave sleep at night and daytime memory performance in a group of older adults.. In a follow-up study, Benloucif et al. (2004) found that morning or evening activity significantly improved both subjective sleep and performance on a neuropsychological battery. These studies, however, were both small, and larger trials are needed to determine if physical activity might improve rhythms and cognitive outcomes.

Restless Legs Syndrome, Periodic Limb Movements in Sleep, and Cognition

Restless legs syndrome (RLS) is characterized by unpleasant sensations in and urges to move the legs that increase while the individual is inactive or at rest, become more severe in the evening, and are relieved by movement (Allen et al., 2003). Restless legs syndrome can interfere significantly with sleep onset. The syndrome is diagnosed on the basis of a clinical interview. Although prevalence estimates differ based on the assessment methods utilized in epidemiologic surveys, between 5% and approximately 9% of the general population of adults can reasonably be estimated to have RLS (Ohayon et al., 2011). The prevalence of RLS is higher in older adults in North American and European populations, but this does not appear to be the case in Asian populations (Ohayon et al., 2011).

Little is currently known about the cognitive correlates of RLS, and most of what is known derives from mixed-aged samples. Patients with RLS have been shown to demonstrate deficits in attention and executive function (Pearson et al., 2006; Fulda et al., 2010). However, a comparison of cognitive performance between patients with RLS and sleep-deprived individuals without RLS found that patients with RLS performed better than controls on tests of executive function and might therefore have adapted to sleep loss (Gamaldo et al., 2008). A study in older adults found that elders with RLS demonstrated relative deficits in executive function when compared to those without RLS (Celle et al., 2010).

In a related area, periodic limb movements in sleep (PLMS) are leg jerks that occur during sleep and often lead to sleep fragmentation. Although RLS and PLMS are separate disorders, most individuals with RLS have an elevated number of PLMS (Allen & Earley, 2001). Unlike RLS, which is assessed through a clinical interview, PLMS are measured using PSG and are commonly quantified using a PLM index (PLMI; mean number of PLMS per hour of sleep), with values of 5 or greater considered elevated. Elevated levels of PLMS are very common among older adults. It is estimated that 45% to approximately 65% of community-dwelling elders have a PLMI of 5 or greater (Ancoli-Israel et al., 1991c; Claman et al., 2006). Currently, we are unaware of any studies that have focused on cognitive correlates of PLMS in older or younger adults.

Sleep Disorders Among Cohorts With Dementia and Mild Cognitive Impairment

A substantial proportion of our knowledge regarding sleep and cognition in older adults comes from studies of sleep disturbances in older adults with dementia. Compared to normal older adults, those with dementia exhibit greater sleep fragmentation (Prinz et al., 1982; Vitiello, 1990). One study found that demented patients in nursing homes are rarely asleep for a full hour and rarely awake for a full hour, suffering from fragmentation of both sleep and wake (Pat-Horenczyk et al., 1998). Family caregivers of older adults with dementia find sleep disturbance particularly hard to tolerate (Sanford, 1975; Pollak & Perlick, 1991) and poor sleep has been identified as a risk factor for nursing home placement in elders with AD (Bianchetti et al., 1995). In an extension of existing research on sleep in dementia, studies have begun to focus on sleep disruption in older adults with MCI (Beaulieu-Bonneau & Hudon, 2009). In one such study, sleep fragmentation was linked to lower executive function and worse memory performance (Naismith et al., 2010), although another study found fewer associations between sleep fragmentation and cognition in this population (Kim et al., 2011). In nursing home residents with cognitive impairment, greater sleep fragmentation and longer objectively measured sleep duration have been linked to lower performance on a measure of general cognitive function (Cole et al., 2009).

Early research on SDB and cognition in older adults focused on the elevated prevalence of SDB among elders with dementia (Ancoli-Israel et al., 1991a; Hoch et al., 1986; Mant et al., 1988). Hoch et al. (1986) found that an apnea index of 5 or greater was more common among older adults with Alzheimer's disease (AD) (42%) than among healthy elders (5%), elders with depression (14%), or a group with mixed depression and cognitive impairment (17%). In a study of nursing home residents, Ancoli-Israel et al. (1991a) found that those with more severe dementia had more severe SDB.

Among older adults with AD, CPAP therapy might produce improvements in multiple cognitive domains, including executive function and memory (Ancoli-Israel et al., 2008). In addition, preliminary findings suggest that long-term use of CPAP may slow the deterioration seen in cognitive function (Cooke et al., 2009). Randomized trials in larger samples of older adults with cognitive impairment are needed to more definitively determine whether CPAP therapy improves cognition in this population.

Relative to healthy older adults, those with dementia exhibit disrupted circadian rhythms. Their sleep/wake rhythm is more fragmented than that of healthy elders, with elevated levels of nocturnal wakefulness and sleep fragmentation and more time spent sleeping during the day (Prinz et al. 1982). The degree of disturbance in rest/activity rhythms (i.e., blunting of rhythm, irregularity) appears to be positively associated with the severity of cognitive impairment (Ancoli-Israel et al., 1997; Witting et al., 1990). Older adults with dementia also have been found to exhibit a phase delay (rather than the expected phase advance) relative to normal elders (Harper et al., 2005), and among nursing home residents, dementia severity has been linked to a greater phase delay (Ancoli-Israel et al., 1997).

The disruption of circadian rhythms observed in older adults with dementia has been attributed to a particularly pronounced loss of SCN volume in this population, compared to that observed in normal elders (Swaab et al., 1985). In addition, institutionalized patients with dementia commonly are exposed to low levels of light. Shochat et al. (2000) studied 66 institutionalized adults, most of whom had dementia, and showed that the median light level was only 52 lux with a median of less than 11 minutes over 1000 lux. In this observational study, higher light levels were associated with fewer awakenings at night, and residents with higher light exposure demonstrated a later peak of activity, suggesting that daytime light exposure affects noctural sleep consolidation and circadian rest/activity rhythms (Shochat et al.).

Evidence suggests that bright light therapy exposure might improve sleep (Sloane et al., 2007) and circadian rhythms (Van Someren et al., 1997, 1999) in older adults with dementia who are institutionalized. Riemersma-van der Lek et al. (2008) found that long-term care residents who were continuously exposed to increased bright light showed improved sleep and less of a decline on the MMSE. Melatonin had some positive effects on sleep but also had some negative effects on mood and behavior; the mood effect was attenuated when melatonin was combined with light (Riemersma-van der Lek et al., 2008).

Summary and Conclusion

Sleep disturbances are common in older adults, as is cognitive impairment. Although findings are mixed, a growing number of studies suggest that short and long sleep duration (as opposed to more intermediate durations), sleep fragmentation, and SDB are associated with cognitive dysfunction in older people and that these disturbances may predict and be causally related to cognitive decline. Although circadian rhythm disruption is pronounced in older adults with dementia, further research is needed to determine the extent to which circadian rhythm disturbances in the general population of older adults predict adverse cognitive outcomes. Similarly, relatively little is known about the association of RLS or PLMS with cognitive performance in older adults.

The evidence supporting an association between late-life sleep disturbance and cognitive impairment or decline among elders raises the critical question of whether treating poor sleep—or preventing the deterioration of good sleep—in older adults would reduce or perhaps even prevent adverse cognitive outcomes in this population. To date, there have been very few studies examining whether treating sleep disturbances in later life has an impact on cognitive function or cognitive trajectories. Those studies that have examined treatments suggest that increased light (Riemersma-van der Lek et al., 2008), increased physical activity (Benloucif et al. 2004; Naylor et al., 2000), and treating SDB (Ancoli-Israel et al., 2008; Cooke et al., 2009) might all have a positive effect on cognitive function. Ironically, we know especially little about the impact of treating insomnia—the most common sleep disturbance in older adults—on cognitive outcomes in elders. Indeed, additional trials of interventions for sleep disorders are needed to determine whether treating disturbed sleep reduces or prevents cognitive decline and to more fully understand whether the association between sleep disturbances and cognitive dysfunction is, in fact, causal. The results of such research could have significant implications for the maintenance of cognitive health, independence, and quality of life within the growing U.S. population of older adults.

References

Alapin, I., C. S. Fichten, E. Libman, L. Creti, S. Bailes, & J. Wright. How Is Good and Poor Sleep in Older Adults and College Students Related to Daytime Sleepiness, Fatigue, and Ability to Concentrate? *J Psychosom Res 49*, no. 5 (2000): 381–390.

Allen, R. P., & C. J. Earley. Restless Legs Syndrome: A Review of Clinical and Pathophysiologic Features. *J Clin Neurophysiol 18*, no. 2 (2001): 128–147.

Allen, R. P., D. Picchietti, W. A. Hening, C. Trenkwalder, A. S. Walters, & J. Montplaisi. Restless Legs Syndrome: Diagnostic Criteria, Special Considerations, and Epidemiology. A Report from the Restless Legs Syndrome Diagnosis and Epidemiology Workshop at the National Institutes of Health. *Sleep Med 4*, no. 2 (2003): 101–119.

Aloia, M. S., J. T. Arnedt, J. D. Davis, R. L. Riggs, & D. Byrd. Neuropsychological Sequelae of Obstructive Sleep Apnea-Hypopnea Syndrome: A Critical Review. *Journal of the International Neuropsychological Society 10*, no. 5 (2004): 772–785.

Aloia, M. S., N. Ilniczky, P. Di Dio, M. L. Perlis, D. W. Greenblatt, & D. E. Giles. "Neuropsychological Changes and Treatment Compliance in Older Adults with Sleep Apnea." *J Psychosom Res 54*, no. 1 (2003): 71–76.

American Academy of Sleep Medicine. ICSD-2 – International Classification of Sleep Disorders, 2nd Ed.: Diagnostic and Coding Manual. Westchester, IL: *American Academy of Sleep Medicine*, (2005).

American Psychiatric Association. Diagnostic and Statistical Manual of Mental Disorders: DSM-IV-TR. 4th ed. Washington, DC: American Psychiatric Association, (2000)

Ancoli-Israel, S., R. Cole, C. Alessi, M. Chambers, W. Moorcroft, & C. P. Pollak. The Role of Actigraphy in the Study of Sleep and Circadian Rhythms. *Sleep 26*, no. 3 (2003): 342–392.

Ancoli-Israel, S., & J. R. Cooke. "Prevalence and Comorbidity of Insomnia and Effect on Functioning in Elderly Populations." *J Am Geriatr Soc 53*, no. 7 Suppl (2005): S264–S271.

Ancoli-Israel, S., M. R. Klauber, N. Butters, L. Parker, & D. F. Kripke. Dementia in Institutionalized Elderly: Relation to Sleep Apnea. *J Am Geriatr Soc 39*, no. 3 (1991a): 258–263.

Ancoli-Israel, S., M. R. Klauber, D. W. Jones, D. F. Kripke, J. Martin, W. Mason, et al. Variations in Circadian Rhythms of Activity, Sleep, and Light Exposure Related to Dementia in Nursing-Home Patients. *Sleep 20*, no. 1 (1997): 18–23.

Ancoli-Israel, S., D. F. Kripke, M. R. Klauber, W. J. Mason, R. Fell, & O. Kaplan. Sleep-Disordered Breathing in Community-Dwelling Elderly. *Sleep 14*, no. 6 (1991b): 486–495.

Ancoli-Israel, S., D. F. Kripke, M. R. Klauber, W. J. Mason, R. Fell, & O. Kaplan. Periodic Limb Movements in Sleep in Community-Dwelling Elderly. *Sleep, 14*, no. 6 (1991c): 496–500.

Ancoli-Israel, S., B. W. Palmer, J. R. Cooke, J. Corey-Bloom, L. Fiorentino, L. Natarajan, et al. Cognitive effects of treating obstructive sleep apnea in Alzheimer's disease: a randomized controlled study. *J Am Geriatr Soc no. 56*, no. 11 (2008): 2076–2081.

Bastien, C. H., E. Fortier-Brochu, I. Rioux, M. LeBlanc, M. Daley, & C. M. Morin. Cognitive Performance and Sleep Quality in the Elderly Suffering from Chronic Insomnia. Relationship between Objective and Subjective Measures. *J Psychosom Res 54*, no. 1 (2003): 39–49.

Beaulieu-Bonneau, S., & C. Hudon. Sleep Disturbances in Older Adults with Mild Cognitive Impairment. *Int Psychogeriatr 21*, no. 4 (2009): 654–666.

Beebe, D. W., L. Groesz, C. Wells, A. Nichols, & K. McGee. The Neuropsychological Effects of Obstructive Sleep Apnea: A Meta-Analysis of Norm-Referenced and Case-Controlled Data. *Sleep 26*, no. 3 (2003): 298–307.

Benloucif, S., L. Orbeta, R. Ortiz, I. Janssen, S. I. Finkel, J. Bleiberg, et al. "Morning or Evening Activity Improves Neuropsychological Performance and Subjective Sleep Quality in Older Adults." *Sleep 27*, no. 8 (2004): 1542–1551.

Berry, D. T., B. A. Phillips, Y. R. Cook, F. A. Schmitt, N. A. Honeycutt, A. A. Arita, et al. Geriatric Sleep Apnea Syndrome: A Preliminary Description. [In eng]. *J Gerontol 45*, no. 5 (1990): M169–M174.

Berry, D. T., B. A. Phillips, Y. R. Cook, F. A. Schmitt, R. L. Gilmore, R. Patel, et al. Sleep-Disordered Breathing in Healthy Aged Persons: Possible Daytime Sequelae. *J Gerontol 42*, no. 6 (1987): 620–626.

Bianchetti, A., A. Scuratti, O. Zanetti, G. Binetti, G.B. Frisoni, E. Magni, et al. Predictors of Mortality and Institutionalization in Alzheimer Disease Patients 1 Year after Discharge from an Alzheimer Dementia Unit. *Dementia 6*, no. 2 (1995): 108–112.

Blackwell, T., K. Yaffe, S. Ancoli-Israel, S. Redline, K. E. Ensrud, M. L. Stefanick, et al. Association of Sleep Characteristics and Cognition in Older Community-Dwelling Men: The Mros Sleep Study." *Sleep 34*, no. 10 (2011): 1347–1356.

Blackwell, T., K. Yaffe, S. Ancoli-Israel, S. Redline, K. E. Ensrud, M. L. Stefanick, et al. Associations between Sleep Architecture and Sleep-Disordered Breathing and Cognition in Older Community-Dwelling Men: The Osteoporotic Fractures in Men Sleep Study. *J Am Geriatr Soc 59*, no. 12 (2011): 2217–2225.

Blackwell, T., K. Yaffe, S. Ancoli-Israel, J. L. Schneider, J. A. Cauley, T. A. Hillier, et al. Poor Sleep Is Associated with Impaired Cognitive Function in Older Women: The Study of Osteoporotic Fractures. *The Journals of Gerontology: Series A: Biological Sciences and Medical Sciences 61A*, no. 4 (2006): 405–410.

Buysse, D. J., C. F. Reynolds, T. H. Monk, S. R. Berman, & Kupfer, D.J. The Pittsburgh Sleep Quality Index: A New Instrument for Psychiatric Practice and Research. *Psychiatry Research 28*, no. 2 (1989): 193–213.

Celle, S., F. Roche, J. Kerleroux, C. Thomas-Anterion, B. Laurent, I. Rouch, et al. Prevalence and Clinical Correlates of Restless Legs Syndrome in an Elderly French Population: The Synapse Study. *The Journals of Gerontology. Series A, Biological sciences and medical sciences 65*, no. 2 (2010): 167–173.

Claman, D.M., S Redline, T. L. Blackwell, S. Ancoli-Israel, S. Surovec, N. Scott, et al. Prevalence and Correlates of Periodic Limb Movements in Older Women. *JCSM 2*, no. 4 (2006): 438–445.

Cohen-Zion, M., C. Stepnowsky, S. Johnson, M. Marler, J. E. Dimsdale, & S. Ancoli-Israel. Cognitive Changes and Sleep Disordered Breathing in Elderly: Differences in Race. *J Psychosom Res 56*, no. 5 (2004): 549–553.

Cohen-Zion, M, C Stepnowsky, M. R. Marler, T. Shochat, D. F. Kripke, & S. Ancoli-Israel. Changes in Cognitive Function Associated with Sleep Disordered Breathing in Older People. *J Am Geriatr Soc 49*, no. 12 (2001): 1622–1627.

Cole, C. S., K. C. Richards, C. C. Beck, P. K. Roberson, C. Lambert, A. Furnish, et al. Relationships among Disordered Sleep and Cognitive and Functional Status in Nursing Home Residents. *Res Gerontol Nurs 2*, no. 3 (2009): 183–191.

Cooke, J. R., L. Ayalon, B. W. Palmer, J. S. Loredo, J. Corey-Bloom, L. Natarajan, et al. Sustained Use of Cpap Slows Deterioration of Cognition, Sleep, and Mood in Patients with Alzheimer's Disease and Obstructive Sleep Apnea: A Preliminary Study. *Journal of clinical sleep medicine 5*, no. 4 (2009): 305–309.

Cricco, M., E. M. Simonsick, & D. J. Foley. The Impact of Insomnia on Cognitive Functioning in Older Adults. *Journal of the American Geriatrics Society 49*, no. 9 (2001): 1185–1189.

Czeisler, C. A., M. Dumont, J. F. Duffy, J. D. Steinberg, G. S. Richardson, E. N. Brown, et al. Association of Sleep-Wake Habits in Older People with Changes in Output of Circadian Pacemaker. *Lancet 340*, no. 8825 (1992): 933–936.

Duffy, J. F., D. J. Dijk, E. B. Klerman, & C. A. Czeisler. Later Endogenous Circadian Temperature Nadir Relative to an Earlier Wake Time in Older People. *Am J Physiol 275*, no. 5 Pt 2 (Nov 1998): R1478–R1487.

Engleman, H. M., R. N. Kingshott, S. E. Martin, & N. J. Douglas. Cognitive Function in the Sleep Apnea/Hypopnea Syndrome (Sahs). *Sleep 23* Suppl 4 (2000): S102–S108.

Faubel, R., E. Lopez-Garcia, P. Guallar-Castillon, A. Graciani, J. R. Banegas, & F. Rodriguez-Artalejo. Usual Sleep Duration and Cognitive Function in Older Adults in Spain. *J Sleep Res 18*, no. 4 (2009): 427–435.

Foley, D. J., A. A. Monjan, S. L. Brown, E. M. Simonsick, R. B. Wallace, & D. G. Blazer. Sleep Complaints among Elderly Persons: An Epidemiologic Study of Three Communities. *Sleep 18*, no. 6 (1995): 425–432.

Foley, D. J., K. Masaki, L. White, E. K. Larkin, A Monjan, & S. Redline. Sleep-Disordered Breathing and Cognitive Impairment in Elderly Japanese-American Men. *Sleep 26*, no. 5 (2003): 596–599.

Frisoni, G. B., D. De Leo, R. Rozzini, & M. Bernardini. Psychic Correlates of Sleep Symptoms in the Elderly. *International Journal of Geriatric Psychiatry 7*, no. 12 (1992): 891–898.

Fulda, S., M. E. Beitinger, S. Reppermund, J. Winkelmann, & T. C. Wetter. Short-Term Attention and Verbal Fluency Is Decreased in Restless Legs Syndrome Patients. *Movement disorders: official journal of the Movement Disorder Society 25*, no. 15 (2010): 2641–2648.

Gamaldo, C. E., A. R. Benbrook, R. P. Allen, O. Oguntimein, & C. J. Earley. A Further Evaluation of the Cognitive Deficits Associated with Restless Legs Syndrome (RLS). *Sleep Med 9*, no. 5 (2008): 500–505.

Ganguli, M., C. F. Reynolds, & J. E. Gilby. Prevalence and Persistence of Sleep Complaints in a Rural Older Community Sample: The Movies Project. *J Am Geriatr Soc 44*, no. 7 (1996): 778–784.

Haimov, I. Association Between Memory Impairment and Insomnia Among Older Adults. *European Journal of Aging 3* (2006): 107–115.

Haimov, I., E. Hanuka, & Y. Horowitz. Chronic Insomnia and Cognitive Functioning among Older Adults. [In eng]. *Behav Sleep Med 6*, no. 1 (2008): 32–54.

Harper, D. G., L. Volicer, E. G. Stopa, A. C. McKee, M. Nitta, & A. Satlin. Disturbance of Endogenous Circadian Rhythm in Aging and Alzheimer Disease. *Am J Geriatr Psychiatry 13*, no. 5 (May 2005): 359–368.

Hart, R. P., C. M. Morin, & A. M. Best. Neuropsychological Performance in Elderly Insomnia Patients. *Aging Cognit 2*, no. 4 (1995): 268–278.

Hoch, C. C., C. F. Reynolds, D. J. Kupfer, P. R. Houck, S.R. Berman, & J.A. Stack. Sleep-Disordered Breathing in Normal and Pathologic Aging. *Journal of Clinical Psychiatry 47*, no. 10 (1986): 499–503.

Hoch, C. C., C. F. Reynolds, 3rd, R. D. Nebes, D. J. Kupfer, S. R. Berman, & D. Campbell. Clinical Significance of Sleep-Disordered Breathing in Alzheimer's Disease. Preliminary Data. *J Am Geriatr Soc 37*, no. 2 (1989): 138–144.

Iber, C., S. Ancoli-Israel, A. Chesson, & S. F. Quan for the American Academy of Sleep Medicine. *The AASM Manual for the Scoring of Sleep and Associated Events: Rules, Terminology, and Technical Specifications.* 1st ed. Westchester, Illinois: American Academy of Sleep Medicine, 2007.

Jelicic, M., H. Bosma, R. W. Ponds, M. P. Van Boxtel, P. J. Houx, & J. Jolles. Subjective Sleep Problems in Later Life as Predictors of Cognitive Decline. Report from the Maastricht Ageing Study (Maas). *Int J Geriatr Psychiatry 17*, no. 1 (2002): 73–77.

Jorm, A. F., & D. Jolley. The Incidence of Dementia: A Meta-Analysis. *Neurology 51*, no. 3 (1998): 728–733.

Kang, J. E., M. M. Lim, R. J. Bateman, J. J. Lee, L. P. Smyth, J. R. Cirrito, et al. Amyloid-Beta Dynamics Are Regulated by Orexin and the Sleep-Wake Cycle. *Science 326*, no. 5955 (2009): 1005–1007.

Kim, S. J., J. H. Lee, D. Y. Lee, J. H. Jhoo, & J. I. Woo. Neurocognitive Dysfunction Associated with Sleep Quality and Sleep Apnea in Patients with Mild Cognitive Impairment. *The American Journal of Geriatric Psychiatry 19*, no. 4 (2011): 374–381.

Knight, H., R. P. Millman, R. C. Gur, A. J. Saykin, J. U. Doherty, & A. I. Pack. Clinical Significance of Sleep Apnea in the Elderly. *Am Rev Respir Dis 136*, no. 4 (1987): 845–850.

Lichstein, K. L., H. H. Durrence, B. W. Riedel, D. J. Taylor, & A. J. Bush. *Epidemiology of sleep: Age, gender, and ethnicity*. Mahwah, New Jersey: Lawrence Erlbaum Associates, 2004.

Lim, A. S., & C. B. Saper. Sleep, Circadian Rhythms, and Dementia. *Ann Neurol 70*, no. 5 (2011): 677–679.

Loerbroks, A., D. Debling, M. Amelang, & T. Sturmer. Nocturnal Sleep Duration and Cognitive Impairment in a Population-Based Study of Older Adults. *Int J Geriatr Psychiatry 25*, no. 1 (2010): 100–109.

Maggi, S., J. A. Langlois, N. Minicuci, F. Grigoletto, M. Pavan, D. J. Foley, et al. Sleep Complaints in Community-Dwelling Older Persons: Prevalence, Associated Factors, and Reported Causes. *J Am Geriatr Soc 46*, no. 2 (1998): 161–168.

Mant, A., N. A. Saunders, A. E. Eyland, C. D. Pond, A. H. Chancellor, & I. W. Webster. Sleep-Related Respiratory Disturbance and Dementia in Elderly Females. *J Gerontol 43*, no. 5 (Sep 1988): M140–M144.

Mehra, R., K. L. Stone, T. Blackwell, S. Ancoli-Israel, T-T L. Dam, M. L. Stefanick, et al. Prevalence and correlates of sleep-disordered breathing in older men: Osteoporotic Fractures in Men Sleep Study. *Journal of the American Geriatrics Society* no. 55 (2007):1356–1364.

Mellinger, G. D., M. B. Balter, & E. H. Uhlenhuth. Insomnia and Its Treatment: Prevalence and Correlates. *Archives of General Psychiatry 42*, no. 3 (1985): 225–232.

Moldofsky, H., R. Goldstein, W. T. McNicholas, F. Lue, N. Zamel, & E. A. Phillipson. 1983. Disordered breathing during sleep and overnight deterioration in patients with pathological aging. In C. Guilleminault & E. Lugaresi (eds.). *Sleep/Wake Disorders: Natural History, Epidemiology, and Long-Term Evaluation*, . New York: Raven Press.

Naismith, S. L., N. L. Rogers, I. B. Hickie, J. Mackenzie, L. M. Norrie, & S. J. Lewis. Sleep Well, Think Well: Sleep-Wake Disturbance in Mild Cognitive Impairment. *J Geriatr Psychiatry Neurol 23*, no. 2 (2010): 123–130.

Naylor, E., P. D. Penev, L. Orbeta, I. Janssen, R. Ortiz, E. F. Colecchia, et al. Daily Social and Physical Activity Increases Slow-Wave Sleep and Daytime Neuropsychological Performance in the Elderly. *Sleep 23*, no. 1 (2000): 87–95.

Nebes, R. D., D. J. Buysse, E. M. Halligan, P. R. Houck, & T. H. Monk. Self-Reported Sleep Quality Predicts Poor Cognitive Performance in Healthy Older Adults. *J Gerontol B Psychol Sci Soc Sci 64*, no. 2 (2009): 180–187.

O'Hara, R., C.M Schroeder, H.C. Kraemer, N. Kryla, C. Cao, E. Miller, et al. 2005. Nocturnal sleep apnea/hypopnea is associated with lower memory performance in APOE ε4 carriers. *Neurology* no. 65:642–644.

Ohayon, M. M., M. A. Carskadon, C. Guilleminault, & M. V. Vitiello. Meta-Analysis of Quantitative Sleep Parameters from Childhood to Old Age in Healthy Individuals: Developing Normative Sleep Values across the Human Lifespan. *Sleep 27*, no. 7 (2004): 1255–1273.

Ohayon, M. M., R. O'Hara, & M. V. Vitiello. Epidemiology of restless legs syndrome: A synthesis of the literature. *Sleep Med Rev 16*, no. 4 (2012): 283–295.

Ohayon, Maurice M., & M-F Vecchierini. Daytime Sleepiness and Cognitive Impairment in the Elderly Population. *Arch Intern Med 162* (2002): 201–208.

Ohayon, M. M., & M. F. Vecchierini. Normative Sleep Data, Cognitive Function and Daily Living Activities in Older Adults in the Community. *Sleep 28*, no. 8 (2005): 981–989.

Oosterman, J. M., E. J. van Someren, R. L. Vogels, B. Van Harten, & E. J. Scherder. Fragmentation of the Rest-Activity Rhythm Correlates with Age-Related Cognitive Deficits. *J Sleep Res 18*, no. 1 (2009): 129–135.

Pat-Horenczyk, R., M. R. Klauber, T. Shochat, & S. Ancoli-Israel. Hourly Profiles of Sleep and Wakefulness in Severely Versus Mild-Moderately Demented Nursing Home Patients. *Aging (Milano) 10*, no. 4 (1998): 308–315.

Pearson, V. E., R. P. Allen, T. Dean, C. E. Gamaldo, S. R. Lesage, & C. J. Earley. Cognitive Deficits Associated with Restless Legs Syndrome (Rls). *Sleep Med 7*, no. 1 (2006): 25–30.

Plassman, B. L., K. M. Langa, G. G. Fisher, S. G. Heeringa, D. R. Weir, M. B. Ofstedal, et al. Prevalence of Cognitive Impairment without Dementia in the United States. *Ann Intern Med 148*, no. 6 (2008): 427–434.

Plassman, B. L., K. M. Langa, G. G. Fisher, S. G. Heeringa, D. R. Weir, M. B. Ofstedal, et al. Prevalence of Dementia in the United States: The Aging, Demographics, and Memory Study. *Neuroepidemiology 29*, no. 1-2 (2007): 125–132.

Pollak, Charles P., & Deborah Perlick. Sleep Problems and Institutionalization of the Elderly. *Journal of Geriatric Psychiatry & Neurology 4*, no. 4 (1991): 204–210.

Prinz, P. N., E. R. Peskind, P. P. Vitaliano, M. A. Raskind, C. Eisdorfer, N. Zemcuznikov, et al. Changes in the Sleep and Waking Eegs of Nondemented and Demented Elderly Subjects. *J Am Geriatr Soc 30*, no. 2 (1982): 86–93.

Richardson, G. S. The Human Circadian System in Normal and Disordered Sleep. *The Journal of Clinical Psychiatry 66* (Suppl 9) (2005): 3–9.

Riemann, D., U. Voderholzer, K. Spiegelhalder, M. Hornyak, D. J. Buysse, C. Nissen, et al. Chronic Insomnia and Mri-Measured Hippocampal Volumes: A Pilot Study. *Sleep 30*, no. 8 (2007): 955–958.

Riemersma-van der Lek, R. F., D. F. Swaab, J. Twisk, E. M. Hol, W. J. Hoogendijk, & E. J. Van Someren. Effect of Bright Light and Melatonin on Cognitive and Noncognitive Function in Elderly Residents of Group Care Facilities: A Randomized Controlled Trial. *JAMA 299*, no. 22 (2008): 2642–2655.

Ritchie, K., D. Kildea, & J. M. Robine. The Relationship between Age and the Prevalence of Senile Dementia: A Meta-Analysis of Recent Data. *International Journal of Epidemiology 21*, no. 4 (1992): 763–769.

Sanchez, A. I., P. Martinez, E. Miro, W. A. Bardwell, & G. Buela-Casal. Cpap and Behavioral Therapies in Patients with Obstructive Sleep Apnea: Effects on Daytime Sleepiness, Mood, and Cognitive Function. *Sleep Medicine Reviews 13*, no. 3 (2009): 223–233.

Sanford, JRA. Tolerance of Debility in Elderly Dependants by Supporters at Home: Its Significance for Hospital Practice. *British Medical Journal 3* (1975): 471–473.

Schmutte, T., S. Harris, R. Levin, R. Zweig, M. Katz, & R. Lipton. The Relation between Cognitive Functioning and Self-Reported Sleep Complaints in Nondemented Older Adults: Results from the Bronx Aging Study. *Behavioral Sleep Medicine 5*, no. 1 (2007): 39–56.

Sforza, E., F. Roche, C. Thomas-Anterion, J. Kerleroux, O. Beauchet, S. Celle, et al. Cognitive Function and Sleep Related Breathing Disorders in a Healthy Elderly Population: The Synapse Study. *Sleep 33*, no. 4 (2010): 515–521.

Shochat, T., J. Martin, M. Marler, & S. Ancoli-Israel. Illumination Levels in Nursing Home Patients: Effects on Sleep and Activity Rhythms. *Journal of Sleep Research 9*, no. 4 (2000): 373–379.

Sloane, P. D., C. S. Williams, C. M. Mitchell, J. S. Preisser, W. Wood, A. L. Barrick, et al. High-Intensity Environmental Light in Dementia: Effect on Sleep and Activity. *J Am Geriatr Soc 55*, no. 10 (2007): 1524–1533.

Spira, A. P., T. Blackwell, K. L. Stone, S. Redline, J. A. Cauley, S. Ancoli-Israel, et al. Sleep Disordered Breathing and Cognition in Community-Dwelling Older Women. *J Am Geriatr Soc 56* (2008): 45–50.

Stone, J., C. M. Morin, R. P. Hart, S. Remsberg, & J. Mercer. Neuropsychological Functioning in Older Insomniacs with or without Obstructive Sleep Apnea. *Psychol Aging 9*, no. 2 (1994): 231–236.

Swaab, D. F., E. Fliers, & T. S. Partiman. The Suprachiasmatic Nucleus of the Human Brain in Relation to Sex, Age and Senile Dementia. *Brain Research 342*, no. 1 (1985): 37–44.

Tranah, G. J., T. Blackwell, K. L. Stone, S. Ancoli-Israel, M. L. Paudel, K. E. Ensrud, et al. Circadian Activity Rhythms and Risk of Incident Dementia and Mild Cognitive Impairment in Older Women. *Ann Neurol 70*, no. 5 (2011): 722–732.

Tworoger, S. S., S. Lee, E. S. Schernhammer, & F. Grodstein. The Association of Self-Reported Sleep Duration, Difficulty Sleeping, and Snoring with Cognitive Function in Older Women. *Alzheimer Dis Assoc Disord 20*, no. 1 (2006): 41–48.

Van Den Berg, J. F., F. J. Van Rooij, H. Vos, J. H. Tulen, A. Hofman, H. M. Miedema, et al. Disagreement between Subjective and Actigraphic Measures of Sleep Duration in a Population-Based Study of Elderly Persons. *J Sleep Res 17*, no. 3 (2008): 295–302.

Van Someren, E. J., A. Kessler, M. Mirmiran, & D. F. Swaab. Indirect Bright Light Improves Circadian Rest-Activity Rhythm Disturbances in Demented Patients. *Biol Psychiatry 41*, no. 9 (1997): 955–963.

Van Someren, E. J., D. F. Swaab, C. C. Colenda, W. Cohen, W. V. McCall, & P. B. Rosenquist. Bright Light Therapy: Improved Sensitivity to Its Effects on Rest-Activity Rhythms in Alzheimer Patients by Application of Nonparametric Methods. *Chronobiol Int 16*, no. 4 (1999): 505–518.

Vignola, A., C. Lamoureux, C. H. Bastien, & C. M. Morin. Effects of Chronic Insomnia and Use of Benzodiazepines on Daytime Performance in Older Adults. *J Gerontol B Psychol Sci Soc Sci 55*, no. 1 (2000): P54–P62.

Vitiello, M.. Sleep in Normal Aging. *Sleep Medicine Clinics* no. *1* (2) (2006): 171–176.

Vitiello, M. V., P. N. Prinz, D. E. Williams, M. S. Frommlet, & R. K. Ries. Sleep Disturbances in Patients with Mild-Stage Alzheimer's Disease. *J Gerontol 45*, no. 4 (1990): M131–M138.

Weitzman, E. D., M. L. Moline, C. A. Czeisler, & J. C. Zimmerman. Chronobiology of Aging: Temperature, Sleep-Wake Rhythms and Entrainment. *Neurobiology of Aging 3*, no. 4 (1982): 299–309.

Wellman, A., & D. P. White. Central Sleep Apnea and Periodic Breathing. (2011). In M. H. Sanders (ed.). *Principles and Practice of Sleep Medicine* (pp. 1140–1152). St. Louis, MO: Elsevier.

Witting, W., I. H. Kwa, P. Eikelenboom, M. Mirmiran, & D. F. Swaab. Alterations in the Circadian Rest-Activity Rhythm in Aging and Alzheimer's Disease. *Biol Psychiatry 27*, no. 6 (1990): 563–572.

Yaffe, K., T. Blackwell, D. E. Barnes, S. Ancoli-Israel, & K. L. Stone. Preclinical Cognitive Decline and Subsequent Sleep Disturbance in Older Women. *Neurology 69*, no. 3 (2007): 237–242.

Yaffe, K., A. M. Laffan, S. L. Harrison, S. Redline, A. P. Spira, K. E. Ensrud, et al. Sleep-Disordered Breathing, Hypoxia, and Risk of Mild Cognitive Impairment and Dementia in Older Women. *JAMA 306*, no. 6 (2011): 613–619.

Yaffe, K., L. E. Middleton, L. Y. Lui, A. P. Spira, K. Stone, C. Racine, et al. Mild Cognitive Impairment, Dementia, and Their Subtypes in Oldest Old Women. [In eng]. *Archives of Neurology 68*, no. 5 (2011): 631–636.

Yesavage, J., D. Bliwise, C. Guilleminault, M. Carskadon, & W. Dement. Preliminary Communication: Intellectual Deficit and Sleep-Related Respiratory Disturbance in the Elderly. *Sleep 8*, no. 1 (1985): 30–33.

Young, T., M. Palta, J. Dempsey, J. Skatrud, S. Weber, & S. Badr. The Occurrence of Sleep-Disordered Breathing among Middle-Aged Adults. *N Engl J Med 328*, no. 17 (1993): 1230–1235.

9

Physical Activity and Cognitive Aging

DEBORAH E. BARNES, PHD, MPM AND

NICOLA T. LAUTENSCHLAGER, MD

Introduction

There is growing recognition that physical activity has beneficial effects on the brain as well as the body. In this chapter, we provide an overview of the effects of physical activity on the body and the brain, including summaries of evidence from both observational studies and randomized, controlled trials (RCTs), and we also discuss the hypothesized mechanisms by which physical activity may promote brain health and reduce the risk of dementia. We conclude that although the evidence is not definitive, physical activity is likely to enhance brain function through multiple interrelated mechanisms. Research is critically needed to identify the optimal frequency and type of physical activity for maintaining cognitive function and to develop successful strategies for motivating adults, particularly older adults, to engage in regular physical activity.

Physical Activity and the Body

Physical activity is widely accepted as an important component of health and longevity worldwide. In this section, we briefly review the history and definitions of physical activity and then summarize the effects of physical activity on the body, focusing on conditions that may also play a role in dementia, including cardiovascular disease, diabetes mellitus, and depression.

PHYSICAL ACTIVITY: HISTORY AND DEFINITIONS

Physical activity has been promoted for thousands of years as a critical component of a longer and healthier life. Records from ancient China (approximately

2500 B.C.) describe exercises modeled on the movements of animals as a means for health promotion. Ancient Greek physicians and philosophers such as Hippocrates and Plato also recommended daily exercise as a means of treating and preventing disease and disability. Several epidemiologic studies from the late nineteenth and early twentieth centuries found the first formally documented health benefits of exercise by showing that individuals who engaged in sports had a reduced risk of mortality and cardiovascular disease (MacAuley, 1994).

The modern literature on physical activity includes a wide range of terms to describe different aspects of movement and physiologic responses to movement (Warburton, Nicol, & Breden, 2006). "Physical activity" refers broadly to any leisure or non-leisure body movement that results in increased energy expenditure in comparison to the body at rest. "Physical fitness," on the other hand, refers to a physiologic state of well-being that enables one to meet the physical demands of daily life. "Exercise" refers to a structured and repetitive physical activity program that is performed to maintain or improve physical fitness. Throughout this chapter, we will use the terms *physical activity* and *exercise* somewhat interchangeably to refer to any bodily movement that conveys health benefits.

PHYSICAL ACTIVITY AND CARDIOVASCULAR DISEASE

Since the 1950s, extensive research has supported the beneficial effects of physical activity on the heart (Warburton, Nicol, & Breden, 2006). Longitudinal observational studies have consistently found that individuals who engage in higher levels of physical activity experience a reduced risk of death from any cause and from cardiovascular disease in particular (Kushi et al.,1997; Lee et al., 1995). When comparing the least active to the most active, risk reductions range from 20% to 50%, depending on the study population. Further, there is strong evidence of a dose–response association in which greater levels of physical activity are associated with progressively lower risks.

Randomized, controlled trials have also found that physical activity is effective for the secondary prevention in individuals who already have cardiovascular disease (Taylor et al., 2004). A meta-analysis of 48 RCTs that included 8,940 patients found that compared with usual care, exercise-based cardiac rehabilitation resulted in significantly lower all-cause mortality (odds ratio [OR] = 0.80; 95% confidence interval [CI]: 0.68–0.93) and cardiac mortality (OR = 0.74; 95% CI: 0.61–0.96) as well as greater reductions in total cholesterol, triglycerides, systolic blood pressure, and smoking.

Physical activity also is associated with a reduced risk of cerebrovascular disease. A meta-analysis found a 25% lower risk of stroke or stroke mortality in highly active individuals (OR = 0.75; 95% CI: 0.69–0.82) and a 17% lower risk in moderately active individuals (OR = 0.83; 95% CI: 0.76–0.89) compared to those with low activity levels (Lee Folsom, & Blair, 2003). As discussed in detail in Chapter 1, there is extensive evidence that cerebrovascular disease exacerbates or accelerates the clinical manifestation of dementia symptoms (Snowdon et al., 1997; Vermeer et al., 2003). Therefore, one hypothesis is that the impact of physical activity on the brain may be largely mediated through a vascular mechanism.

PHYSICAL ACTIVITY AND DIABETES MELLITUS

Observational studies also have consistently found that the incidence of type II diabetes is lower in individuals who are physically active compared to those who are not (Bassuk & Manson, 2005; Gill & Cooper, 2008). In particular, these studies have found that moderate intensity exercise performed at least 150 minutes/week is associated with a 20% to 30% reduction in diabetes incidence. As in studies of cardiovascular and cerebrovascular disease, there is evidence of a dose–response association in which more exercise was associated with greater benefits. Some studies have suggested that the benefits of exercise may be greater in women than men or in high-risk (e.g., those who are obese, have a family history, or have impaired glucose tolerance) than low-risk individuals, although these findings have not been consistent across all studies.

Randomized, controlled trials in high-risk populations provide compelling evidence that lifestyle interventions that include greater physical activity are associated with a lower incidence of developing type II diabetes. A review concluded that modest weight loss achieved through diet and exercise reduced diabetes incidence in high-risk individuals by 40% to 60% over 3 to 4 years (Williamson et al., 2004). Similar benefits were observed in both normal weight and overweight individuals.

Both observational studies and RCTs also have found that exercise is associated with better outcomes in those who currently have diabetes, including a reduced risk of all-cause mortality (Warburton, Nicol, & Breden, 2006). A meta-analysis of 14 clinical trials found that exercise resulted in a significant reduction in glycosolated hemoglobin levels beyond that produced by use of oral hypoglycemic agents (Boulé et al., 2001).

As discussed in detail in Chapters 4, 5, and 6, there also is extensive evidence that diabetes mellitus and related conditions, including metabolic syndrome, impaired glucose tolerance, insulin resistance, and obesity (particularly in midlife), are associated with an increased risk of developing dementia (Lu Lin, & Kuo, 2009; Profenno Porsteinsson, & Faraone, 2010). Thus, the effects of physical activity on diabetes as well as glucose metabolism and regulation provide another potential mechanism by which it could impact cognition and risk of dementia.

PHYSICAL ACTIVITY AND DEPRESSION

There also is growing evidence of an association between physical activity and beneficial effects on mental health disorders, particularly depression. A recent meta-analysis identified 13 RCTs that have examined the effects of exercise interventions on depression outcomes in older adults, finding that elders who suffer from clinical depression or elevated depressive symptomatology benefit from exercise (Sjösten & Kivelä, 2006). A review of reviews on exercise and depression also recently concluded that there is evidence from RCTs that exercise is more effective than no treatment and may be as effective as traditional pharmacologic and psychotherapeutic treatments in some settings, although it was acknowledged that the quality of these studies was typically low (Daley, 2008).

Depression, in turn, has been linked to an increased risk of developing cognitive impairment and dementia, with approximately a twofold increase in dementia incidence in depressed compared to non-depressed elders (Jorm, 2001; Ownby et al., 2006). It remains unclear whether depression is a true casual risk factor for dementia or whether it is an early manifestation of an underlying neurodegenerative process. However, there is growing awareness that chronic depression may lead to a variety of adverse consequences including increased risk of vascular disease, lower levels of neuronal growth factors and reduced hippocampal volume (Alexopoulos, 2003).

Physical Activity and the Brain: Observational Studies

Although the beneficial effects of physical activity on the body have been widely accepted for thousands of years, the effects of physical activity on the brain have not been as well recognized until more recently. In this section, we describe the accumulating evidence that physical activity has positive effects on brain health, focusing on findings from longitudinal, observational studies.

RISK OF DEMENTIA AND COGNITIVE IMPAIRMENT

Most longitudinal, observational studies—although not all—have found that physical activity is associated with a reduced risk of developing cognitive impairment or dementia (Hamer & Chida, 2009). A recent meta-analysis identified 16 studies that examined the association between physical activity and risk of either dementia or Alzheimer's disease (AD; Table 9.1). For all-cause dementia, 11 studies that included 23,168 subjects were identified, of which six found a significant association between physical activity and reduced dementia risk (Ho et al., 2001; Abbott et al., 2004; Podewils et al., 2005; Rovio, 2005; Larson et al., 2006; Sumic et al., 2007), and an additional three studies had point estimates suggestive of an association (Fabrigoule et al., 1995; Laurin et al., 2001; Wang et al., 2002). Only two studies suggested no evidence of an association (Verghese, 2003; Wang, 2006). When all of these studies were combined, the risk of dementia was reduced by 28% in the highest versus lowest physical activity groups (RR, 0.72; 95% CI: 0.60–0.86) (Hamer, 2009).

An even stronger association was observed for AD (Table 9.1). A total of six studies that included 13,771 subjects were identified. Four found a statistically significant association between high physical activity and reduced risk of AD (Rovio, 2005; Podewils, 2005; Laurin et al., 2001; Yoshitake, 1995), and a fifth had a point estimate that was suggestive of a protective association (Abbott, 2004). Only one study suggested no association between physical activity and AD (Wilson, 2002). When all of these studies were combined, study participants with the highest levels of physical activity at baseline had approximately a 45% reduction in the risk of AD compared to those with the lowest levels of physical activity (RR, 0.55; 95% CI: 0.36–0.84) (Hamer, 2009).

Although some of these studies suggested that the effects of physical activity were more pronounced in specific subgroups, these findings were inconsistent across studies. In studies that reported results separately by gender, two suggested that the association between physical activity and AD or dementia was stronger in women than men (Sumic et al., 2007; Laurin et al., 2001), whereas a third suggested no difference between women and men (Ho, 2001). These studies also reached differing conclusions about the impact of the apolipoprotein-E (APOE) ε4 allele, with one study finding a stronger association in APOE ε4 carriers (Rovio, 2005) and another finding a stronger association in APOE ε4 noncarriers (Podewils, 2005).

Another recent meta-analysis examined the association between physical activity and vascular dementia (VaD) (Aarsland et al., 2010). A total of five studies (374 people with VaD, 10,108 without dementia) were identified (Yoshitake, 1995; Laurin et al., 2001; Abbott, 2004; Podewils, 2005; Ravaglia, 2008). Although only one of these studies found a significant association between physical activity and VaD (Ravaglia, 2008), there was a statistically significant 38% reduction in the risk of developing VaD when the studies were combined (RR = 0.62; 95% CI: 0.41–0.92).

Many studies also have examined the association between physical activity and cognitive decline or cognitive impairment (Albert et al., 1995; Schuitt, 2001; Yaffe, 2001; Richards, 2003; Lytle, 2004; van Gelder, 2004; Weuve, 2004; Singh-Manoux, 2005; Sturman, 2005; Middleton, 2008a; 2008b). The results of these studies are generally consistent with findings related to dementia in that most—but not all—have found a significant association between engaging in physical activity and experiencing less cognitive deterioration. One of the earlier studies found that older women in the highest quartile of walking experienced a 34% lower odds of cognitive decline over 6 years to 8 years compared to those in the lowest quartile (OR = 0.66; 95% CI: 0.54–0.82) (Yaffe, 2001).

Table 9.1 Longitudinal, Observational Studies of Physical Activity and Risk of Dementia or Alzheimer's Disease

Author (year)	Exposure	Sample size	Outcome	Hazard ratio dementia (95% CI)	Hazard ratio AD (95% CI)
Fabrigoule et al. (1995)	Any sports	2,040	AD/D (MMSE, DSM-III)	0.33 (0.10–1.04)	n/a
Yoshitake et al. (1995)	Daily physical activity	826	AD (MMSE < 21, DSM-II)	n/a	0.20 (0.06–0.68)
Ho et al. (2001)—men	Any exercise	519	Cognitive impairment (CAPE<7)	0.73 (0.53–1.01)	n/a
Ho et al. (2001)—women		469		0.84 (0.71–0.99)	n/a
Laurin et al. (2001)—men	≥3 times/week vigorous	1,831	AD/dementia (3MS < 77, DSM-IV)	0.91 (0.45–1.83)	0.73 (0.27–1.98)
Laurin et al. (2001)—women		2,784		0.55 (0.25–1.21)	0.27 (0.08–0.90)
Wang et al. (2002)	Daily physical activity	732	Dementia (MMSE screen, DSM-IV)	0.41 (0.13–1.31)	n/a
Wilson et al. (2002)	≥5 hours/week	1,249	AD (clinical diagnosis)	n/a	1.04 (0.98–1.10)
Verghese et al. (2003)	Highest quintile	469	AD/dementia (DSM-IV)	1.27 (0.78–2.06)	n/a
Abbott et al. (2004)—men	>2 miles/day walking	2,257	AD/dementia (CASI > 74, DSM-IV)	0.63 (0.43–0.93)	0.61 (0.36–1.02)
Podewils et al. (2005)	≥2 times/week	3,375	AD/dementia (3MS < 80, clinical diagnosis)	0.58 (0.41–0.83)	0.55 (0.34–0.88)

Study		N	Outcome		
Rovio et al. (2005)	≥2 times/week	1,449	AD/dementia (DSM-IV)	0.47 (0.25–0.90)	0.35 (0.16–0.80)
Larson et al. (2006)	≥3 times/week	1,740	AD/dementia (CASI < 86, DSM-IV)	0.69 (0.48–0.96)	n/a
Wang et al. (2006)	Highest quintile	5,437	Cognitive impairment (MMSE < 24)	0.98 (0.95–1.01)	n/a
Sumic et al. (2007)—men	>4 hours/week	27	Cognitive impairment/ dementia (MMSE < 24, CDR ≥ 0.5)	0.91 (0.25–3.40)	n/a
Sumic et al. (2007)—women	>4 hours/week	39	-	0.12 (0.03–0.41)	n/a
Combined		23,168 dementia / 13,771 AD		0.72 (0.60–0.86)	0.55 (0.36–0.84)

Adapted from Hamer and Chida (2008). AD, Alzheimer's disease; CAPE, Clifton Assessment Procedures for the Elderly; CASI, Cognitive Abilities Screening Instrument; CI, confidence interval; D, dementia; DSM, Diagnostic and Statistical Manual of Mental Disorders; MMSE, Mini-Mental State Examination; 3MS, Modified Mini-Mental State Examination.

OPTIMAL AMOUNT OF PHYSICAL ACTIVITY

The U.S. Surgeon General guidelines currently recommend at least 30 minutes/day, 5 days/week of moderate-intensity exercise. These recommendations are largely based on extensive research related to all-cause mortality and cardiovascular mortality. However, the optimal "dose" of physical activity for brain health is less clearly established, and it is possible that the ideal dose will vary based on factors such as age, fitness level, comorbid illnesses, and other factors.

Some studies support a dose–response relationship in which there is a graded association between the duration or intensity of physical activity and the risk of adverse cognitive outcomes (Laurin et al., 2001; van Gelder et al., 2004; Weuve et al., 2004; Schuitt et al., 2001). However, other studies have suggested more of a threshold effect. For example, one study found little difference between subjects engaging in 3 days versus 5 days of exercise per week (Lytle et al., 2004). In many studies, although there is evidence of a dose–response relationship, the greatest difference appears to lie between those who are completely sedentary and those who engage in at least some leisure activity (Middleton et al., 2010), suggesting that all older adults should be encourage to engage in at least a minimal level of physical activity.

LIFE-COURSE STUDIES

One limitation of most observational studies in this area is that follow-up periods have typically ranged from 3 years to 9 years (Hamer & Chida, 2009). It is now widely accepted that the pathological processes underlying AD, VaD, and other dementias begin many years and even decades prior to the manifestation of clinical symptoms. Therefore, it is possible that the observed association between physical activity and risk of dementia reflects a preclinical process in which individuals begin to withdraw from usual activities as they begin to experience subtle cognitive deterioration.

Several studies have addressed this issue by examining the association between physical activity performed in early life or midlife and risk of developing cognitive impairment or dementia in late life. One study found that individuals who engaged in leisure-time physical activity in midlife were significantly less likely than those who were sedentary to develop either dementia (odds ratio [OR] = 0.47; 95% CI: 0.25–0.90) or AD (OR = 0.35; 95% CI: 0.19–0.80) (Rovio, 2005). However, other studies have had mixed results, with some (Andel et al., 2008; Middleton et al., 2010), but not all (Carlson et al., 2008; Yamada et al., 2003), finding an association between midlife physical activity and late-life cognitive impairment.

A handful of studies have also examined the association between physical activity earlier in life (prior to age 30 years) and late-life cognition. Most have found that early life physical activity is associated with less cognitive impairment, better information processing speed, and slower memory decline

(Dik et al., 2003; Middleton et al., 2010; Richards Hardy, & Wadsworth, 2003). In one recent study, 9,344 older women were asked about their physical activity levels as teenagers, at age 30 years, at age 50 years, and in late life. Although participation in physical activity at any age was associated with a reduced risk of cognitive impairment in late life, the strongest association was observed with teenage physical activity (Middleton et al., 2010).

OBJECTIVE ASSESSMENT OF ACTIVITY LEVELS

Another limitation of most observational studies in this area is the use of self-reported measures to assess physical activity levels. This may result in inaccurate reporting, particularly in individuals with poor memory, and could potentially bias the results of these studies. Several studies have addressed this issue by utilizing objective measures of aerobic fitness, movement, or energy expenditure, and these studies have consistently found strong associations between objective measures of activity or fitness levels and cognitive outcomes (Barnes et al., 2003; Barnes et al., 2008; Middleton et al., 2010).

One of the earliest studies examined the association between cardiorespiratory fitness based on maximum oxygen consumption (VO_2-max) during treadmill exercise testing and cognitive decline based on a modified version of the Mini-Mental State Examination (MMSE) and found that higher cardiorespiratory fitness levels were associated with slower rates of cognitive decline over 6 years (Barnes et al., 2003). Notably, objective measures of fitness were much more strongly associated with cognition than self-reported activity levels, suggesting that studies based on self-report may actually be biased toward the null. Another study utilized doubly-labeled water methods—which are generally considered the gold standard for objectively assessing energy expenditure—and found that individuals in the highest tertile of energy expenditure experienced an 81% reduction in the risk of cognitive impairment (OR = 0.19; 95% CI: 0.01–0.79) (Middleton et al., 2010).

SUMMARY OF OBSERVATIONAL STUDIES

Taken together, longitudinal, observational studies have provided consistent evidence that physical activity is associated with a reduced risk of developing cognitive impairment or dementia, including AD and VaD. However, it remains possible that these associations reflect the effects of uncontrolled confounders such as better health status or other lifestyle factors. Furthermore, the optimal dose and type of physical activity for maintaining optimal brain health and function remain poorly understood. Randomized, controlled trials are needed to demonstrate a causal association between engaging in physical activity in late life and lowering risk of cognitive impairment and dementia and for examining the effects of specific exercise regimens.

Physical Activity and the Brain: Randomized, Controlled Trials

Randomized, controlled trials are crucial for providing evidence of a causal association between engaging in physical activity and experiencing better cognitive outcomes. Since the 1980s, numerous RCTs have examined the effects of various exercise interventions on cognitive function in different study populations. In this section, we highlight exercise RCTs that have been performed in healthy elders, "high-risk" populations, and individuals with dementia (Table 9.2).

Table 9.2 **Meta-Analyses of Randomized, Controlled Trials (RCTs) of Physical Activity and Cognitive Change**

Author (year)	Study population	No. RCTs	No. Subjects	Effect size (SE or 95% CI)
Colcombe & Kramer (2003)	Healthy elders	18	197	Overall: 0.32 (0.03)
(exercise vs. control)		—	37	Executive functions: 0.68 (0.05)
		—	74	Controlled processing: 0.46 (0.04)
		—	23	Spatial: 0.43 (0.06)
		—	32	Speed: 0.24 (0.05)
Angevaren et al. (2008)	Healthy elders	6	312	Cognitive speed: 0.24 (0.01, 0.46)
(aerobic vs. any intervention)		4	209	Verbal memory (immediate): 0.17 (−0.10, 0.44)
		2	65	Visual memory (immediate): 0.04 (−1.66, 1.75)
		3	189	Working memory: 0.36 (−0.31, 1.03)
		1	124	Memory (delayed): 0.5 (−0.44, 1.44)
		7	326	Executive functions: 0.16 (−0.20, 0.51)
		3	160	Perception: −0.10 (−0.63, 0.43)
		3	189	Cognitive inhibition: −0.02 (−0.31, 0.26)

(continued)

Tabel 9.2 **(Continued)**

Author (year)	Study population	No. RCTs	No. Subjects	Effect size (SE or 95% CI)
		5	290	Visual attention: 0.26 (0.02, 0.49)
		5	243	Auditory attention: 0.05 (−0.45, 0.54)
		4	237	Motor function: 0.52 (−0.25, 1.30)
Angevaren et al. (2008)	Healthy elders	8	236	Cognitive speed: 0.10 (−0.16, 0.36)
(aerobic vs. no intervention)		6	141	Verbal memory (immediate): 0.06 (−0.30, 0.42)
		3	81	Visual memory (immediate): −0.15 (−0.58, 0.29)
		2	65	Working memory: 0.49 (−0.76, 1.73)
		2	40	Memory (delayed): −0.55 (−2.11, 1.00)
		6	202	Executive functions: 0.23 (−0.09, 0.56)
		4	76	Perception: 0.10 (−0.38, 0.57)
		2	65	Cognitive inhibition: 2.47 (−0.62, 5.55)
		5	176	Visual attention: 0.09 (−0.20, 0.39)
		5	121	Auditory attention: 0.52 (0.13, 0.91)
		3	115	Motor function: 1.17 (0.19, 2.15)
Heyn Beatriz, & Ottenbacher (2004)	Cognitive impairment or dementia	10	820	0.57 (0.38, 0.75)
Forbes et al. (2008)	Dementia	4	280	Could not be calculated

CI, confidence interval; RCTs, randomized controlled trials; SE, standard error.

EXERCISE RANDOMIZED, CONTROLLED TRIALS IN HEALTHY ELDERS

A meta-analysis published in 2003 identified 18 exercise intervention studies with a total of 197 subjects that were published between 1966 and 2001 (Colcombe et al., 2003). Most of the studies included older participants with normal cognition, although three publications were from clinical populations. The primary finding was that cognitive function improved significantly more in intervention group participants (0.48 standard deviations [SDs]) compared to control group participants (0.16 SDs) for an effect size (standardized difference between intervention and control groups) of 0.32 SDs ($p < 0.05$). The largest effect sizes were observed for executive function (0.68 SDs), although significant benefits also were observed for other cognitive outcomes, including controlled processing (0.46 SDs), visuospatial function (0.43 SDs), and speed (0.27 SDs). Interestingly, participants who performed a combined aerobic and strength program experienced greater benefits (0.59 SDs) than aerobic exercise alone (0.41 SDs). In addition, benefits appeared to be greater in studies that had a greater proportion of women (0.60 SDs) than men (0.15 SDs) and for mid-old (66–70 years: 0.69 SDs) and old-old (71–80 years: 0.55 SDs) than young-old (55–65 years: 0.30 SDs) participants.

However, several more recent systematic reviews and meta-analyses have reached more cautious conclusions about the effects of exercise interventions on cognitive outcomes in healthy elders. A Cochrane review published in 2008 focusing on the effects of aerobic physical activity programs identified 11 RCTs that included a total of 625 subjects (Angevaren et al., 2008). The majority of individual trials showed nonsignificant results. However, when comparing aerobic exercise to any other intervention across 11 cognitive domains, the authors reported significant effect sizes for cognitive speed (0.24 SDs) and visual attention (0.26 SDs) but not other domains. When comparing aerobic exercise to no intervention, significant effects sizes were found for motor function (1.17 SDs) and auditory attention (0.50 SDs) but not other domains. The article concluded that these studies provide evidence that aerobic exercise is beneficial for cognitive function in healthy older adults but noted that more trials are needed to determine the effects of non-aerobic exercises and to gain a greater understanding of why the effects of exercise appear to be limited to certain cognitive domains.

Another recent systematic review identified 30 RCTs and concluded that although there were some positive studies, the evidence was insufficient to conclude that physical activity or exercise improved cognition in older adults (Snowden et al., 2011). Similarly, a recent State-of-the-Science report that performed a comprehensive review of factors associated with cognitive decline and AD concluded that there was preliminary evidence that physical activity is associated with preservation of cognitive function but that the overall quality of the evidence was low (Williams et al., 2010).

Although most studies have focused on the effects of aerobic exercise, there also is limited evidence that resistance training is associated with improvements in executive function (Liu-Ambrose et al., 2010a). In one RCT, 155 older, community-dwelling women were randomized to resistance training once or twice a week or a twice-weekly balance and toning control group. Both of the resistance training groups significantly improved their performance on the Stroop test, a standard measure of executive function, compared to the control group, although performance on other tests did not differ.

Most RCTs in healthy elders performed to date have focused on cognitive change as their primary outcome. Unfortunately, none have examined the important question of whether exercise interventions are associated with a reduced risk or delayed onset of dementia, largely because of the large numbers of subjects and lengthy follow-up that would be required to accrue an adequate number of cases (Barnes et al., 2007).

EXERCISE RANDOMIZED, CONTROLLED TRIALS IN "HIGH-RISK" POPULATIONS

A handful of RCTs have examined the effects of exercise interventions on cognitive outcomes in various "high-risk" populations. An Australian group investigated a home-based walking program in 170 participants ages 50 years or older who had subjective memory complaints or mild cognitive impairment (MCI) but were living in the community (Lautenschlager et al., 2008). The 24-week intervention had a target of at least 150 minutes of physical activity per week and was individually tailored. Pedometers were used to provide an objective measure of activity levels. Compliance and adherence were enhanced using a modified behavioral approach based on social cognitive theory (Cox et al., 2003) that included a workshop, manual, newsletters, and regular phone calls. Participants were re-assessed at the end of the active intervention period at 6 months and then again at 12 months and 18 months. The primary outcome measure was the Alzheimer's Disease Assessment Scale-cognitive subscale (ADAS-Cog), which is a 70-point scale (lower scores are better) that is commonly used to assess cognitive function in dementia drug trials. There was a significant difference between the groups over time in which the physical activity group experienced progressive improvement in their ADAS-cog scores (change from baseline: −0.26 points at 6 months, −0.55 points at 12 months, −0.73 points at 18 months), whereas the usual care group did not (change from baseline: 1.04 points at 6 months, 0.04 points at 12 months, −0.04 points at 18 months) ($p = 0.04$).

Another recent RCT focused on older adults with MCI who were sedentary (defined as less than 30 minutes of physical activity, fewer than three times a week in the past 6 months) (Baker et al., 2010a). Thirty-three subjects were randomly assigned to 6 months of either aerobic training or flexibility exercises. The results showed a gender-specific effect, with women in the aerobic group demonstrating improved executive function as well as some changes in biological variables such as an increased glucose disposal and reduced fasting plasma levels of insulin, cortisol, and brain-derived neurotrophic factor (BDNF). Male participants improved on the Trails B test and had increased plasma levels of insulin-like growth factor 1. The authors suggested that these findings might have resulted from gender-specific differences in certain metabolic systems.

A second RCT by this group examined the effects of exercise in an elderly population that was cognitively normal but was "high-risk" because of impaired glucose tolerance (Baker et al., 2010b). They investigated the impact of a 6-month aerobic exercise program compared to a stretching control. Six months of aerobic exercise resulted in significant improvements in executive function ($p = 0.04$), cardiorespiratory fitness ($p = 0.03$), and insulin sensitivity ($p = 0.05$) relative to the control group but not on measures of memory ($p = 0.58$).

However, other RCTs have yielded less consistent findings. One study randomly assigned 126 sedentary elders with subjective cognitive complaints to participate in either aerobic exercise or a stretching and toning control group 3 days/week for 12 weeks and found that although cognitive function improved significantly in both groups, there were no significant differences between the groups (Barnes, 2010). It is not clear whether this negative finding resulted from the relatively brief study duration of 12 weeks or whether a more intensive stretching and toning program may have benefits comparable to aerobic exercise in some settings.

The hypothesis that some non-aerobic forms of exercise may have cognitive benefits has been supported by another recent study. Lam et al. (2011) recruited 389 older adults who were not demented but had a diagnosis of amnestic MCI or a clinical dementia rating (CDR) score of 0.5 from 19 social centers or residential homes. The participating centers were then cluster-randomized either to an intervention or control group. In the intervention group, 24 forms of simplified Tai Chi were practiced for 12 months at least three times a week and at least 30 minutes per session. In the first 8 weeks to 12 weeks (induction phase), participants were taught by Tai Chi masters. After that, in the maintenance phase, they received a training video. The control group performed supervised stretching exercises. Two months after completion of the induction phase, both groups showed significant improvement in both subjective and objective measures of cognition ($p < 0.05$). However, the intervention group showed additional improvement on a balance test (Berg Balance Scale), in visual attention, and on the CDR sum of boxes score. They also showed an independent association with a stable CDR score at follow-up (OR = 0.14; 95% CI: 0.03–0.71, $p = 0.02$). The authors concluded that the improvement in visual attention in the intervention group might be related to the specific cognitive demands of Tai Chi. These results raise the interesting question of whether physical activities that have an integral cognitive component (e.g., Tai Chi or dancing) might have additional benefits.

EXERCISE RANDOMIZED, CONTROLLED TRIALS IN INDIVIDUALS WITH DEMENTIA

A review and meta-analysis by Heyn et al. (2004) identified 30 exercise RCTs that included a total of 2,020 participants with cognitive impairment or dementia published between 1970 and 2003. Of these, 10 studies with 820 participants examined one or more cognitive outcomes and had a significant overall effect size of 0.57 SD (95% CI: 0.38–0.75).

However, a more recent Cochrane review (Forbes et al., 2008) that was restricted to exercise RCTs in individuals with diagnosed dementia identified only four papers published as of September 2007, most of which focused on physical function, behaviors, and psychological symptoms and did not examine cognition as an outcome. Not surprisingly, the authors concluded that there was not enough evidence to determine the effectiveness of physical activity for improving cognitive function or other outcomes among patients with dementia.

Two recent small trials that included participants with dementia in residential care (Kemoun et al., 2010) or who were recruited from a Memory Clinic (Yáguez et al., 2010) reported significant benefits of exercise interventions on cognitive performance compared to the control groups.

There are a number of interesting trials underway where protocols have been published. Cyarto et al. (2010) published a study protocol for a 12-month trial aiming to recruit 230 community-dwelling participants with AD and their caregivers. The study focused on a home-based walking program that included a behavioral intervention based on the stages of change model modified for physical activity (Marcus et al., 1992). The caregiver enrolled into the trial as a "coach" helping the participant to remember to walk and to keep motivated. The control group received standard care, and both groups received educational material on healthy lifestyle and dementia. Outcomes included cognition, psychological symptoms of dementia, quality of life of the patient and caregiver, caregiver burden, functional level, and global clinical impression.

Several research groups also are developing physical activity interventions for specific clinical population. Liu-Ambrose et al. (2010b), for example, published a study protocol for a 12-month RCT focusing on older adults who had mild subcortical ischemic vascular cognitive impairment (SIVCI). The authors reported that their study aimed to include 60 non-demented participants with SIVCI into the study. They were randomized to an aerobic training or usual care control group. Outcome parameters included cognition, biomarkers, physical function and fall risk, quality of life, and health resource utilization.

Pitkala et al. (2010) published a study protocol aiming to recruit 210 community-dwelling participants with AD and their caregivers. This trial had three arms with a home-based physical activity intervention, a group-based physical activity intervention in a rehabilitation center and a control group with usual care and information on exercise and nutrition. The intervention period was 12 months, and outcomes included cognition, physical function, mobility, psychological symptoms, caregiver burden, and quality of life. This trial aimed to perform a follow-up after 24 months to measure the rate of institutionalization and an additional outcome related to health economics.

One group has recently begun development of a novel integrative exercise program called Preventing Loss of Independence through Exercise (PLIÉ) that incorporates elements of Tai Chi, yoga, and Feldenkrais with traditional exercises. The goal of the program is to improve cognitive function, physical function, dementia-related behaviors, and quality of life through simple, gentle exercises that promote body awareness and well-being (clinicaltrials.gov: NCT01371214).

SUMMARY OF EXERCISE RANDOMIZED, CONTROLLED TRIALS

Taken together, these RCTs suggest that exercise interventions are associated with significant improvements in some aspects of cognitive function in healthy elders as well as elders with cognitive impairment, although there is a lack of consistency across the trials. Most trials published to date have been limited by small sample sizes, and synthesis of results across trials is difficult because of differences in the nature of the exercise interventions and outcome measures. Further, RCTs have not yet determined definitively whether exercise can prevent or delay dementia onset, and the most effective types and amounts of exercise for enhancing cognitive function remain poorly understood. Several trials that are underway should provide more evidence in the near future. For example, the Lifestyle Interventions and Independence for Elders (LIFE) study is a phase 3 RCT comparing a supervised, moderate intensity physical activity program with a successful aging education control group in 1,600 sedentary elders with cognitive decline as one of the outcomes (Fielding et al., 2011).

Potential Mechanisms

There are currently several different mechanisms by which physical activity could lead to better brain function and a reduced risk of dementia. These can be broadly classified as mechanisms that operate through indirect effects on the body—including reduced risk of vascular and metabolic disorders or reduced impact of stress, oxidation, and inflammation—and mechanisms that have

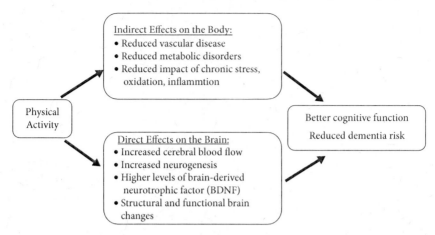

Figure 9.1 Hypothesized mechanisms underlying the effects of physical activity on brain health and function.

direct effects on the brain—including increased cerebral blood flow, increased neurogenesis, increased levels of BDNF, increased hippocampal volume, and reduced AD pathology (Fig. 9.1). Most current hypotheses are based on animal research. However, increasingly, physical activity studies with humans contribute useful data on potential mechanisms.

REDUCED RISK OF VASCULAR AND METABOLIC DISORDERS

As discussed earlier in this chapter, physical activity has many well-documented effects on the body, including reduced risk of vascular events and metabolic disorders such as diabetes mellitus. Further, as described in detail in other chapters, there is ample evidence that vascular and metabolic disorders, in turn, have profound effects on the brain. Therefore, one of the most plausible mechanisms by which physical activity may affect brain health is by lowering the risk of micro- and macrovascular events and metabolic dysregulation. However, most of the observational studies that have examined the association between physical activity and risk of cognitive decline or dementia have adjusted for comorbid medical conditions and have found a consistent, independent effect of physical activity. Although it is difficult to fully adjust for vascular and metabolic factors, these findings suggest that other mechanisms are likely to play an important role in the effects of physical activity on the brain.

INCREASED CEREBRAL BLOOD FLOW

Another commonly hypothesized mechanism underlying the effects of exercise is an increase in cerebral blood flow or general improvement of vascularization.

Rhyu et al. (2010), for example, presented results of an animal study with female cynomolgus monkeys who underwent a 5-month intervention of treadmill running (1 hour/day for 5 days for 5 months), which was compared to the sedentary lifestyle of a control group. Both middle-aged (10–12 years) as well as mature (15–17 years) monkeys benefitted from the intervention, showing improved cognitive performance ($p = 0.05$) as well as an increase in their vascular volume fraction in the motor cortex ($p = 0.03$) compared to the control group. Unfortunately, this increase was not maintained when the animals returned to a sedentary lifestyle after another 3 months, suggesting that it may be important to continue exercising to maintain cognitive benefits.

An interesting observational study in humans also supports the hypothesis that an increase in cerebral blood flow may underlie some of the cognitive benefits of physical activity (Rogers Meyer, & Mortel, 1990). This study examined three groups of elderly individuals who were approaching the age of retirement: 30 continued to work, 30 retired but engaged in regular physical activity, and 30 retired but did not engage in regular physical activity. Retirees who were physically inactive experienced significant declines in cerebral blood flow over 4 years of follow-up and also performed more poorly on cognitive tests at the study endpoint, suggesting that a post-retirement sedentary lifestyle may lead to a decline in cerebral blood flow that results in more rapid cognitive deterioration over time.

INCREASED NEUROGENESIS

One of the most exciting developments over the past several decades has been the discovery that the human brain is highly plastic and continues to generate new neurons (neurogenesis) in specific areas of the brain, including the hippocampus, throughout life. In a recent review on neurogenesis and aging, physical activity was examined as one of the environmental factors that could contribute to neurogenesis in the aging brain (Lazarov et al., 2010a). The authors highlighted that age-dependent reduction of neurogenesis can be minimized (Kronenberg et al., 2006) and even be partially reversed (van Praag et al., 2005) when rodents are exposed to physical activity. However, this effect was dependent on the biological age of the animals. Eighteen-month-old (equivalent to middle-age) mice that were exposed to a running wheel showed benefit, but this was not replicated when the mice were 22 months old (equivalent to older age) (Creer et al., 2010). This review also has emphasized that the results of physical activity and neurogenesis are more inconsistent in the literature when it comes to AD rodent models, with some studies showing increased neurogenesis and improved cognition with exercise (Hu et al., 2010; Lazarov & Marr, 2010b) and other studies showing no association (Feng et al., 2001; Levi & Michaelson, 2007; Choi et al., 2008; Mirochnic et al., 2009).

INCREASED BRAIN-DERIVED NEUROTROPHIC FACTOR

Brain-derived neurotrophic factor is considered to be an important biological marker for brain plasticity. Berchthold and colleagues (2010) investigated BDNF levels in mice immediately after completion of a 3-week running period compared to a 1- or 2-week delay after completion of the exercise period. Significant elevations of BDNF were reported immediately after completion of the 3-week physical activity period and 1 and 2 weeks after completion, returning to baseline levels after 3 to 4 weeks. These elevations also correlated with cognitive improvements in the radial water maze. This finding is of significance because it demonstrates that the benefits of physical activity on brain plasticity can extend beyond the physical activity period before returning to pre-exercise levels.

STRUCTURAL AND FUNCTIONAL BRAIN CHANGES

Several RCTs have recently found that aerobic exercise interventions in sedentary elders resulted in structural brain changes. In one study, 59 healthy sedentary elders ages 60 years to 79 years were randomized to a 6-month aerobic walking program or stretching and toning control group. Invention group participants experienced significant increases in both gray and white matter volume (Colcombe et al., 2006).

A more recent study from the same group compared the effects of aerobic walking to stretching and toning in 120 healthy, sedentary elders over 12 months (Erickson et al., 2011). The intervention group experienced a 2% gain in hippocampal volume, which the authors suggested was equivalent to reversing age-related atrophy by 1 year to 2 years. This volume gain was also associated with improved spatial memory and an increase in serum levels of BDNF. The control group experienced a hippocampal volume decline of 1.43% during the study period. Further, functional magnetic resonance imaging (fMRI) studies showed that the walking group experienced significant gains in functional connectivity that were correlated with greater improvements in executive function (Voss et al., 2010). Another recent RCT demonstrated changes in functional plasticity with twice-weekly resistance training over 12 months in sedentary elders (Liu-Ambrose et al., 2011).

REDUCED ALZHEIMER'S DISEASE PATHOLOGY

Several studies have shown impressive results, demonstrating a direct effect of physical activity on AD pathology in animal models. Specifically, in these studies, physical activity was associated with a reduction of amyloid deposition (Adlard et al., 2005; Lazarov & Marr, 2010b) and Aβ-dependent neuronal cell death in the hippocampus (Um et al., 2011). These findings are exciting because they suggest that physical activity may have a direct impact on the AD pathological process.

REDUCED IMPACT OF CHRONIC STRESS, OXIDATION, AND INFLAMMATION

Nakajima and colleagues (2010) looked at a different component of neurogenesis, focusing on the impact of chronic stress on the brain by impairing hippocampal neurogenesis via an increase of oxidative stress and an increase of lipid peroxide. In a chronic restraint stress (CRS) model, mice were exposed for 5 weeks, 6 days a week, to 12 hours of immobilization daily by being house in a very small cage. Half the mice had access to a running wheel for the 5 days prior to the immobilization phase compared to a control group that had no access to physical activity. The prior access to the running wheel reduced CRS-induced cognitive impairment and improved cell proliferation in the dentate gyrus.

In another study with an AD mouse model, the impact of physical activity on AD-related oxidative damage was investigated (Herring et al., 2010). For 4 months, mice were either housed in standard housing or environmentally enriched housing that included access to physical activity. In this experiment, physical activity was associated with multiple anti-oxidative defense mechanisms in the brain activated via several pathways such as reduction of oxidative stress biomarkers and downregulation of pro-inflammatory and pro-oxidative mediators, amongsothers. This finding suggests that physical activity may positively impact on the cerebral inflammatory reactions to AD pathology.

SUMMARY OF POTENTIAL MECHANISMS

There are a wide range of plausible mechanism by which physical activity could impact brain health, cognitive function, and the risk of developing dementia. These include indirect effects mediated through vascular disease, metabolic disorders, stress, oxidative damage, and inflammation. In addition, physical activity appears to have a variety of direct beneficial effects on the brain, including reduced development of AD pathology as well as BDNF-induced neurogenesis, increased hippocampal volume, and increased cerebral blood flow. These studies, when combined with evidence from observational studies and RCTs, provide compelling evidence in favor of the hypothesis that physical activity enhances brain health and function.

Conclusions and Next Steps

As we have described in this chapter, the beneficial effects of physical activity on the body have been widely accepted for thousands of years, and there is growing recognition that these benefits extend to the brain. There is evidence from observational studies that individuals who are physically active are less likely to develop cognitive impairment and dementia, and RCTs have found that exercise interventions are associated with improvements in at least some aspects of cognitive function as well as increases in brain volume, particularly hippocampal volume, and functional brain connectivity. Animal studies have identified several potential mechanisms that may underlie these findings in humans, including both indirect and direct effects of physical activity on neuronal health and function.

Despite this knowledge, approximately one-third of adults in the United States are sedentary, including more than half of those age 75 years or older (Centers for Disease Control and Prevention, 2010). A recent study estimated that 1 in 5 cases of AD (more than 1.1 million) in the United States are potentially attributable to physical inactivity and that a 10% reduction in the prevalence of physical inactivity could potentially prevent nearly 90,000 cases (Barnes & Yaffe, 2011). Given the looming dementia epidemic, it is imperative that we identify strategies for encouraging all adults, particularly high-risk elders, to engage in physical activity as part of their daily routine.

References

Aarsland D, Sardahaee FS, Anderssen S, Ballard C, & Alzheimer's Society Systematic Review Group. (2010). Is physical activity a potential preventive factor for vascular dementia? A systematic review. *Aging Mental Health 14*, 386–395.

Abbott RD, White LR, Ross GW, Masaki KH, Curb JD, & Petrovitch J. (2004). Walking and dementia in physically capable elderly men. *J Am Med Assn 292*, 1447–1453.

Adlard PA, Perreau VM, Pop V, & Cotman CW. (2005). Voluntary exercise decreases amyloid load in a transgenic model of Alzheimer's disease. *J Neurosci 25*, 4217–4221.

Albert MS, Jones K, Savage CR, Berkman L, Seeman T, Blazer D, et al. (1995). Predictors of cognitive change in older persons: MacArthur studies of successful aging. *Psychol Aging 10*, 578–589.

Alexopoulos GS. (2003). Vascular disease, depression and dementia. *J Am Geriatr Soc 51*, 1178–1180.

Andel R, Crowe M, Pedersen NL, Fratiglioni L, Johansson B, & Gatz M (2008). Physical exercise at mid-life and risk of dementia three decades later: A population-based study of Swedish twins. *J Gerontol Med Sci 63*, 62–66.

Angevaren M, Aufdemkampe G, Verhaar HJJ, Aleman A, & Vanhees L. (2008). Physical activity and enhanced fitness to improve cognitive function in older people without known cognitive impairment. *Cochrane Database Syst Rev. 3*(CD005381. DOI: 10.1002/14651858. CD005381.pub3.

Baker LD, Frank LL, Foster-Schubert K, Green PS, Wilkinson CW, McTiernan A, et al. (2010a). Effects of aerobic exercise on mild cognitive impairment: A controlled trial. *Arch Neurol 67*, 71–79.

Baker LD, Frank LL, Foster-Schubert K, Green PS, Wilkinson CW, McTiernan A, et al. (2010b). Aerobic exercise improves cognition for older adults with glucose intolerance, a risk factor for Alzheimer's disease. *J Alzheimers Dis 22*, 569–579.

Barnes DE, Blackwell T, Stone KL, Goldman SE, Hillier T, Yaffe K. (2008) Cognition in older women: the importance of daytime movement. *J Am Geriatr Soc. 56*(9),1658–1664.

Barnes DE, Whitmer RA, & Yaffe K. (2007). Physical activity and dementia: The need for prevention trials. *Exerc Sport Sci Rev. 35*(1), 24–29.

Barnes DE, Yaffe K, Satariano WA, & Tager IB. (2003) A longitudinal study of cardiorespiratory fitness and cognitive function in healthy older adults. *J Am Geriatr Soc. 51*(4), 459–465.

Barnes DE (2010). The Mental Activity and eXercise (MAX) Trial: A randomized, controlled trial to enhance cognitive function in older adults with cognitive complaints. International Conference on Alzheimer's Disease. Honolulu, HI.

Barnes DE & Yaffe K. (2011). The projected effect of risk factor reduction on Alzheimer's disease prevalence. *Lancet Neurology 10*, 819–828.

Bassuk SS & Manson JE. (2005). Epidemiologic evidence for the role of physical activity in reducing risk of type 2 diabetes and cardiovascular disease. *J Appl Physiol 99*, 1193–1204.

Berchtold NC, Castello N, & Cotman DW. (2010). Exercise and time-dependent benefits to learning and memory. *Neuroscience 167*, 588–597.

Boulé NG, Haddad E, Kenny GP, Wells GA, & Sigal RJ. (2001). Effects of exercise on glycemic control and body mass in type 2 diabetes mellitus: A meta-analysis of controlled clinical trials. *J Am Med Assn 286*, 1218–1227.

Carlson MC, Helms MJ, Steffens DC, Burke JR, Potter GG, & Plassman BL. (2008). Midlife activity predicts risk of dementia in older male twin pairs. *Alzheimer's Dementia 4*, 324–331.

Centers for Disease Control and Prevention (2010). Vital and health statistics: summary health statistics for US adults, National Health Interview Survey, 2009. Hyattsville, MD: US Department of Health and Human Services, Centers for Disease Control and Prevention, National Center for Health Statistics.

Choi SH, Veeraraghavalu K, Lazarov O, Marler S, Ransohoff RM, Ramirez JM, et al. (2008). Non-cell-autonomous effects of presenilin 1 variants on enrichment-mediated hippocampal progenitor cell proliferation and differentiation. *Neuron 59*, 568–580.

Colcombe S & Kramer AF. (2003). Fitness effects on the cognitive function of older adults: A meta-analytic study. *Psychol Sci 14*, 125–130.

Colcombe SJ, Erickson KI, Scalf PE, Kim JS, Prakash R, McAuley E, et al. (2006). Aerobic exercise training increases brain volume in aging humans. *J Gerontol A Biol Sci Med Sci 61*, 1166–1170.

Cox KL, Burke V, Beilin TJ, & Puddey IB. (2003). Controlled comparison of retention and adherence in home- vs center-initiated exercise interventions in women ages 40-65 years: the S.W.E.A.T Study. *Prev Med 36*, 17–29.

Creer DJ, Romberg C, Saksida LM, van Pragg H, & Bussey TJ. (2010). Running enhances spatial pattern separation in mice. *Proc Natl Acad Sci 107*, 2367–2372.

Cyarto EV, Cox KL, Almeida OP, Flicker L, Ames D, Byrne G, et al. (2010). The Fitness for the Ageing Brain Study II (FABSII): protocol for a randomized controlled clinical trial evaluating the effect of physical activity on cognitive function in patients with Alzheimer's disease. *Trials 11*, 120.

Daley A. (2008). Exercise and depression: A review of reviews. *J Clin Psychol Med Settings 15*, 140–147.

Dik M, Deeg DJ, Visser M, & Jonker C. (2003). Early life physical activity and cognition at old age. *J Clin Exp Neuropsychol 25*, 643–653.

Erickson KI, Voss MW, Prakash RS, Basak C, Szabo A, Chaddock L, et al. (2011). Exercise training increases size of hippocampus and improves memory. *Proc Natl Acad Sci U S A 108*, 3017–3022.

Fabrigoule C, Letenneur L, Dartigues JF, Zarrouk M, Commenges D, & Barberger-Gateau P. (1995). Social and leisure activities and risk of dementia: A prospective longitudinal study. *J Am Geriatr Soc 43*, 485–490.

Fielding RA, Rejeski WJ, Blair S, Church T, Espeland MA, Gill TM, et al. (2011). The Lifestyle Interventions and Independence for Elders Study: design and methods. *J Gerontol A Biol Sci Med Sci 66*, 1226–1237.

Feng R, Rampon C, Tang Y-P, Shrom D, Jin J, Kyin M, et al. (2001). Deficient neurogenesis in forebrain-specific presenilin-1 knockout mice is associated with reduced clearance of hippocampal memory traces. *Neuron 32*, 911–926.

Forbes D, Forbes S, Morgan DG, Markle-Reid M, Wood J, & Culum I. (2008). Physical activity programs for persons with dementia. *Cochrane Database Syst Rev. 3* (CD006489. DOI: 10.1002/14651858.CD006489.pub2).

Geda YE, Roberts RO, Knopman DS, Christianson TJ, Pankratz VS, Ivnik RJ, et al. (2010). Physical exercise, aging, and mild cognitive impairment: A population-based study. *Arch Neurol 67*, 80–86.

Gill JM & Cooper AR. (2008). Physical activity and prevention of type II diabetes mellitus. *Sports Med 38*, 807–824.

Hamer M & Chida Y. (2009). Physical activity and risk of neurodegenerative disease: A systematic review of prospective evidence. *Psychol Med 39*, 3–11.

Herring A, Blome M, Ambree O, Sachser N, Paulus W, & Keyvani K. (2010). Reduction of cerebral oxidative stress following environmental enrichment in mice with Alzheimer-like pathology. *Brain Pathol 20*, 166–175.

Heyn P, Beatriz CA, & Ottenbacher KJ. (2004). The effects of exercise training on elderly persons with cognitive impairment and dementia: A meta-analysis. *Arch Phys Med Rehabil 85*, 1694–1704.

Ho SC, Woo J, Sham A, Chan SG, & Yu AL. (2001). A 3-year follow-up study of social, lifestyle and health predictors of cognitive impairment in a Chinese older cohort. *Int J Epidemiol 30*, 1389–1396.

Hu Y, Xu P, Pigino G, Brady ST, Larson J, & Lazarov O. (2010). Complex environment experience rescues impaired neurogenesis, enhances synaptic plasticity, and attenuates neuropatholoy in familial Alzheimer's disease-linked APPswe/PS1Δ E9 mice. *FASEBJ 24*, 1667–1681.

Jorm AF. (2001). History of depression as a risk factor for dementia: An updated review. *Aust N Z J Psychiatry 35*, 776–781.

Kemoun G, Thibaud M, Roumagne N, Carette P, Albinet C, Toussaint L, et al. (2010). Effects of a physical training programme on cognitive function and walking efficiency in elderly persons with dementia. *Dement Geriatr Cogn Disord 29*, 109–114.

Kronenberg G, Bick-Sander A, Bunk E, Wolf C, Ehninger D, & Kempermann G. (2006). Physical exercise prevents age-related decline in precursor cell activity in the mouse dentate gyrus. *Neurobiol Aging 27*, 1505–1513.

Kushi L, Fee R, Folsom A, Mink P, Anderson K, & Sellers T. (1997). Physical activity and mortality in postmenopausal women. *J Am Med Assn 277*, 1287–1292.

Lam LCW, Chau RCM, Wong BML, Fung AWT, Liu VWC, Tam CCW, et al. (2011). Interim follow-up of a randomized controlled trial comparing Chinese style mind body (Tai Chi) and stretching exercises on cognitive function in subjects at risk of progressive cognitive decline. *Int J Geriatr Psychiatry 26*, 733–740.

Larson EB, Wang L, Bowen JD, McCormick WC, Teri L, Crane P, et al. (2006). Exercise is associated with reduced risk for incident dementia among persons 65 years of age and older. *Ann Intern Med 144*, 73–81.

Laurin D, Verreault R, Lindsay J, MacPherson K, & Rockwood K. (2001). Physical activity and risk of cognitive impairment and dementia in elderly persons. *Arch Neurol 58*, 498–504.

Lautenschlager NT, Cox KL, Flicker L, Foster JK, Van Bockxmeer F, Xiao J, et al. (2008). Effects of physical activity on cognitive function in older adults at risk for Alzheimer Disease. *J Am Med Assn 300*, 1027–1037.

Lazarov O, Mattson MP, Peterson DA, Pimplikar SW, & van Praag H. (2010a). When neurogenesis encounters aging and disease. *Trends Neurosci 33*, 569–579.

Lazarov O & Marr RA. (2010b). Neurogenesis and Alzheimer's disease: At the crossroads. *Exp Neurol 223*, 267–281.

Lee I, Hsieh C, & Paffenbarger R. (1995). Exercise intensity and longevity in men. *J Am Med Assn 273*, 1179–1184.

Lee CD, Folsom AR, & Blair SN. (2003). Physical activity and stroke risk: A meta-analysis. *Stroke 34*, 2475–2481.

Levi O & Michaelson DM. (2007). Environmental enrichment stimulates neurogenesis in apo-lipoprotein E3 and neuronal apoptosis in apolipoprotein E4 transgenic mice. *J Neurochem* 100, 202–210.

Liu-Ambrose T, Nagamatsu LS, Graf P, Beattie L, Ashe MC, & Handy TC. (2010a). Resistance training and executive functions: A 12-month randomized controlled trial. *Arch Intern Med* 170, 170–178.

Liu-Ambrose T, Eng JJ, Boyd LA, Jacova C, Davis JC, Bryan S, et al. (2010b). Promotion of the Mind through Exercise (PROMoTE): A proof-of-concept randomized, controlled trial of aerobic exercise training in older persons with vascular cognitive impairment. *BMC Neurol* 10:14.

Liu-Ambrose T, Nagamatsu LS, Voss MW, Khan KM, & Handy TC. (2012). Resistance training and functional plasticity of the aging brain: A 12-month randomized, controlled trial. *Neurobiol Aging*, 33(8), 1690–1698.

Lu FP, Lin KP, & Kuo HK. (2009). Diabetes and the risk of multi-system aging phenotypes: a systematic review and meta-analysis. *PLoS One* 4, e4144.

Lytle ME, Vander Bilt J, Pandav RS, Dodge HH, & Ganguli M. (2004). Exercise level and cognitive decline: The MoVIES project. *Alzheimer Dis Assoc Disord* 18, 57–64.

MacAuley D. (1994). A history of physical activity, health and medicine. *J Royal Soc Med* 87, 32–35.

Marcus BH, Banspach SW, Lefebvre RC, Rossi JS, Carleton RA, & Abrams DB. (1992). Using the stages of change model to increase the adoption of physical activity among community participants. *Am J Health Promotion* 6, 424–429.

Middleton LE, Barnes DE, Lui LY, & Yaffe K. (2010). Physical activity over the lifecourse and its association with cognitive performance and impairment in old age. *J Am Geriatr Soc* 58, 1322–1326.

Middleton LE, Mitnitski A, Fallah N, Kirkland SA, & Rockwood K. (2008a). Changes in cognition and mortality in relation to exercise in late life: A population based study. *PLoS One* 3, e3124.

Middleton LE, Kirkland S, & Rockwood K. (2008b). Prevention of CIND by physical activity: different impact on VCI-ND compared with MCI. *J Neurol Sci* 269, 80–84.

Middleton LE, Manini TM, Simonsick EM, Harris TB, Barnes DE, Tylavsky F, et al. (2011). Activity energy expenditure and incident cognitive impairment in older adults. *Arch Intern Med* 171, 1251–1257.

Mirochnic S, Wolf S, Staufenbiel M, & Kempermann G. (2009). Age effects on the regulation of adult hippocampal neurogenesis by physical activity and environmental enrichment in the APP23 mouse model of Alzheimers disease. *Hippocampus* 19, 1008–1018.

Nakajima S, Ohsawa I, Ohta S, Ohno M, & Mikame T. (2010). Regular voluntary exercise cures stress-induced impairment of cognitive function and cell proliferation accompanied by increases in cerebral IGF-1 and GST activity in mice. *Elsevier* 211, 178–184.

Ownby RL, Crocco E, Acevedo A, John V, & Loewenstein D. (2006). Depression and risk for Alzheimer disease: Systematic review, meta-analysis, and metaregression analysis. *Arch Gen Psychiatry* 63, 530–538.

Pitkala KH, Raivio MM, Laakkonenn M, Tilvis RS, Kautiainen H, & Strandberg TE. (2010). Exercise rehabilitation on home-dwelling patients with Alzheimer's disease—a randomized, controlled trial. *Study protocol, Trials* 11, 92.

Podewils LJ, Guallar E, Kuller LH, Fried LP, Lopez OL, Carlson M, et al. (2005). Physical activity, APOE genotype, and dementia risk: Findings from the Cardiovascular Health Cognition Study. *Am J Epidemiol* 161, 639–651.

Profenno LA, Porsteinsson AP, & Faraone SV. (2010). Meta-analysis of Alzheimer's disease risk with obesity, diabetes, and related disorders. *Biol Psychiatry* 67, 505–512.

Ravaglia G, Forti P, Lucicesare A, Pisacane N, Rietti E, & Bianchin M. (2008). Physical activity and dementia risk in the elderly: Findings from a prospective Italian study. *Neurology* 70, 1786–1794.

Rhyu IJ, Bytheway JA, Kohler SJ, Lange H, Lee KJ, Boklewski J, et al. (2010). Effects of aerobic exercise training on cognitive function and cortical vascularity in monkeys. *Neuroscience* 167, 1239–1248.

Richards M, Hardy R, & Wadsworth ME. (2003). Does active leisure protect cognition? Evidence from a national birth cohort. *Soc Sci Med* 56, 785–792.

Rogers RL, Meyer JS, & Mortel KF. (1990). After reaching retirement age physical activity sustains cerebral perfusion and cognition. *J Am Geriatr Soc 38*, 123–128.

Rovio S, Kareholt I, Helkala EL, Viitanen M, Winblad B, Tuomilehto J, et al. (2005). Leisure-time physical activity at midlife and the risk of dementia and Alzheimer's disease. *Lancet Neurol 4*, 705–711.

Schuitt AJ, Feskens EJ, Launer LJ, & Kromhaut D. (2001). Physical activity and cognitive decline, the role of the apolipoprotein E e4 allele. *Med Sci Sports Exer 33*, 772–777.

Shephard RJ. (2009). Independence: a new reason for recommending regular exercise to your patients. *Phys Sports Med 37*, 115–118.

Singh-Manoux A, Hillsdon M, Brunner E, & Marmot M. (2005). Effects of physical activity on cognitive functioning in middle age: Evidence from the Whitehall II prospective cohort study. *Am J Publ Health 95*, 2252–2258.

Sjösten N & Kivelä S-L (2006). The effects of physical exercise on depressive symptoms among the aged: A systematic review. *Int J Geriatr Psychiatry 21*, 410–418.

Snowden M, Steinman L, Mochan K, Grodstein F, Prohaska TR, Thurman DJ, et al. (2011). Effect of exercise on cognitive performance in community-dwelling older adults: Review of intervention trials and recommendations for public health practice and research. *J Am Geriatr Soc 59*, 704–716.

Snowdon DA, Greiner LH, Mortimer JA, Riley KP, Greiner PA, & Markesbery WR. (1997). Brain infarction and the clinical expression of Alzheimer disease. *The nun study. J Am Med Assn 277*, 813–817.

Sturman MT, Morris JC, Mendes de Leon CF, Bienias JL, Wilson RS, & Evans DA. (2005). Physical activity, cognitive activity and cognitive decline in a biracial community population. *Arch Neurol 62*, 1750–1754.

Sumic A, Michael YL, Carlson NE, Howieson DB, & Kaye JA. (2007). Physical activity and risk of dementia in oldest old. *J Aging Health 19*, 242–259.

Sun Q, Townsend MK, Okercke OI, Franco OH, Hu FB, & Grodstein F. (2010). Physical activity at midlife in relation to successful survival in women at age 70 years or older. *Arch Intern Med 170*, 194–201.

Taylor RS, Brown A, Ebrahim S, Jolliffe J, Noorani H, Rees K, et al. (2004). Exercise-based rehabilitation for patients with coronary heart disease: Systematic review and meta-analysis of randomized, controlled trials. *Am J Med 116*, 682–692.

Um H-S, Kang E-B, Koo J-H, Kim H-T, Jin-Lee, Kim E-J, et al. (2011). Treadmill exercise represses neuronal cell death in an aged transgenic mouse model of Alzheimer's disease. *Elsevier 69*, 161–173.

van Gelder BM, Tijhuis MA, Kalmijn S, Giampaoli S, Nissinen A, & Kromhout D. (2004). Physical activity in relation to cognitive decline in elderly men: The FINE study. *Neurology 63*, 2316–2321.

van Praag H, Christie BR, Sejnowski TJ, & Gage FH. (2005). Running enhances neurogenesis, learning, and long-term potentiation in mice. *Proc Natl Acad Sci 96*, 13,427–13,431.

Verghese J, Lipton RB, Katz MJ, Hall CB, Derby CA, Kuslansky G, et al. (2003). Leisure activities and the risk of dementia in the elderly. *New Engl J Med 348*, 2508–2516.

Vermeer SE, Prins ND, den Heijer T, Hofman A, Koudstaal PJ, & Breteler MM. (2003). Silent brain infarcts and the risk of dementia and cognitive decline. *N Engl J Med 348*, 1215–1222.

Vogel T, Brechat P-H, Leprêtre P-M, Kaltenbach G, Bertel M, & Lonsdorfer J. (2009). Health benefits of physical activity in older patients: A review. *Int J Clin Pract 63*, 303–320.

Voss MW, Prakash RS, Erickson KI, Basak C, Chaddock L, Kim JS, et al. (2010). Plasticity of brain networks in a randomized intervention trial of exercise training in older adults. *Front Aging Neurosci 2*, pii 32.

Wang HX, Karp A, Winblad B, Fratiglioni L.(2002) Late-life engagement in social and leisure activities is associated with a decreased risk of dementia: a longitudinal study from the Kungsholmen project. *Am J Epidemiol 155*(12), 1081–1087.

Wang JY, Zhou DH, Li J, Zhang M, Deng J, Tang M, et al. (2006). Leisure activity and risk of cognitive impairment: The Chongqing aging study. *Neurology 66*, 911–913.

Warburton DER, Nicol CW, & Bredin SSD. (2006). Health benefits of physical activity: The evidence. *CMAJ 174*, 801–809.

Weuve J, Kang JH, Manson JE, Breteler MM, Ware JH, & Grodstein F. (2004). Physical activity, including walking, and cognitive function in older women. *J Am Med Assn 292*, 1454–1461.

Williams JW, Plassman BL, Burke J, Holsinger T, & Benjamin S. (2010). Preventing Alzheimer's Disease and Cognitive Decline. Evidence Report/Technology Assessment No. 193. AHRQ Publication No. 10-E005. Rockville, MD: Agency for Healthcare Research and Quality.

Williamson DF, Vinicor F, Bowman BA, Centers for Disease Control and Prevention Primary Prevention Working Group. (2004). Primary prevention of type 2 diabetes mellitus by lifestyle intervention: implications for health policy. *Ann Inter Med 140*, 951–957.

Wilson RS, Bennett DA, Bienias JL, Aggarwal NT, Mendes De Leon CF, Morris MC, et al. (2002). Cognitive activity and incident AD in a population-basesd sample of older persons. *Neurology 59*, 1910–1914.

Yágüez L, Shaw K, Morris R, & Matthews D. (2010). The effects on cognitive functions of a movement-based intervention in patients with Alzheimer's type dementia: A pilot study. *Int J Geriatr Psychiatry 26*, 173–181.

Yaffe K, Barnes D, Nevitt M, Lui LY, & Covinsky K. (2001). A prospective study of physical activity and cognitive decline in elderly women: Women who walk. *Arch Intern Med 161*, 1703–1708.

Yamada M, Kasagi F, Sasaki H, Masunari N, Mimori Y, & Suzuki G. (2003). Association between dementia and midlife risk factors: The Radiation Effects Research Foundation adult health study. *J Am Geriatr Soc 51*, 410–414.

Yoshitake T, Kiyohara Y, Kato I, Ohmura T, Iwamoto H, Nakayama K, et al. (1995). Incidence and risk factors of vascular dementia and Alzheimer's disease in a defined elderly Japanese population: the Hisayama study. *Neurology 45*, 1161–1168.

10

Dietary Patterns and Dementia

PASCALE BARBERGER-GATEAU, MD, PHD, CATHERINE FÉART, PHD,

CÈCILIA SAMIERI, PHD, AND LUC LETENNEUR, PHD

Introduction

As a consequence of population aging, the prevalence of dementia is increasing worldwide (Wimo et al., 2003; Ferri et al., 2005; Kalaria et al., 2008). However, cognitive decline is preceded by a long phase of silent accumulation of neuropathological abnormalities leading to neurodegeneration (Jack Jr et al., 2010). Late-onset dementia results from a complex interaction between genetic predisposition and environmental protective or risk factors, including vascular and metabolic disorders (Fotuhi et al., 2009a). A recent systematic review of factors associated with cognitive decline concluded that the current literature did not provide adequate evidence to make recommendations for interventions for the prevention of dementia (Plassman et al., 2010). However, areas that were considered to offer potential leads included nutritional patterns such as a Mediterranean diet or diets high in vegetables or omega-3 fatty acids (Filley et al., 2011). Indeed, many risk factors for cognitive decline, such as hypertension, dyslipidemia, metabolic syndrome, diabetes, and obesity, may be modified by diet. Strongly linked to nutritional status, hyperinsulinemia, hyperglycemia, and insulin resistance are associated with a higher risk of dementia (Luchsinger, 2010). In addition, diet may have general effects on inflammation (Fung et al., 2005) and oxidative stress (Deschamps et al., 2001) that accompany brain aging and neurodegeneration (Parachikova et al., 2007; Querfurth et al., 2010). More specifically, several classes of nutrients could exert neuroprotective effects (Joseph et al., 2009). Thus, it is reasonable to hypothesize that the risk of dementia itself could be modified by diet. Healthy dietary patterns such as the Mediterranean diet combine several classes of nutrients that could work in synergy to slow down cognitive decline.

This chapter discusses the potential mechanisms linking diet to cognitive decline or risk for dementia and examines evidence from epidemiological studies and randomized clinical trials (RCTs) to support a protective effect of some nutrients and dietary patterns against brain aging.

Mechanisms Linking Diet and Dementia

The two main causes of late-life dementia are Alzheimer's disease (AD) and vascular dementia (VaD), including many mixed forms. In late-onset dementia, cognitive impairment results from genetic predisposing factors for sporadic AD (the ε4 allele of the apolipoprotein E gene [APOE4] and recently discovered genes such as CLU, CR1, or PICALM) but also from many acquired chronic conditions (Fotuhi et al., 2009a). These factors interact with inflammation and oxidative stress that are associated with brain aging and accumulation of β-amyloid (Aβ) protein in neuritic plaques and aggregation of hyperphosphorylated tau protein, the neuropathological hallmarks of AD. Thus, cognitive impairment results from nonmodifiable risk factors such as aging and genetics but also from an imbalance between deleterious and protective factors among which nutrition may play a major role (Fig. 10.1). In addition, subtle deficiencies in specific nutrients could contribute to worsen the neurodegenerative process.

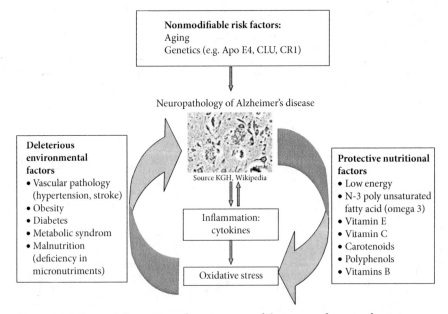

Figure 10.1 Impact of genetic and environmental factors on the aging brain.

ENERGY INTAKE

Being overweight results from a chronic imbalance between energy intake and energy expenditure. Obesity, especially visceral fat, is associated with higher levels of inflammation (Zajacova et al., 2011) and insulin resistance (Nomura et al., 2010), lower brain volume (Debette et al., 2010), poorer cognitive performance (Sabia et al., 2009), and higher risk of AD (Profenno et al., 2010). Higher caloric intake is associated with increased risk of AD, especially among individuals carrying the APOE4 allele (Luchsinger et al., 2002; Luchsinger et al., 2007). Conversely, caloric restriction (CR) is associated with an attenuation of oxidative damage and a modulation of insulin levels (Mattson et al., 2001; Heilbronn et al., 2006).

Few data are available to support a beneficial effect of CR on cognitive performance in humans. A small RCT assessed the effect of 6 months of CR on cognitive functioning in 48 overweight adults ages 25 years to 50 years (Martin et al., 2007). Daily energy deficit was not significantly associated with change in cognitive test performance over 6 months. To our knowledge, a single intervention study assessed the impact of CR on cognitive performance in elderly humans (Witte et al., 2009). In this trial, 50 normal-to-overweight elderly participants ages 50years to 80 years were assigned either to a CR diet, a diet enriched with unsaturated fatty acids, or to a control diet based on their age, sex, and body mass index (BMI). After 3 months, subjects assigned to a CR diet had a significant improvement in memory performance that was not observed in the other two groups. Moreover, memory improvement was correlated with decreases in fasting insulin and inflammation. Nevertheless, the results of this non-randomized trial should be considered as preliminary and certainly not generalized to the whole elderly population, where many individuals are at risk of under-nutrition. Although CR has some benefits in overweight individuals, its utility for the prevention of dementia, especially in older individuals, is not supported by current knowledge.

GLYCEMIC INDEX AND GLYCEMIC LOAD

The glycemic index (GI) is a measure of blood glucose elevation after consumption of a given food expressed relatively to that observed with a reference food, usually the same amount of glucose (Foster-Powell et al., 2002). The glycemic load (GL) of a typical serving of food is the product of the amount of available carbohydrate in that serving and the GI of the food (Foster-Powell et al., 2002). Diets rich in fruits, vegetables, and legumes such as the Mediterranean diet are related positively to GL but negatively to GI (Mendez et al., 2009).

Both GI and GL are related to some risk factors of dementia or cognitive decline. Low-GI or low-GL diets are independently associated with a reduced risk of type 2 diabetes and coronary heart disease (Barclay et al., 2008) and lower insulin levels (Shai et al., 2008). Obese adults assigned to a low-GL diet significantly decreased their triglyceride levels (Shai et al., 2008), a component of the metabolic syndrome associated with a higher risk of dementia (Raffaitin et al., 2009) and cognitive decline (Raffaitin et al., 2011).

However, energy-adjusted GL was not associated with risk of AD in a cohort of elderly community dwellers in New York (Luchsinger et al., 2007). A small RCT assessed the effects of low- and high-GL energy-restricted diets on mood and cognitive performance over 6 months in 42 overweight adults (Cheatham et al., 2009). Worsening mood outcome over time was observed in the high-GL diet group compared to the low-GL group. There was no significant change over time in cognitive performance in the subsample of 28 participants who completed the neuropsychological testing. Hence, the few available data do not support the practice of low-GL diets for the prevention of AD in the elderly (Luchsinger et al., 2007). Larger RCTs with longer follow-up are required.

DIETARY FAT

Fatty acids are classified according to their number of double bonds as saturated fatty acids (SFAs), mono-unsaturated fatty acids (MUFAs), or poly-unsaturated fatty acids (PUFAs). There are two families of PUFA: the omega-3 (or n-3) and the omega-6 (or n-6). In each family, the precursor cannot be synthesized by human beings and must therefore be found in the diet, mainly in vegetable oils and seeds. From these precursors, animals and human beings can synthesize long-chain derivatives. In the n-3 series, the precursor is alpha-linolenic acid (ALA) found in canola, walnut and soya oils, and in flaxseed and nuts. The main long-chain n-3 derivatives are eicosapentaenoic acid (EPA) and docosahexaenoic acid (DHA). However, the rate of conversion of ALA to EPA and then to DHA is very low (Burdge et al., 2005). A dietary supply of EPA and DHA by fatty fish (e.g., salmon, tuna, herring, mackerel, etc.) is therefore necessary. In the n-6 family, the precursor is linoleic acid mainly found in sunflower and grape seed oils, from which arachidonic acid is synthesized. n-3 and n-6 PUFAs come in competition for the biosynthesis of eicosanoids that have respective opposite effects (Schmitz et al., 2008). Indeed, long-chain n-3 PUFAs exert protective effects on the cardiovascular system including lowering triglyceride levels, anti-arrhythmic effects, vasodilatation, lower blood pressure, decreased inflammatory response, and decreased platelet aggregation (Jung et al., 2008), whereas n-6 PUFAs mainly have reverse effects. Moreover, fatty acids can modulate the expression of gene receptors because they are potent ligands for nuclear receptors (Schmitz et al., 2008). Eicosapentaenoic acid, DHA, and some eicosanoids are activators of peroxisome proliferator activated receptors (PPARs). The PPARs inhibit NFκB, a transcription factor that plays an important role in various inflammatory processes.

Long-chain n-3 PUFAs, especially DHA, have a major role in the brain. Docosahexaenoic acid is an absolute requirement for the development of the human central nervous system (Lukiw et al., 2008). Indeed, DHA is a major component of neuronal membranes under the form of phospholipids, contributing to membrane fluidity and synaptic plasticity (Gomez-Pinilla, 2008; Chytrova et al., 2010). Free unesterified DHA, undetectable in the brain under basal conditions, increases during brain injury, cerebral ischemia, and other pathological conditions (Lukiw et al., 2008). Unesterified DHA can be further metabolized to neuroprotective metabolites such as neuroprotectine D1 (NPD1), which exerts potent antioxidant, anti-inflammatory, and anti-apoptotic functions (Bazan, 2007; Lukiw et al., 2008).

Several longitudinal epidemiological studies have reported that people with high dietary intake of fish or long-chain n-3 PUFAs (Kalmijn et al., 1997b; Pascale Barberger-Gateau et al., 2002; Morris et al., 2003a; Morris et al., 2005a; van Gelder et al., 2007; Vercambre et al., 2009; Kesse-Guyot et al., 2011a) or higher blood levels of n-3 PUFAs (Schaefer et al., 2006; Beydoun et al., 2007; Samieri et al., 2008; Lopez et al., 2011) have lower risk of dementia or cognitive decline, although some contradictory results exist as well (Laurin et al., 2003; Devore et al., 2009; Kroger et al., 2009; van de Rest et al., 2009; Kesse-Guyot et al., 2011a; for reviews, *see* (Cunnane et al., 2009; Fotuhi et al., 2009b). This protective effect seems to be more pronounced in individuals who are not APOE4 carriers (Huang et al., 2005; Barberger-Gateau et al., 2007) with some inconsistent findings (Beydoun et al., 2007; Samieri et al., 2011a). The mechanisms underlying this gene–diet interaction are still speculative (Barberger Gateau et al., 2011).

Based on these promising data from observational studies, several recent RCTs of n-3 PUFAs for the prevention of dementia or cognitive decline have been conducted, but most of them have yielded disappointing results (Table 10.1). A notable exception is the MIDAS trial, which showed some efficacy of 900 mg/d of DHA for 24 weeks in middle-aged adults (55 years and older) with cognitive complaints and very mild age-related cognitive impairment (Yurko-Mauro et al., 2010). A small exploratory RCT of DHA (800 mg/d) supplementation associated or not with lutein during 4 months also showed a significant impact of DHA on verbal fluency and some memory items but not on other tasks (Johnson et al., 2008).

Mono-unsaturated fatty acids, or their dietary source in the form of olive oil, have also been associated with slower cognitive decline (Solfrizzi et al., 2006; Berr et al., 2009). Conversely, higher SFA intake at midlife was associated with poorer global cognitive function and prospective memory and with an increased risk of MCI (Eskelinen et al., 2008) and dementia (Laitinen et al., 2006) later in life. Higher intakes of SFA were also associated with cognitive decline (Morris et al., 2004) and higher risk of AD (Morris et al., 2003b) in older persons. Eventually, high consumption of trans-unsaturated fat also

Table 10.1 Randomized Controlled Trials With Omega-3 Polyunsaturated Fatty Acids for the Prevention of Cognitive Decline or Dementia

Study	Duration, Sample	Population	Intervention	Main cognitive outcomes	Results
MEMO (van de Rest et al., 2008)	26 weeks $n = 302$	≥ 65 years non-demented, volunteers, MMSE > 21	■ EPA+DHA (fish oil) (400 mg/d, ratio EPA/DHA=1,2) ■ EPA+DHA (1800 mg/d, ratio EPA/DHA=1,2) ■ Placebo (olive oil)	Four primary composite endpoints on several cognitive domains: attention, memory, sensorimotor speed and executive function, computed from five psychometric tests	No significant difference between treatment and placebo in any cognitive domain Post hoc analyses: improvement of attention in APOE4 carriers
Johnson et al. (2008)	4 months $n = 49$	60–80 years non-demented, women, volunteers	■ DHA (800 mg/d) ■ lutein (12 mg/d) ■ DHA+lutein ■ Placebo	Nine psychometric tests assessing verbal fluency, memory, processing speed, and attention	Improvement of verbal fluency in the three intervention arms compared to placebo; improvement of memory and learning in the DHA + lutein arm compared to placebo
OPAL (Dangour et al., 2010)	24 months $n = 867$	70–79 years non-demented, from general practices, MMSE > 24	■ EPA (200 mg/d) + DHA (500 mg/d), ratio EPA/DHA=0.4 ■ Placebo (olive oil)	California verbal learning test, Wechsler Memory Scale, spatial memory, three processing speed tests, digit span, verbal fluency, three tests of prospective memory	No significant difference between treatment and placebo
MIDAS (Yurko-Mauro et al., 2010)	24 months $n = 465$	≥ 55 years non-demented, with a subjective memory complaint and age-related cognitive decline, MMSE > 26	■ DHA (900 mg/d) ■ Placebo (corn + soy oils)	Cambridge Neuropsychological Test Automated Battery including Paired Associate Learning (PAL) test, PAL 6 pattern errors score	Improvement of episodic memory (PAL) in the treatment arm Secondary outcomes: improvement of verbal recognition memory score; no improvement of working memory or executive function

increases risk of AD (Morris et al., 2003b). However, no association with any type of dietary fat was observed in the Rotterdam study after 6 years of follow-up (Engelhart et al., 2002a) in contradiction with their previous finding (Kalmijn et al., 1997b).

Improving both the carbohydrate and lipid content of the diet might produce significant beneficial effects on cognition. A recent RCT assessed the impact of a LOW diet (low in fat, especially SFA, and low GI) in 48 older adults either healthy or with amnestic MCI (Bayer-Carter et al., 2011). The isocaloric control diet was high in fat and SFA and had a high GI. All food was delivered to the homes of participants for 4 weeks. The LOW diet had a significant impact on several biomarkers. In plasma, the LOW diet decreased insulin and cholesterol concentration. In CSF, the LOW diet increased $A\beta 42$ in participants with amnestic MCI but decreased $A\beta 42$ in normal controls; the LOW diet decreased F2-isoprostanes, a marker of oxidative stress. Finally, the LOW diet also had a small impact on cognition, with a significant improvement of delayed visual recall, but not on other measures of delayed memory or executive domains.

ANTIOXIDANT VITAMINS E AND C

Long-chain PUFAs are particularly vulnerable to lipid peroxidation in a situation of oxidative stress because of their multiple double-bonds. Hence, dietary antioxidants could contribute to protect these molecules and enhance the potential benefits of n-3 PUFAs. Oxidative stress results from an imbalance between production of free radicals and antioxidant defense mechanisms. The brain is particularly vulnerable to oxidative stress because of its high content of easily peroxidizable long-chain PUFAs and the high *in situ* production of free radicals coming from oxygen and glucose metabolism (Floyd et al., 2002). Paradoxically, the brain is not highly enriched in antioxidant defense mechanisms (Floyd et al., 2002). Moreover, accumulation of $A\beta$ is associated with increased production of free radicals leading to increased lipid peroxidation (Montine et al., 2002). In turn, lipid peroxidation directly damages neuronal membranes and contributes to the progression of neurodegeneration (Montine et al., 2005).

Vitamin E is a generic term for eight compounds including tocopherols and tocotrienols found in vegetable oils, seeds, and nuts. Vitamin E represents the major lipid-soluble antioxidant found in cells. The main function of vitamin E is to prevent the peroxidation of membrane phospholipids (Lucarini et al., 2007). Several longitudinal epidemiological studies have found an inverse association between dietary intake of vitamin E and risk of AD or cognitive decline (Engelhart et al., 2002b; Morris et al., 2005b; Wengreen et al., 2007; Devore et al., 2010), whereas no association was evidenced in other studies (Kalmijn et al., 1997a; Luchsinger et al., 2003; Laurin et al., 2004). Low plasma vitamin E was also linked to increased risk of incident dementia or cognitive decline in

Table 10.2 Randomized Controlled Trials With Antioxidants for the Prevention of Cognitive Decline or Dementia

Study	Design	Inclusion criteria	Interventions	Cognitive outcomes	Results
Vitamin E					
Substudy from the Women's Health Study (Kang et al., 2006)	$n = 6,377$ in the cognitive substudy (initiated 5.6 years after randomization) 10 years treatment, 4 years follow-up	≥ 65 years Women, non-demented, volunteers	■ α-tocopherol 600 IU on alternate day ■ Placebo	Telephone cognitive battery of five tests measuring general cognition (Telephone Interview of Cognitive Status), verbal memory and category fluency	No significant difference between treatment and placebo *Post hoc* analyses: improvement among women with dietary intake of vitamin E < 6.1 mg/d, among those practicing exercise less than once a week, among women without diabetes, and among compliant subjects
Alzheimer's Disease Cooperative Study Group (Petersen et al., 2005)	$n=769$ 3 y	55–90 years Amnestic mild cognitive impairment (MCI) of degenerative nature	■ Vitamin E 2000 IU/d ■ Donepezil 10 mg/d ■ Placebo	Incident AD (possible or probable)	No significant difference between any treatment and placebo
β-carotene					
Substudy from the The Physician's Health Study II (Grodstein et al., 2007)	$n = 5,956$ men Two groups:- long-term supplementation ($n = 4,052$ participants from the Physician's Health Study), 18 years; - short-term supplementation ($n = 1,904$ new recruits in 1998), 1 year	Long-term supplementation group:≥55 y at randomization, mean age > 70 years at cognitive assessment Short-term supplementation group:mean age >70 years All volunteers	■ β-carotene 50 mg on alternate day ■ Placebo	Telephone cognitive battery of five tests measuring general cognition (Telephone Interview of Cognitive Status), verbal memory and category fluency	Long-term supplementation group: improvement of global cognition in the treatment arm compared to placebo. Short-term supplementation group: no significant difference between treatment and placebo

Vitamins E + C + β-carotene

MRC / BHF Heart protection study (Heart Protection Study Collaborative Group, 2002)	$n = 20,536$ 5 years	40–80 years Coronary heart disease, other occlusive arterial disease or diabetes	■ vitamin C 250mg/d + vitamin E 600 mg/d + β-carotene 20 mg/d ■ Placebo	Telephone Interview for Cognitive Status	No significant difference between any treatment and placebo for cognitive performances
Smith et al. (1999)	$n = 185$ 12 months	60–80 years Volunteers	■ vitamin C 500mg/d + α-tocopherol 400 mg/d + β carotene 12 mg/d ■ Placebo	Psychometric tests assessing episodic memory, recognition memory, reaction time and vigilance, logical reasoning, attention	No significant difference between treatment and placebo in any psychometric test

Vitamins E + C + β-carotene + Zn + Cu

Substudy from the Age-Related Eye Disease Study (AREDS) (Yaffe et al., 2004)	$n = 2,166$ in the cognitive substudy 6.9 years in median	Mean age 75 years Non-demented Volunteers	■ Antioxidants:vitamin C 500mg/d + vitamin E 400 IU/d + β carotene 15 mg/d ■ Zn 80mg/d + Cu oxide 2mg/d ■ Antioxidants + Zn + Cu ■ Placebo	Performances on six psychometric tests	No significant difference between treatment and placebo in any psychometric test

(continued)

Table 10.2 **(Continued)**

Study	Design	Inclusion criteria	Interventions	Cognitive outcomes	Results
Zn					
ZENITH (Maylor et al., 2006)	$n = 387$ 6 months	55–87 years BMI between 20 and 30 kg/m² Good health MMSE > 23 Not depressed	▪ Zn 15 mg/d ▪ Zn 30 mg/d ▪ Placebo	Cambridge Neuropsychological Test Automated Battery	Beneficial effect of both doses of Zn on spatial working memory at 3 months Detrimental effect of 15 mg/d for matching to sample visual search latency

several studies (Helmer et al., 2003; Cherubini et al., 2005; Mangialasche et al., 2010), whereas other studies found no significant relationship (Kang et al., 2008; Ravaglia et al., 2008). Interestingly, in the Chicago Health and Aging Project (CHAP) the protective effect of dietary vitamin E was observed only among individuals without the APOE4 allele (Morris et al., 2002). However, most studies examined only the role of α-tocopherol, whereas each form exhibits specific biological functions, including anti-inflammatory activity and modulation of different signaling pathways that could have an impact on brain aging (Mangialasche et al., 2010). Hence various tocopherol forms may be important in the protective association with AD (Morris et al., 2005b; Mangialasche et al., 2010).

Vitamin C is a water-soluble compound found in many fruits and vegetables. Vitamin C exerts strong antioxidant effects because of its reducing capacities. However, there is little epidemiological evidence that higher dietary intake of vitamin C is associated with better cognitive performances over time (Engelhart et al., 2002b; Wengreen et al., 2007), whereas most studies did not find such an association (Kalmijn et al., 1997a; Commenges et al., 2000; Morris et al., 2002; Luchsinger et al., 2003; Laurin et al., 2004; Devore et al., 2010).

Randomized controlled trials have been conducted with various doses of vitamin E either alone (Petersen et al., 2005; Kang et al., 2006) or in combination with other antioxidants (Smith et al., 1999; Heart Protection Study Collaborative Group, 2002; Yaffe et al., 2004) for the prevention of dementia or cognitive decline, mostly in cognitively normal volunteers except one in patients with MCI (Petersen et al., 2005) and another in participants with vascular risk factors (Heart Protection Study Collaborative Group, 2002) (Table 10.2). There was no significant difference between any treatment arm with vitamins C or E and placebo, except in the Women's Health Study among women with dietary intake of vitamin E below the median (6.1 mg/d), among those practicing exercise less than once a week, among women without diabetes, and among compliant subjects, with the methodological limitations inherent to such *post hoc* analyses (Kang et al., 2006). Notably, all these RCTs used vitamin E doses far above the recommended intake (15 mg/day for adults).

CAROTENOIDS

Carotenoids are a vast family of fat-soluble anti-oxidant molecules including pro-vitamin A carotenoids (α- and β-carotene, β-cryptoxanthin) but also lycopene and xanthophylls (e.g., lutein, zeaxanthin), which have no vitamin A activity. Carotenes are found in colored fruits and vegetables, whereas xanthophylls are found in green vegetables, corn, and egg yolk and lycopene in tomato.

Cohort studies linking carotenoids and cognitive decline have provided conflicting results. Two cohort studies with 7 years of follow-up observed a slower cognitive decline in participants who had higher serum β-carotene levels but only among APOE4 carriers (Hu et al., 2006) or in those with higher total dietary intake of carotene, yet this protective association was limited to the first 3 years of follow-up (Wengreen et al., 2007). Conversely, in the Etude du Vieillissement Arteriel (EVA) study and in a subsample of the Nurses' Health Study, plasma levels of total carotenoids or levels of specific carotenoids were not associated with rate of cognitive decline (Berr et al., 2000; Kang et al., 2008). Regarding risk of dementia, dietary intake of carotenoids was not related to a decreased risk of AD in the Washington Heights-Inwood Columbia Aging Project (WHICAP) (Luchsinger et al., 2003). Similarly, midlife dietary intake of β-carotene was not related to the incidence of late-life dementia in the Honolulu-Asia Aging Study (Laurin et al., 2004). Conversely, intake of β-carotene was associated with lower risk of AD in the Rotterdam study but only among current smokers with a mean follow-up of 6 years (Engelhart et al., 2002b) and not after 10 years of follow-up (Devore et al., 2010).

Five RCTs have evaluated the impact of a supplementation with carotenoids—either alone or in combination—on cognition, and two have yielded partially positive results (Tables 10.1 and 10.2). In the Physicians' Health Study, older participants in the β-carotene arm (50 mg on alternate days) had a significantly higher mean cognitive score at the end of the trial than the placebo arm but only in the continuing participants with mean treatment duration of 18 years and not in newer recruits (Grodstein et al., 2007). A small RCT showed a significant impact of lutein (12 mg/d), administered during 4 months either alone or in combination with DHA, on verbal fluency (Johnson et al., 2008). Interestingly, this trial also evidenced an impact of the supplementation on some memory tests but only in the combined arm, suggesting a synergy between DHA and lutein (Table 10.1). Other combinations of carotene with various antioxidants did not have any impact on cognition in RCTs (Smith et al., 1999; Heart Protection Study Collaborative Group, 2002; Yaffe et al., 2004).

POLYPHENOLS

Polyphenolic compounds are the most abundant antioxidants in the diet. The main dietary sources of polyphenols are fruits, vegetables, plant-derived beverages (such as tea, coffee, and wine), and virgin olive oil. Polyphenols show an important chemical diversity and can broadly be divided into two categories—that is, flavonoids and non-flavonoid polyphenols. In vivo and in vitro studies have demonstrated the antioxidant activity of phenolic compounds (Singh et al., 2008). Moreover, catechins, a subclass of flavonoids, have shown anti-inflammatory and anti-apoptosis properties in animal models (Singh et al., 2008). Another polyphenol, curcumin, also showed anti-inflammatory effects and prevented Aβ peptide aggregation (Singh et al., 2008). Resveratrol is a non-flavonoid polyphenol found in grapes, red wine, and berries. Resveratrol improved several cognitive functions in adult primates in a similar manner as CR (Dal-Pan et al., 2011). Administration of resveratrol improved cerebral blood flow in healthy adults but had no impact on cognitive function (Kennedy et al., 2010).

Few epidemiological studies have examined the association between polyphenol intake and cognitive performance. In the Zutphen Elderly Study, decline on the MMSE over 3 years was not associated with dietary intake of flavonoids (Kalmijn et al., 1997a). However, the follow-up was probably too short to capture a significant decline of cognitive performance. In the French PAQUID study, individuals in the highest quartile of flavonoid intake had a significantly slower cognitive decline on the MMSE over 10 years (Letenneur et al., 2007). Moreover, a gradient in cognitive decline was observed according to flavonoid intake since cognitive decline worsened as dietary flavonoid intake decreased. Dietary intake of flavonoids in the two highest tertiles was also associated with a 50% reduction in risk of incident dementia in the same cohort (Commenges et al., 2000). In the Rotterdam Study, a high intake of flavonoids was associated with reduced risk of AD but only in current smokers (Engelhart et al., 2002b) and not confirmed in a longer follow-up of the cohort (Devore et al., 2010). Similarly, in the Honolulu-Asia Aging Study, midlife dietary intake of flavonoids did not modify the risk of late-life dementia (Laurin et al., 2004). Interestingly, tea (Ng et al., 2008) and coffee (Ritchie et al., 2007) consumption have been inversely associated with cognitive decline, maybe in part because of their polyphenol content. Indeed, the major phenolic compound of green tea extract is able to prevent memory impairment in transgenic mice by reducing Aβ levels through a modification of secretase activities (Lee et al., 2009). However, convincing arguments for a protective role of polyphenols in cognitive aging in humans are still lacking, mainly because of the huge variety of molecules and the difficulty of assessment of their intake and bioavailability (Manach et al., 2004; Perez-Jimenez et al., 2010). To our knowledge, no published RCT is available to assess the impact of various classes of polyphenols on cognition in humans yet.

SELENIUM AND ZINC

Cofactors of the antioxidant enzymatic defence systems glutathione peroxidase, Cu/Zn superoxide dismutase and catalase such as selenium, zinc, and manganese are also found in the diet. Interestingly, zinc deficiency impairs whole-body accumulation of PUFAs, suggesting a beneficial synergy between zinc and PUFA for the brain (Jayasooriya et al., 2005; Bourre, 2006). In the EVA study, low selenium levels in plasma were associated with a higher risk of cognitive decline (Berr et al., 2000).

However, the two RCTs assessing the impact of zinc supplementation on cognitive function have yielded disappointing results. An ancillary study of the Age-Related Eye Disease Study did not show any significant effect of treatment with zinc (80 mg) and copper (cupric oxide, 2 mg) either alone or in combination with antioxidants on cognitive endpoints (Table 10.2) (Yaffe et al., 2004). The ZENITH study comparing two levels of zinc supplementation (15 mg/d or 30 mg/d) with placebo showed only a modest impact of both doses on spatial working memory at 3 months but a detrimental effect of 15 mg/d for matching to sample visual search latency (Maylor et al., 2006).

B VITAMINS

B vitamins play an important role in risk of cardiovascular disease and brain development. Folate (vitamin B9), along with vitamins B6 and B12, is required for the metabolism of homocysteine (Mattson et al., 2003). In the brain, homocysteine promotes excitotoxicity via stimulation of NMDA receptors and damages neuronal DNA (Mattson et al., 2003). Folate deprivation and increased homocysteine interact synergistically with several factors that contribute to the development of AD, including Aβ neurotoxicity, oxidative stress, and apoptosis (Mattson et al., 2003). Hyperhomocysteinemia is also associated with high circulating concentrations of pro-inflammatory cytokines (Gori et al., 2005). Moreover, elevated concentration of homocysteine in serum is a major risk factor of cardiovascular disease (Wald et al., 2002; de Ruijter et al., 2009).

Homocysteine concentration is mainly determined by folate intake (Fairfield et al., 2002). Folate is found in green leafy vegetables, liver, and wheat germ. Vitamin B6 is found in a wide variety of foods including beans, meat, poultry, fish, and some fruits and vegetables. Vitamin B12 is found in animal products, especially liver. Many manufactured foods are fortified with folic acid (the synthetic form of folate) or vitamins B6 or B12.

Prospective cohort studies have shown that hyperhomocysteinemia was a strong independent risk factor for dementia and AD (Seshadri et al., 2002), raising the hope that lowering homocysteine concentration could prevent dementia (Morris, 2003). In addition, epidemiological studies have provided support for a protective effect of B vitamins against neurodegenerative disorders, with nevertheless some inconsistent findings (Raman et al., 2007; Clarke et al., 2008). However, most RCTs examining the impact of various B vitamins—either alone or in combination—on cognitive decline have been extremely disappointing despite a strong effect on homocysteine concentration (Clarke et al., 2008). A recent meta-analysis concluded that trials of folic acid, with or without other B vitamins, have shown no effect on cognitive function within 3 years of the start of treatment (Wald et al., 2010).

There are, however, three promising exceptions to this general lack of impact of B vitamins on cognitive function in RCTs. The Folic Acid and Carotid Intima-media Thickness (FACIT) trial evidenced that a 3-year supplementation with folic acid (0.8 mg/d) was associated with better global cognitive function, memory, and information processing speed compared to placebo in participants ages 50 years to 70 years with raised homocysteine concentration (Durga et al., 2007). Recently, the VITACOG trial showed that treatment with folic acid (0.8 mg/d), vitamin B12 (0.5 mg/d), and vitamin B6 (20 mg/d) for 2 years significantly slowed the rate of brain atrophy by 30% compared to placebo in participants age 70 years and older with a diagnosis of MCI (Smith et al., 2010a). Although such quantities cannot be achieved by diet alone, these trials support a role of B vitamins in brain aging. The interaction between B vitamins and n-3 PUFA on cognitive functions has been tested in an ancillary study of the SUFOLOM3 (SUpplementation with FOLate, vitamins B-6 and B-12, and/or OMega-3 fatty acids) RCT (Andreeva et al., 2011). There was no overall effect of treatment on cognition but less decline on the temporal orientation task in the subgroup with prior stroke receiving the combined treatment.

POTENTIAL ROLE OF OTHER NUTRIENTS: VITAMIN D

Vitamin D is found in fatty fish along with long-chain n-3 PUFA and could thus contribute to the protective relationship of fish consumption to cognitive decline. The prevalence of vitamin D deficiency is very high in older adults (Holick, 2007; Cashman et al., 2009). There is ample biological evidence to suggest an important role for vitamin D in brain development and function (McCann et al., 2008) but epidemiological evidence is still lacking. Several cross-sectional studies have found an association between vitamin D deficiency and cognitive impairment (Oudshoorn et al., 2008; Buell et al., 2009; Wilkins et al., 2009; Annweiler et al., 2010b; Annweiler et al., 2010a; Seamans et al., 2010; Llewellyn et al., 2011). More convincingly, participants in the InCHIANTI cohort study who were severely serum 25hydroxy-vitamin D-deficient (<25 nmol/L) had a significantly increased risk of decline on neuropsychological tests of global and executive cognitive functions over 6 years (Llewellyn et al., 2010). Yet this association was not reproduced in another longitudinal study (Slinin et al., 2010). More research is therefore needed on the role of vitamin D in brain aging (Miller, 2010) before implementing RCTs.

LIMITS OF A "SINGLE-NUTRIENT" APPROACH

In summary, experimental and epidemiological data suggest a protective role of n-3 PUFA, some antioxidants, and B vitamins against cognitive aging. However, most RCT of supplementation with high doses of single nutrients for the prevention of dementia or cognitive decline have been disappointing. Several explanations may account for these discrepancies. First, the timing and length of the supplementation in RCTs may be inadequate—that is, too short in duration or too late in the course of the disease. Indeed, diet measured at a single point in time in most observational studies may reflect lifelong habits, providing a longlasting protective environment for the brain. Second, most RCTs used dosages of nutrients far above the recommended intakes, which may be inappropriate for the prevention of cognitive decline in healthy, non-deficient individuals. Moreover, high-dose supplements may be more harmful than beneficial (Bjelakovic et al., 2007). Eventually, most RCTs administered single nutrients, whereas these are consumed in combination in the diet where they can exert additional or synergistic effects. It is therefore difficult to pinpoint any single nutrient that contributes the most to the observed protective effects (Voutilainen et al., 2006).

We can therefore make the assumption that healthy dietary patterns combining nutrients in adequate amounts and proportions would be more efficient than single nutrients to slow down cognitive decline and postpone the onset of dementia. This assumption is supported by the promising results of a RCT of a medical food combining several nutrients, including EPA; DHA; vitamins A, B, C, D and E; zinc; and many other trace elements in patients with mild AD (Scheltens et al., 2010; Kamphuis et al., 2011). Although these data need to be replicated in other ongoing RCTs, they suggest that balanced diets could contribute to slow down cognitive decline in older persons. The second part of this chapter will focus on healthy dietary patterns and their relationship with cognition.

Dietary Patterns and Cognitive Decline

OVERALL DIET QUALITY

Several indices have been proposed to assess overall diet quality, but few longitudinal studies have examined their association with cognitive performances. The Healthy Eating Index (HEI) is a measure of compliance to the key recommendations of the Dietary Guidelines for Americans. A revised version was developed and validated to take into account the 2005 Dietary Guidelines (Guenther et al., 2008a; Guenther et al., 2008b). The HEI-2005 is composed of 12 food groups or nutrients including fruits, vegetables, whole grain, milk, meat, beans, oils, sodium, saturated fat, and calories from solid fat, alcohol, and sugar. A scoring system gives points according to quantities actually consumed expressed as a ratio to energy intake. The score increases with increasing adherence to the recommendations. To our knowledge, the single study examining the link between the HEI and cognition showed no association between the HEI-2005 score and the rate of cognitive decline over 7.6 years in the CHAP participants (Tangney et al., 2011).

In the Cache County Study on Memory and Aging, a recommended food score (RFS) was derived by summing the number of foods recommended by current dietary guidelines, based on 57 food items (Wengreen et al., 2009). Conversely, a non-RFS was computed by summing the number of non-recommended highly processed, energy-dense foods consumed at least three times/week. Higher

RFS was associated with better modified MMSE score at baseline but also with slower cognitive decline over 11 years of follow-up. The non-RFS was not associated with cognitive performance.

Adherence to the French nutritional guidelines was assessed on a score based on 13 recommendations (Kesse-Guyot et al., 2011b). A higher score was associated with better cognitive performances for memory, and semantic and phonemic fluency evaluated 13 years later in adults participating in the Supplementation with Antioxidant Vitamins and Minerals (SUVIMAX) study.

THE DASH DIET

The Dietary Approaches to Stop Hypertension (DASH) diet tried to combine protective nutrients in a diet rich in fruits, vegetables, and low-fat dairy foods and containing reduced amounts of saturated fat, total fat, and cholesterol (Appel et al., 1997). Higher adherence to the DASH diet is associated with lower blood pressure (Appel et al., 1997; Schulze et al., 2003).

The Exercise and Nutritional Interventions for Cardiovascular Health (ENCORE) RCT was designed to examine the effects of the DASH diet (alone or in combination with weight management through exercise and CR) on blood pressure in overweight adults with high blood pressure (Blumenthal et al., 2010). Besides its beneficial effects on blood pressure and insulin sensitivity (the latter only if combined with weight management), the DASH diet was associated with a significantly improved psychomotor speed relative to controls (Smith et al., 2010b). Interestingly, an improvement of executive functions was also observed when the DASH diet was associated with weight management, suggesting a favorable impact of CR combined with a healthy diet on cognitive functions in this specific population.

THE MEDITERRANEAN DIET

The traditional Mediterranean diet is characterized by a high consumption of fruits and nuts, vegetables, legumes, cereals, and olive oil, a moderate consumption of fish and wine, but a low-to-moderate intake of dairy products and a low intake of meat as sources of saturated fat (Trichopoulou et al., 2003). Adherence to a Mediterranean diet is usually assessed by the Mediterranean diet (MeDi)-score based on eight food groups and the MUFA-to-SFA ratio in the diet (Trichopoulou et al., 2003). High adherence to a Mediterranean-style diet was associated with longer survival, reduced risk for cardiovascular mortality and cancer incidence, and mortality in meta-analyses (Sofi et al., 2008; Sofi et al., 2010).

Recently, several longitudinal epidemiological studies have shown that higher adherence to a Mediterranean diet was associated with a lower risk of global cognitive decline (Feart et al., 2009; Tangney et al., 2011), MCI

(Scarmeas et al., 2009a), or AD (Scarmeas et al., 2006b), but inconsistent results exist as well regarding incidence of all-cause dementia (Feart et al., 2009; Roberts et al., 2010) or MCI (Roberts et al., 2010). The association between the MeDi-score and cognition was independent of physical activity level (Scarmeas et al., 2009b) and vascular risk factors (Scarmeas et al., 2006a; Feart et al., 2009). A meta-analysis combining data from the first two studies, the WHICAP in the United States and the 3C study in France, estimated that the overall risk of neurodegenerative disease was decreased by 13% for a 2-point increase of adherence score to the Mediterranean diet (Sofi et al., 2010). In the WHICAP, higher adherence to a Mediterranean diet was also associated with reduced cerebrovascular disease burden—notably infarcts—whereas no association was found with white matter hyperintensities (Scarmeas et al., 2011).

Many mechanisms could explain the beneficial effects of the Mediterranean diet on cognition. Indeed, the Mediterranean diet combines several foods and nutrients that might interact to protect the brain: olive oil (Berr et al., 2009; Samieri et al., 2011b), fruits and vegetables (Kang et al., 2005; Morris et al., 2006; Hughes et al., 2010). However, in most studies there was no association with any single component of the score, confirming that composite dietary patterns can capture dimensions of nutrition that may be missed by individual components. A combination of dietary sources of n-3 PUFA and antioxidants as provided by the Mediterranean diet seems necessary to achieve protection against dementia (Barberger-Gateau et al., 2007).

Vascular factors are possible mediators to explain the relationship of the Mediterranean diet to cognition although nonvascular biological mechanisms, such as inflammation, oxidative, and metabolic responses, could also be involved (Frisardi et al., 2010). Indeed, a RCT evidenced that individuals consuming a Mediterranean diet had a decreased lipid oxidative and inflammatory status in plasma and a decreased expression of genes related to inflammatory processes and oxidative stress, an effect that was attributed to virgin olive oil polyphenols (Konstantinidou et al., 2010). Higher adherence to a Mediterranean diet was also associated with decreased lipid peroxidation (Gaskins et al., 2010) and higher plasma n-3 PUFA concentrations (Feart et al., 2011). A RCT showed that polyphenols from olive oil had a beneficial effect on biomarkers of oxidative stress (Covas et al., 2006). A recent meta-analysis of 50 epidemiological studies and RCTs totalling 534,906 participants suggested that higher adherence to a Mediterranean diet was significantly associated with a decreased risk of metabolic syndrome and an improvement of all its components (Kastorini et al., 2011). The Prevencion con Dieta Mediterranea (PREDIMED) RCT demonstrated that it was able to reduce the incidence of type 2 diabetes by 50% (Salas-Salvado et al., 2011). Moreover, the Mediterranean diet may prevent weight gain (Beunza et al., 2010; Romaguera et al., 2010) and obesity (Buckland et al., 2008) and reduce body weight, as recently demonstrated by a meta-analysis

(Esposito et al., 2011). However, the association of the MeDi score with AD risk was independent of inflammation (Gu et al., 2010) and fasting insulin (Gu et al., 2010), suggesting other underlying mechanisms.

Conclusion

Taken altogether, these data suggest that healthy diets such as the Mediterranean diet may contribute to slow down cognitive aging, in addition to many other benefits. Healthy diets can improve cardiovascular and metabolic profiles and over the long term might lead to lower incidence of AD (Barnes, 2011). Because dementia is a multifactorial disease, diets combining adequate energy intake, low GI, and several classes of protective nutrients brought by fruits, vegetables, and fish are probably the most efficient for prevention.

However, these data must be confirmed by RCTs before specific dietary recommendations can be made for the prevention of cognitive decline and dementia. Importantly, residual confounding cannot be excluded and inter-action with other components of lifestyle should be considered, especially physical activity. Exercise can enhance the impact of DHA supplementation in animals, thanks in particular to improved synaptic plasticity (Chytrova et al., 2010). Large RCTs with long follow-up are needed to definitely rule out resid-ual confounding and examine the interaction between different components of the diet and physical activity.

Given that many factors of dementia act at midlife, healthy diets should prob-ably be started early and sustained for many years, which may be impossible to evidence by RCTs. Indeed, cognitive benefits of healthy diets may be achieved only over the long term. Nevertheless, RCTs should assess the impact of shift-ing to a healthy diet on trajectories of cognitive decline in older persons, all the more because lifestyle interventions such as promoting a Mediterranean diet are exceptionally low risk with a high potential for gain (Barnes, 2011).

References

Andreeva, V.A., E. Kesse-Guyot, P. Barberger-Gateau, L. Fezeu, S. Hercberg, & P. Galan. 2011. Cognitive function after supplementation with B vitamins and long-chain omega-3 fatty acids: ancillary findings from the SU.FOL.OM3 randomized trial, *American Journal of Clinical Nutrition, 94* (1), 278–286.

Annweiler, C., A.M. Schott, Y. Rolland, H. Blain, F.R. Herrmann, & O. Beauchet. 2010a. Dietary intake of vitamin D and cognition in older women, *Neurology, 75* (20), 1810–1816.

Annweiler, C., A.M. Schott, G. Allali, S.A. Bridenbaugh, R.W. Kressig, P. Allain, et al. 2010b. Association of vitamin D deficiency with cognitive impairment in older women. Cross-sectional study, *Neurology, 74* (1), 27–32.

Appel, L.J., T.J. Moore, E. Obarzanek, W.M. Vollmer, L.P. Svetkey, F.M. Sacks, et al. 1997. A clinical trial of the effects of dietary patterns on blood pressure, *New England Journal of Medicine, 336* (16), 1117–1124.

Barberger-Gateau, P., L. Letenneur, V. Deschamps, K. Peres, J.-F. Dartigues, & S. Renaud. 2002. Fish, meat, and risk of dementia: cohort study, *British Medical Journal, 325* (7370), 932–3.

Barberger-Gateau, P., C. Raffaitin, L. Letenneur, C. Berr, C. Tzourio, J.F. Dartigues et al. 2007. Dietary patterns and risk of dementia: the Three-City cohort study, *Neurology, 69* (20), 1921–1930.

Barberger Gateau, P., C. Samieri, C. Feart, & M. Plourde. 2011. Dietary omega 3 polyunsaturated fatty acids and Alzheimer's disease: Interaction with apolipoprotein E genotype, *Current Alzheimer Research, 8* (5), 479–491.

Barclay, A.W., P. Petocz, J. McMillan-Price, V.M. Flood, T. Prvan, P. Mitchell et al. 2008. Glycemic index, glycemic load, and chronic disease risk – a meta-analysis of observational studies, *American Journal of Clinical Nutrition, 87* (3), 627–637.

Barnes, D.E. 2011. The mediterranean diet: Good for the heart = good for the brain?, *Annals of Neurology, 69* (2), 226–228.

Bayer-Carter, J.L., P.S. Green, T.J. Montine, B. VanFossen, L.D. Baker, G.S. Watson, et al. 2011. Diet intervention and cerebrospinal fluid biomarkers in amnestic Mild Cognitive Impairment, *Archives of Neurology, 68* (6), 743–752.

Bazan, N.G. 2007. Omega-3 fatty acids, pro-inflammatory signaling and neuroprotection, *Current Opinion in Clinical Nutrition and Metabolic Care, 10* (2), 136–141.

Berr, C., B. Balansard, J. Arnaud, A.M. Roussel, & A. Alperovitch. 2000. Cognitive decline is associated with systemic oxidative stress: the EVA study. Etude du Vieillissement Arteriel, *Journal of the American Geriatrics Society, 48* (10), 1285–1291.

Berr, C., F. Portet, C. Carriere, N.T. Akbaraly, C. Feart, V. Gourlet, et al. 2009. Olive oil and cognition: results from the Three-City study, *Dementia and Geriatric Cognitive Disorders, 28*, 357–364.

Beunza, J.-J., E. Toledo, F.B. Hu, M. Bes-Rastrollo, M. Serrano-Martinez, A. Sanchez-Villegas, et al. 2010. Adherence to the Mediterranean diet, long-term weight change, and incident overweight or obesity: the Seguimiento Universidad de Navarra (SUN) cohort, *American Journal of Clinical Nutrition, 92* (6), 1484–1493.

Beydoun, M.A., J.S. Kaufman, J.A. Satia, W. Rosamond, & A.R. Folsom. 2007. Plasma n-3 fatty acids and the risk of cognitive decline in older adults: the Atherosclerosis Risk in Communities Study, *American Journal of Clinical Nutrition, 85* (4), 1103–1111.

Bjelakovic, G., D. Nikolova, L.L. Gluud, R.G. Simonetti, & C. Gluud. 2007. Mortality in randomized trials of antioxidant supplements for primary and secondary prevention: systematic review and meta-analysis, *JAMA, 297* (8), 842–857.

Blumenthal, J.A., M.A. Babyak, A. Hinderliter, L.L. Watkins, L. Craighead, P.-H. Lin, et al. 2010. Effects of the DASH Diet Alone and in Combination With Exercise and Weight Loss on Blood Pressure and Cardiovascular Biomarkers in Men and Women With High Blood Pressure: The ENCORE Study, *Archives of Internal Medicine, 170* (2), 126–135.

Bourre, J.M. 2006. Effects of nutrients (in food) on the structure and function of the nervous system: Update on dietary requirements for brain. Part 1: Micronutrients, *Journal of Nutrition Health and Aging, 10* (5), 377–385.

Buckland, G., A. Bach, & L. Serra-Majem. 2008. Obesity and the Mediterranean diet: a systematic review of observational and intervention studies, *Obesity Reviews, 9* (6), 582–593.

Buell, J.S., T.M. Scott, B. Dawson-Hughes, G.E. Dallal, I.H. Rosenberg, M.F. Folstein, et al. 2009. Vitamin D is associated with cognitive function in elders receiving home health services, *Journal of Gerontology A Biological Sciences Medical Sciences, 64*(8), 888–895.

Burdge, G.C. & P.C. Calder. 2005. Conversion of alpha-linolenic acid to longer-chain polyunsaturated fatty acids in human adults, *Reproduction Nutrition Develoment, 45* (5), 581–597.

Cashman, K.D., J.M.W. Wallace, G. Horigan, T.R. Hill, M.S. Barnes, A.J. Lucey, et al. 2009. Estimation of the dietary requirement for vitamin D in free-living adults >=64 y of age, *American Journal of Clinical Nutrition, 89* (5), 1366–1374.

Cheatham, R.A., S.B. Roberts, S.K. Das, C.H. Gilhooly, J.K. Golden, R. Hyatt, et al. 2009. Long-term effects of provided low and high glycemic load low energy diets on mood and cognition, *Physiology & Behavior, 98* (3), 374–379.

Cherubini, A., A. Martin, C. Andres Lacueva, A. Di Iorio, M. Lamponi, P. Mecocci, et al. 2005. Vitamin E levels, cognitive impairment and dementia in older persons: the InCHIANTI study, *Neurobiology of Aging, 26* (7), 987–994.

Chytrova, G., Z. Ying, & F. Gomez-Pinilla. 2010. Exercise contributes to the effects of DHA dietary supplementation by acting on membrane-related synaptic systems, *Brain Research, 1341*, 32–40.

Clarke, R.J. & D.A. Bennett. 2008. B vitamins for prevention of cognitive decline - Insufficient evidence to justify treatment, *JAMA, 300* (15), 1819–1821.

Commenges, D., V. Scotet, S. Renaud, H. Jacqmin-Gadda, P. Barberger-Gateau, & J.-F. Dartigues. 2000. Intake of flavonoids and risk of dementia, *European Journal of Epidemiology, 16* (4), 357–363.

Covas, M.-I., K. Nyyssonen, H.E. Poulsen, J. Kaikkonen, H.-J.F. Zunft, H. Kiesewetter, et al. 2006. The effect of polyphenols in olive oil on heart disease risk factors: a randomized trial, *Annals of Internal Medicine, 145* (5), 333–341.

Cunnane, S.C., M. Plourde, F. Pifferi, M. Bégin, C. Féart, & P. Barberger-Gateau. 2009. Fish, docosahexaenoic acid and Alzheimer's disease, *Progress in Lipid Research, 48* (5), 239–256.

Dal-Pan, A., F. Pifferi, J. Marchal, J.-L. Picq, F. Aujard, & R.C. on behalf of RESTRIKAL Consortium. 2011. Cognitive performances are selectively enhanced during chronic caloric restriction or resveratrol supplementation in a primate, *PLoS ONE, 6* (1), e16581.

de Ruijter, W., R.G.J. Westendorp, W.J.J. Assendelft, W.P.J. den Elzen, A.J.M. de Craen, S. le Cessie et al. 2009. Use of Framingham risk score and new biomarkers to predict cardiovascular mortality in older people: population based observational cohort study, *BMJ, 338* (jan08_2), a3083–.

Debette, S., A. Beiser, U. Hoffmann, C. DeCarli, C.J. O'Donnell, J.M. Massaro, et al. 2010. Visceral fat is associated with lower brain volume in healthy middle-aged adults, *Annals of Neurology, 68* (2), 136–144.

Deschamps, V., P. Barberger-Gateau, E. Peuchant, & J.M. Orgogozo. 2001. Nutritional factors in cerebral aging and dementia: epidemiological arguments for a role of oxidative stress, *Neuroepidemiology, 20* (1), 7–15.

Devore, E.E., F. Grodstein, F.J.A. van Rooij, A. Hofman, B. Rosner, M.J. Stampfer, et al. 2009. Dietary intake of fish and omega-3 fatty acids in relation to long-term dementia risk, *American Journal of Clinical Nutrition, 90* (1), 170–6.

Devore, E.E., F. Grodstein, F.J. van Rooij, A. Hofman, M.J. Stampfer, J.C. Witteman, et al. 2010. Dietary antioxidants and long-term risk of dementia, *Archives of Neurology, 67* (7), 819–825.

Durga, J., M.P. van Boxtel, E.G. Schouten, F.J. Kok, J. Jolles, M.B. Katan, et al. 2007. Effect of 3-year folic acid supplementation on cognitive function in older adults in the FACIT trial: a randomised, double blind, controlled trial, *Lancet, 369* (9557), 208–216.

Engelhart, M.J., M.I. Geerlings, A. Ruitenberg, J.C. van Swieten, A. Hofman, J.C.M. Witteman, et al.. 2002a. Diet and risk of dementia: Does fat matter? The Rotterdam Study, *Neurology, 59* (12), 1915–1921.

Engelhart, M.J., M.I. Geerlings, A. Ruitenberg, J.C. vanSwieten, A. Holman, J.C.M. Witteman, et al. 2002b. Dietary intake of antioxidants and risk of Alzheimer disease, *JAMA, 287* (24), 3223–3229.

Eskelinen, M.H., T.Ngandu, E-L. Helkala, J. Tuomilehto, A. Nissinen, H. Soininen, et al. 2008. Fat intake at midlife and cognitive impairment later in life: a population-based CAIDE study, *International Journal of Geriatric Psychiatry, 23* (7), 741–747.

Esposito, K., C.M. Kastorini, D.B. Panagiotakos, & D. Giugliano. 2011. Mediterranean diet and weight loss: meta-analysis of randomized controlled trials, *Metabolic Syndrome and Related Disorders, 9* (1), 1–12.

Fairfield, K.M. & R.H. Fletcher. 2002. Vitamins for chronic disease prevention in adults – Scientific review, *JAMA, 287* (23), 3116–3126.

Feart, C., C. Samieri, V. Rondeau, H. Amieva, F. Portet, J.-F. Dartigues, et al. 2009. Adherence to a Mediterranean diet, cognitive decline, and risk of dementia, *JAMA, 302* (6), 638–648.

Feart, C., M.J. Torres, C. Samieri, M.A. Jutand, E. Peuchant, A.P. Simopoulos, et al. 2011. Adherence to a Mediterranean Diet and plasma fatty acids: data from the Bordeaux sample of the Three-City study, *British Journal of Nutrition, 106* (1), 149–158.

Ferri, C.P., M. Prince, C. Brayne, H. Brodaty, L. Fratiglioni, M. Ganguli, et al. 2005. Global prevalence of dementia: a Delphi consensus study, *Lancet, 366* (9503), 2112–2117.

Filley, C.M. & C.A. Anderson. 2011. Dementia: five new things, *Neurology, 76* (7 Supplement 2), S26–S30.

Floyd, R.A. & K. Hensley. 2002. Oxidative stress in brain aging. Implications for therapeutics of neurodegenerative diseases, *Neurobiology of Aging, 23* (5), 795–807.

Foster-Powell, K., S.H. Holt, & J.C. Brand-Miller. 2002. International table of glycemic index and glycemic load values: 2002, *American Journal of Clinical Nutrition, 76* (1), 5–56.

Fotuhi, M., V. Hachinski, & P.J. Whitehouse. 2009a. Changing perspectives regarding late-life dementia, *Nature Reviews Neurology, 5* (12), 649–658.

Fotuhi, M., P. Mohassel, & K. Yaffe. 2009b. Fish consumption, long-chain omega-3 fatty acids and risk of cognitive decline or Alzheimer disease: a complex association, *Nature Clinical Practice Neurology, 5* (3), 140–152.

Frisardi, V., F. Panza, D. Seripa, B.P. Imbimbo, G. Vendemiale, A. Pilotto, & V. Solfrizzi. 2010. Nutraceutical properties of Mediterranean diet and cognitive decline: possible underlying mechanisms, *Journal of Alzheimers Disease, 22* (3), 715–740.

Fung, T.T., M.L. McCullough, P.K. Newby, J.E. Manson, J.B. Meigs, N. Rifai, et al. 2005. Diet-quality scores and plasma concentrations of markers of inflammation and endothelial dysfunction, *American Journal of Clinical Nutrition, 82* (1), 163–173.

Gaskins, A.J., A.J. Rovner, S.L. Mumford, E. Yeung, R.W. Browne, M. Trevisan, et al. 2010. Adherence to a Mediterranean diet and plasma concentrations of lipid peroxidation in premenopausal women, *American Journal of Clinical Nutrition, 92* (6), 1461–1467.

Gomez-Pinilla, F. 2008. Brain foods: the effects of nutrients on brain function, *Nature Reviews Neuroscience, 9* (7), 568.

Gori, A.M., A.M. Corsi, S. Fedi, A. Gazzini, F. Sofi, B. Bartali, et al. 2005. A proinflammatory state is associated with hyperhomocysteinemia in the elderly, *American Journal of Clinical Nutrition, 82* (2), 335–341.

Grodstein, F., J.H. Kang, R.J. Glynn, N.R. Cook, & J.M. Gaziano. 2007. A randomized trial of beta carotene supplementation and cognitive function in men: the Physicians' Health Study II, *Archives of Internal Medicine, 167* (20), 2184–2190.

Gu, Y., J.A. Luchsinger, Y. Stern, & N. Scarmeas. 2010. Mediterranean diet, inflammatory and metabolic biomarkers, and risk of Alzheimer's disease, *Journal of Alzheimers Disease, 22* (2), 483–492.

Guenther, P.M., J. Reedy, & S.M. Krebs-Smith. 2008a. Development of the Healthy Eating Index-2005, *Journal of the American Dietetic Association, 108* (11), 1896–1901.

Guenther, P.M., J. Reedy, S.M. Krebs-Smith, & B.B. Reeve. 2008b. Evaluation of the Healthy Eating Index-2005, *Journal of the American Dietetic Association,, 108* (11), 1854–1864.

Heart Protection Study Collaborative Group. 2002. MRC/BHF Heart Protection Study of antioxidant vitamin supplementation in high-risk individuals: a randomised placebo-controlled trial, *Lancet, 360* (9326), 23–33.

Heilbronn, L.K., L. de Jonge, M.I. Frisard, J.P. DeLany, D.E. Larson-Meyer, J. Rood, et al. 2006. Effect of 6-Month Calorie Restriction on Biomarkers of Longevity, Metabolic Adaptation, and Oxidative Stress in Overweight Individuals, *JAMA, 295* (13), 1539–1548.

Helmer, C., E. Peuchant, L. Letenneur, I. Bourdel-Marchasson, S. Larrieu, J.F. Dartigues, et al. 2003. Association between antioxidant nutritional indicators and the incidence of dementia: results from the PAQUID prospective cohort study, *European Journal of Clinical Nutrition, 57* (12), 1555–1561.

Holick, M.F. 2007. Vitamin D deficiency, *New England Journal of Medicine, 357* (3), 266–281.

Hu, P., P. Bretsky, E.M. Crimmins, J.M. Guralnik, D.B. Reuben, & T.E. Seeman. 2006. Association between serum beta-carotene levels and decline of cognitive function in high-functioning older persons with or without apolipoprotein E 4 alleles: MacArthur studies of successful aging, *J Gerontol A Biol Sci Med Sci*, 61 (6), 616–620.

Huang, T.L., P.P. Zandi, K.L. Tucker, A.L. Fitzpatrick, L.H. Kuller, L.P. Fried, et al. 2005. Benefits of fatty fish on dementia risk are stronger for those without APOE epsilon4, *Neurology*, 65 (9), 1409–1414.

Hughes, T.F., R.F. Andel, B.J. Small, A.R. Borenstein, J.A. Mortimer, A. Wolk, et al. 2010. Midlife fruit and vegetable consumption and risk of dementia in later life in Swedish twins, *American Journal of Geriatric Psychiatry*, 18 (5), 413–420.

Jack Jr, C.R., D.S. Knopman, W.J. Jagust, L.M. Shaw, P.S. Aisen, M.W. Weiner, et al. 2010. Hypothetical model of dynamic biomarkers of the Alzheimer's pathological cascade, *Lancet Neurology*, 9 (1), 119–128.

Jayasooriya, A.P., M.L. Ackland, M.L. Mathai, A.J. Sinclair, H.S. Weisinger, R.S. Weisinger, et al. 2005. Perinatal omega-3 polyunsaturated fatty acid supply modifies brain zinc homeostasis during adulthood, *Proceedings of the National Academy of Sciences of the United States of America*, 102 (20), 7133–7138.

Johnson, E.J., K. McDonald, S.M. Caldarella, H.Y. Chung, A.M. Troen, & D.M. Snodderly. 2008. Cognitive findings of an exploratory trial of docosahexaenoic acid and lutein supplementation in older women, *Nutrition Neuroscience*, 11 (2), 75–83.

Joseph, J., G. Cole, E. Head, & D. Ingram. 2009. Nutrition, Brain Aging, and Neurodegeneration, *Journal of Neuroscience*, 29 (41), 12795–12801.

Jung, U.J., C. Torrejon, A.P. Tighe, & R.J. Deckelbaum. 2008. n-3 Fatty acids and cardiovascular disease: mechanisms underlying beneficial effects, *American Journal of Clinical Nutrition*, 87 (6), 2003S–2009S.

Kalaria, R.N., G.E. Maestre, R. Arizaga, R.P. Friedland, D. Galasko, K.T. Hall, et al. 2008. Alzheimer's disease and vascular dementia in developing countries: prevalence, management, and risk factors, *Lancet Neurology*, 7 (9), 812–826.

Kalmijn, S., E.J.M. Feskens, L.J. Launer, & D. Kromhout. 1997a. Polyunsaturated fatty acids, antioxidants, and cognitive function in very old men, *American Journal of Epidemiology*, 145 (1), 33–41.

Kalmijn, S., L.J. Launer, A. Ott, J.C.M. Witteman, A. Hofman, & M.M.B. Breteler. 1997b. Dietary fat intake and the risk of incident dementia in the Rotterdam study, *Annals of Neurology*, 42, 776–782.

Kamphuis, P., F. Verhey, M. Olde Rikkert, J. Twisk, S. Swinkels, & P. Scheltens. 2011. Efficacy of a medical food on cognition in Alzheimer's Disease: Results from secondary analyses of a randomized, controlled trial, *The Journal of Nutrition, Health & Aging*, 15 (8), 720–724.

Kang, J.H. & F. Grodstein. 2008. Plasma carotenoids and tocopherols and cognitive function: A prospective study, *Neurobiology of Aging*, 29 (9), 1394–1403.

Kang, J.H., A. Ascherio, & F. Grodstein. 2005. Fruit and vegetable consumption and cognitive decline in aging women, *Annals of Neurology*, 57 (5), 713–720.

Kang, J.H., N. Cook, J. Manson, J.E. Buring, & F. Grodstein. 2006. A randomized trial of vitamin E supplementation and cognitive function in women, *Archives of Internal Medicine*, 166 (22), 2462–2468.

Kastorini, C.-M., H.J. Milionis, K. Esposito, D. Giugliano, J.A. Goudevenos, & D.B. Panagiotakos. 2011. The effect of Mediterranean diet on metabolic syndrome and its components: a meta-analysis of 50 studies and 534,906 individuals, *Journal of the American College of Cardiology*, 57 (11), 1299–1313.

Kennedy, D.O., E.L. Wightman, J.L. Reay, G. Lietz, E.J. Okello, A. Wilde et al. 2010. Effects of resveratrol on cerebral blood flow variables and cognitive performance in humans: a double-blind, placebo-controlled, crossover investigation, *American Journal of Clinical Nutrition*, 91 (6), 1590–1597.

Kesse-Guyot, E., S. Péneau, C. Ferry, C. Jeandel, S. Hercberg, & P. Galan. 2011a. Thirteen-year prospective study between fish consumption, long-chain N-3 fatty acids intakes and cognitive function, *Journal of Nutrition, Health and Aging*, 15 (2), 115–120.

Kesse-Guyot, E., H. Amieva, K. Castetbon, A. Henegar, M. Ferry, C. Jeandel, et al. 2011b. Adherence to nutritional recommendations and subsequent cognitive performance:

findings from the prospective Supplementation with Antioxidant Vitamins and Minerals 2 (SU.VI.MAX 2) study, *American Journal of Clinical Nutrition*, 93, 200–210.

Konstantinidou, V., M.-I. Covas, D. Muñoz-Aguayo, O. Khymenets, R. de la Torre, G. Saez, et al. 2010. In vivo nutrigenomic effects of virgin olive oil polyphenols within the frame of the Mediterranean diet: a randomized controlled trial, *The FASEB Journal*, 24 (7), 2546–2557.

Kroger, E., R. Verreault, P.-H. Carmichael, J. Lindsay, P. Julien, E. Dewailly, et al. 2009. Omega-3 fatty acids and risk of dementia: the Canadian Study of Health and Aging, *American Journal of Clinical Nutrition*, 90 (1), 184–192.

Laitinen, M.H., T. Ngandu, S. Rovio, E.L. Helkala, U. Uusitalo, M. Viitanen, et al. 2006. Fat intake at midlife and risk of dementia and Alzheimer's disease: a population-based study, *Dementia and Geriatric Cognitive Disorders*, 22 (1), 99–107.

Laurin, D., R. Verreault, J. Lindsay, E. Dewailly, & B.J. Holub. 2003. Omega-3 fatty acids and risk of cognitive impairment and dementia, *Journal of Alzheimers Disease*, 5 (4), 315–322.

Laurin, D., K.H. Masaki, D.J. Foley, L.R. White, & L.J. Launer. 2004. Midlife dietary intake of antioxidants and risk of late-life incident dementia: The Honolulu-Asia Aging Study, *American Journal of Epidemioogy*, 159 (10), 959–967.

Lee, J.W., Y.K. Lee, J.O. Ban, T.Y. Ha, Y.P. Yun, S.B. Han, et al. 2009. Green Tea (-)-Epigallocatechin-3-Gallate Inhibits {beta}-Amyloid-Induced Cognitive Dysfunction through Modification of Secretase Activity via Inhibition of ERK and NF-{kappa}B Pathways in Mice, *Journal of Nutrition*, 139 (10), 1987–1993.

Letenneur, L., C. Proust-Lima, A. Le Gouge, J. Dartigues, & P. Barberger-Gateau. 2007. Flavonoid Intake and Cognitive Decline over a 10-Year Period, *American Journal of Epidemioogy*, 165 (12), 1364–1371.

Llewellyn, D.J., I.A. Lang, K.M. Langa, & D. Melzer. 2011. Vitamin D and cognitive impairment in the elderly U.S. population, *Journal of Gerontology A Biological Sciences Medical Sciences*, 66 (1), 59–65.

Llewellyn, D.J., I.A. Lang, K.M. Langa, G. Muniz-Terrera, C.L. Phillips, A. Cherubini, et al. 2010. Vitamin D and Risk of Cognitive Decline in Elderly Persons, *Archives of Internal Medicine*, 170 (13), 1135–1141.

Lopez, L., D. Kritz-Silverstein, & E. Barrett-Connor. 2011. HIgh dietary and plasma levels of the omega-3 fatty acid docosahexaenoic acid are associated with decreased dementia risk: the rancho bernardo study, *Journal of Nutrition, Health and Aging*, 15 (1), 25–31.

Lucarini, M. & G. Pedulli. 2007. Overview of antioxidant activity of vitamin E. In VR Preedy & RR Watson (eds.), *The Encyclopedia of Vitamin E* (pp. 3–10). Wallingford, UK: CAB International.

Luchsinger, J.A. 2010. Insulin resistance, type 2 diabetes, and AD: Cerebrovascular disease or neurodegeneration? *Neurology*, 75 (9), 758–759.

Luchsinger, J.A., M.X. Tang, & R. Mayeux. 2007. Glycemic load and risk of Alzheimer's disease, *Journal of Nutrition Health and Aging*, 11 (3), 238–241.

Luchsinger, J.A., M.X. Tang, S. Shea, & R. Mayeux. 2002. Caloric intake and the risk of Alzheimer disease, *Archives of Neurology*, 59 (8), 1258–1263.

Luchsinger, J.A., M.X. Tang, S. Shea, & R. Mayeux. 2003. Antioxidant vitamin intake and risk of Alzheimer disease, *Archives of Neurology*, 60 (2), 203–208.

Lukiw, W.J. & N.G. Bazan. 2008. Docosahexaenoic acid and the aging brain, *J Nutr*, 138 (12), 2510–2514.

Manach, C., A. Scalbert, C. Morand, C. Remesy, & L. Jimenez. 2004. Polyphenols: food sources and bioavailability, *American Journal of Clinical Nutrition*, 79 (5), 727–747.

Mangialasche, F., M. Kivipelto, P. Mecocci, D. Rizzuto, K. Palmer, B. Winblad et al. 2010. High plasma levels of vitamin E forms and reduced Alzheimer's disease risk in advanced age, *Journal of Alzheimers Disease*, 20 (4), 1029–1037.

Martin, C.K., S.D. Anton, H. Han, E. York-Crowe, L.M. Redman, E. Ravussin, & D.A. Williamson. 2007. Examination of cognitive function during six months of calorie restriction: results of a randomized controlled trial, *Rejuvenation Research*, 10 (2), 179–190.

Mattson, M.P., W.Z. Duan, J. Lee, & Z.H. Guo. 2001. Suppression of brain aging and neuro-degenerative disorders by dietary restriction and environmental enrichment: molecular mechanisms, *Mechanisms of Ageing and Development*, 122 (7), 757–778.

Mattson, M.P. & T.B. Shea. 2003. Folate and homocysteine metabolism in neural plasticity and neurodegenerative disorders, *Trends in Neuroscience*, 26 (3), 137–146.

Maylor, E.A., E.E.A. Simpson, D.L. Secker, N. Meunier, M. Andriollo Sanchez, A. Polito, et al. 2006. Effects of zinc supplementation on cognitive function in healthy middle-aged and older adults: the ZENITH study, *British Journal of Nutrition*, 96 (4), 752–760.

McCann, J.C. & B.N. Ames. 2008. Is there convincing biological or behavioral evidence linking vitamin D deficiency to brain dysfunction?, *FASEB J.*, 22 (4), 982–1001.

Mendez, M.A., M.I. Covas, J. Marrugat, J. Vila, H. Schröder, on the behalf of the REGICOR and HERMES investigators. 2009. Glycemic load, glycemic index, and body mass index in Spanish adults, *American Journal of Clinical Nutrition*, 89 (1), 316–322.

Miller, J.W. 2010. Vitamin D and cognitive function in older adults. Are we concerned about vitamin D-mentia? *Neurology*, 74 (1), 13–15.

Montine, T.J. & J.D. Morrow. 2005. Fatty acid oxidation in the pathogenesis of Alzheimer's disease, *American Journal of Pathology*, 166 (5), 1283–1289.

Montine, T.J., M.D. Neely, J.F. Quinn, M.F. Beal, W.R. Markesbery, L.J. Roberts et al. 2002. Lipid peroxidation in aging brain and Alzheimer's disease, *Free Radical Biology and Medicine*, 33 (5), 620–626.

Morris, M.C., D.A. Evans, J.L. Bienias, C.C. Tangney, & R.S. Wilson. 2004. Dietary fat intake and 6-year cognitive change in an older biracial community population, *Neurology*, 62 (9), 1573–1579.

Morris, M.C., D.A. Evans, C.C. Tangney, J.L. Bienias, & R.S. Wilson. 2005a. Fish consumption and cognitive decline with age in a large community study, *Archives of Neurology*, 62 (12), 1849–1853.

Morris, M.C., D.A. Evans, C.C. Tangney, J.L. Bienias, R.S. Wilson, N.T. Aggarwal et al. 2005b. Relation of the tocopherol forms to incident Alzheimer disease and to cognitive change, *American Journal of Clinical Nutrition*, 81 (2), 508–514.

Morris, M.C., D.A. Evans, C.C. Tangney, J.L. Bienias, & R.S. Wilson. 2006. Associations of vegetable and fruit consumption with age-related cognitive change, *Neurology*, 67 (8), 1370–1376.

Morris, M.C., D.A. Evans, J.L. Bienias, C.C. Tangney, D.A. Bennett, N. Aggarwal, et al. 2002. Dietary intake of antioxidant nutrients and the risk of incident Alzheimer disease on a biracial community study, *JAMA*, 287 (24), 3230–3237.

Morris, M.C., D.A. Evans, J.L. Bienias, C.C. Tangney, D.A. Bennett, R.S. Wilson, et al. 2003a. Consumption of fish and n-3 fatty acids and risk of incident Alzheimer disease, *Archives of Neurology*, 60 (7), 940–946.

Morris, M.C., D.A. Evans, J.L. Bienias, C.C. Tangney, D.A. Bennett, N. Aggarwal, et al. 2003b. Dietary fats and the risk of incident Alzheimer disease, *Archives of Neurology*, 60 (2), 194–200.

Morris, M.S. 2003. Homocysteine and Alzheimer's disease, *Lancet Neurology*, 2 (7), 425–428.

Ng, T.-P., L. Feng, M. Niti, E.-H. Kua, & K.-B. Yap. 2008. Tea consumption and cognitive impairment and decline in older Chinese adults, *American Journal of Clinical Nutrition*, 88 (1), 224–231.

Nomura, K., M. Eto, T. Kojima, S. Ogawa, K. Iijima, T. Nakamura, et al. 2010. Visceral fat accumulation and metabolic risk factor clustering in older adults, *Journal of the American Geriatrics Society*, 58 (9), 1658–1663.

Oudshoorn, C., F.U.S. Mattace Raso, N. van der Velde, E.M. Colin, & T.J.M. van der Cammen. 2008. Higher serum vitamin D-3 levels are associated with better cognitive test performance in patients with Alzheimer's disease, *Dementia and Geriatric Cognitive Disorders*, 25 (6), 539–543.

Parachikova, A., M.G. Agadjanyan, D.H. Cribbs, M. Blurton Jones, V. Perreau, J. Rogers, et al. 2007. Inflammatory changes parallel the early stages of Alzheimer disease, *Neurobiology of Aging*, 28 (12), 1821–1833.

Perez-Jimenez, J., J. Hubert, L. Hooper, A. Cassidy, C. Manach, G. Williamson, et al. 2010. Urinary metabolites as biomarkers of polyphenol intake in humans: a systematic review, *American Journal of Clinical Nutrition*, 92 (4), 801–809.

Petersen, R.C., R.G. Thomas, M. Grundman, D. Bennett, R. Doody, S. Ferris, et al. 2005. Vitamin E and donepezil for the treatment of mild cognitive impairment, *New England Journal of Medicine*, 352 (23), 2379–2388.

Plassman, B.L., J.W. Williams, J.R. Burke, T. Holsinger, & S. Benjamin. 2010. Systematic Review: Factors Associated With Risk for and Possible Prevention of Cognitive Decline in Later Life, *Annals of Internal Medicine*, 153 (3), 182–193.

Profenno, L.A., A.P. Porsteinsson, & S.V. Faraone. 2010. Meta-analysis of Alzheimer's disease risk with obesity, diabetes, and related disorders, *Biological Psychiatry*, 67 (6), 505–512.

Querfurth, H.W. & F.M. LaFerla. 2010. Alzheimer's Disease, *New England Journal of Medicine*, 362 (4), 329–344.

Raffaitin, C., C. Féart, M. Le Goff, H. Amieva, C. Helmer, T.N. Akbaraly, et al. 2011. Metabolic syndrome and cognitive decline in French elders. the Three-City study, *Neurology*, 76 518–525.

Raffaitin, C., H. Gin, J.P. Empana, C. Helmer, C. Berr, C. Tzourio, et al. 2009. Metabolic syndrome and risk for incident Alzheimer's disease or vascular dementia: the Three - City study, *Diabetes Care*, 32 (1), 169–174.

Raman, G., A. Tatsioni, M. Chung, I.H. Rosenberg, J. Lau, A.H. Lichtenstein et al. 2007. Heterogeneity and lack of good quality studies limit association between folate, vitamins B-6 and B-12, and cognitive function, *Journal of Nutrition*, 137 (7), 1789–1794.

Ravaglia, G., P. Forti, A. Lucicesare, N. Pisacane, E. Rietti, F. Mangialasche, et al. 2008. Plasma tocopherols and risk of cognitive impairment in an elderly Italian cohort, *American Journal of Clinical Nutrition*, 87 (5), 1306–1313.

Ritchie, K., I. Carriere, A. de Mendonca, F. Portet, J.F. Dartigues, O. Rouaud, et al. 2007. The neuroprotective effects of caffeine: A prospective population study (the Three City Study), *Neurology*, 69 (6), 536–545.

Roberts, R.O., Y.E. Geda, J.R. Cerhan, D.S. Knopman, R.H. Cha, T.J.H. Christianson, et al. 2010. Vegetables, unsaturated fats, moderate alcohol intake, and Mild Cognitive Impairment, *Dementia and Geriatric Cognitive Disorders*, 29 (5), 413–423.

Romaguera, D., T. Norat, A.-C. Vergnaud, T. Mouw, A.M. May, A. Agudo, et al. 2010. Mediterranean dietary patterns and prospective weight change in participants of the EPIC-PANACEA project, *American Journal of Clinical Nutrition*, 92, 912–921.

Sabia, S., M. Kivimaki, M.J. Shipley, M.G. Marmot, & A. Singh-Manoux. 2009. Body mass index over the adult life course and cognition in late midlife: the Whitehall II Cohort Study, *American Journal of Clinical Nutrition*, 89 (2), 601–607.

Salas-Salvado, J., M. Bullo, N. Babio, M.A. Martinez-Gonzalez, N. Ibarrola-Jurado, J. Basora, et al. 2011. Reduction in the incidence of type 2 diabetes with the Mediterranean diet: results of the PREDIMED-Reus nutrition intervention randomized trial, *Diabetes Care*, 34 (1), 14–19.

Samieri, C., C. Feart, C. Proust-Lima, E. Peuchant, J. Dartigues, H. Amieva et al. 2011a. Omega-3 fatty acids and cognitive decline: modulation by ApoEepsilon4 allele and depression, *Neurobiology of Aging*, 32 (12), 2317.e13–e22.

Samieri, C., C. Feart, C. Proust-Lima, E. Peuchant, C. Tzourio, C. Stapf, et al. 2011b. Olive oil consumption, plasma oleic acid and stroke incidence. The Three-City Study, *Neurology*, 77 (5), 418–425.

Samieri, C., C. Feart, L. Letenneur, J.-F. Dartigues, K. Peres, S. Auriacombe, et al. 2008. Low plasma eicosapentaenoic acid and depressive symptomatology are independent predictors of dementia risk, *American Journal of Clinical Nutrition*, 88 (3), 714–721.

Scarmeas, N., Y. Stern, R. Mayeux, & J.A. Luchsinger. 2006a. Mediterranean diet, Alzheimer disease, and vascular mediation, *Archives of Neurology*, 63 (12), 1709–1717.

Scarmeas, N., Y. Stern, M.X. Tang, R. Mayeux, & J.A. Luchsinger. 2006b. Mediterranean diet and risk for Alzheimer's disease, *Annals of Neurology*, 59 (6), 912–921.

Scarmeas, N., Y. Stern, R. Mayeux, J.J. Manly, N. Schupf, & J.A. Luchsinger. 2009a. Mediterranean diet and mild cognitive impairment, *Archives of Neurology*, 66 (2), 216–225.

Scarmeas, N., J.A. Luchsinger, N. Schupf, A.M. Brickman, S. Cosentino, M.X. Tang et al. 2009b. Physical activity, diet, and risk of Alzheimer disease, *JAMA, 302* (6), 627–637.

Scarmeas, N., J.A. Luchsinger, Y. Stern, Y. Gu, J. He, C. DeCarli, et al. 2011. Mediterranean diet and magnetic resonance imaging–assessed cerebrovascular disease, *Annals of Neurology, 69* (2), 257–268.

Schaefer, E.J., V. Bongard, A.S. Beiser, S. Lamon-Fava, S.J. Robins, R. Au, et al. 2006. Plasma phosphatidylcholine docosahexaenoic acid content and risk of dementia and Alzheimer disease: The Framingham Heart Study, *Archives of Neurology, 63* (11), 1545–1550.

Scheltens, P., P.J.G.H. Kamphuis, F.R.J. Verhey, M.G.M. Olde Rikkert, R.J. Wurtman, D. Wilkinson, et al. 2010. Efficacy of a medical food in mild Alzheimer's disease: A randomized, controlled trial, *Alzheimer's and Dementia, 6* (1), 1–10.e1.

Schmitz, G. & J. Ecker. 2008. The opposing effects of n-3 and n-6 fatty acids, *Progress in Lipid Research, 47* (2), 147.

Schulze, M.B., K. Hoffmann, A. Kroke, & H. Boeing. 2003. Risk of hypertension among women in the EPIC-Potsdam study: comparison of relative risk estimates for exploratory and hypothesis-oriented dietary patterns, *American Journal of Epidemiology, 158* (4), 365–373.

Seamans, K.M., T.R. Hill, L. Scully, N. Meunier, M. Andrillo-Sanchez, A. Polito, et al. 2010. Vitamin D status and measures of cognitive function in healthy older European adults, *European Journal of Clinical Nutrition, 64* (10), 1172–1178.

Seshadri, S., A. Beiser, J. Selhub, P.F. Jacques, I.H. Rosenberg, R.B. D'Agostino, et al. 2002. Plasma homocysteine as a risk factor for dementia and Alzheimer's disease, *New England Journal of Medicine, 346* (7), 476–483.

Shai, I., D. Schwarzfuchs, Y. Henkin, D.R. Shahar, S. Witkow, I. Greenberg, et al. 2008. Weight loss with a low-carbohydrate, Mediterranean, or low-fat diet, *New England Journal of Medicine, 359* (3), 229–241.

Singh, M., M. Arseneault, T. Sanderson, V. Murthy, & C. Ramassamy. 2008. Challenges for research on polyphenols from foods in Alzheimer's disease: bioavailability, metabolism, and cellular and molecular mechanisms, *Journal of Agricultural and Food Chemistry, 56* (13), 4855–4873.

Slinin, Y., M.L. Paudel, B.C. Taylor, H.A. Fink, A. Ishani, M.T. Canales, et al. 2010. 25-Hydroxyvitamin D levels and cognitive performance and decline in elderly men, *Neurology, 74* (1), 33–41.

Smith, A., R. Clark, D. Nutt, J. Haller, S. Hayward, & K. Perry. 1999. Anti-oxidant vitamins and mental performance of the elderly, *Human Psychopharmacology Clinical and Experimental, 14* (7), 459–471.

Smith, A.D., S.M. Smith, C.A. de Jager, P. Whitbread, C. Johnston, G. Agacinski, et al. 2010a. Homocysteine-Lowering by B Vitamins Slows the Rate of Accelerated Brain Atrophy in Mild Cognitive Impairment: A Randomized Controlled Trial, *PLoS ONE, 5* (9), e12244.

Smith, P.J., J.A. Blumenthal, M.A. Babyak, L. Craighead, K.A. Welsh-Bohmer, J.N. Browndyke, et al. 2010b. Effects of the Dietary Approaches to Stop Hypertension diet, exercise, and caloric restriction on neurocognition in overweight adults with high blood pressure, *Hypertension, 55* (6), 1331–1338.

Sofi, F., R. Abbate, G.F. Gensini, & A. Casini. 2010. Accruing evidence on benefits of adherence to the Mediterranean diet on health: an updated systematic review and meta-analysis, *American Journal of Clinical Nutrition, 92* (5), 1189–1196.

Sofi, F., F. Cesari, R. Abbate, G.F. Gensini, & A. Casini. 2008. Adherence to Mediterranean diet and health status: meta-analysis, *British Medical Journal, 337* (sep11_2), a1344–.

Solfrizzi, V., A.M. Colacicco, A.D. Introno, C. Capurso, F. Torres, C. Rizzo, et al. 2006. Dietary intake of unsaturated fatty acids and age-related cognitive decline: A 8.5-year follow-up of the Italian Longitudinal Study on Aging, *Neurobiology of Aging, 27* (11), 1694–1704.

Tangney, C.C., M.J. Kwasny, H. Li, R.S. Wilson, D.A. Evans, & M.C. Morris. 2011. Adherence to a Mediterranean-type dietary pattern and cognitive decline in a community population, *American Journal of Clinical Nutrition, 93*, 601–607.

Trichopoulou, A., T. Costacou, C. Bamia, and D. Trichopoulos. 2003. Adherence to a Mediterranean diet and survival in a Greek population, *New England Journal of Medicine, 348* (26), 2599–2608.

van de Rest, O., A. Spiro, III, E. Krall-Kaye, J.M. Geleijnse, L.C.P.G.M. de Groot, and K.L. Tucker. 2009. Intakes of (n-3) fatty acids and fatty fish are not associated with cognitive performance and 6-year cognitive change in men participating in the Veterans Affairs Normative Aging Study, *Journal of Nutrition*, *139* (12), 2329–2336.

van Gelder, B.M., M. Tijhuis, S. Kalmijn, & D. Kromhout. 2007. Fish consumption, n-3 fatty acids, and subsequent 5-y cognitive decline in elderly men: the Zutphen Elderly Study, *American Journal of Clinical Nutrition*, *85* (4), 1142–1147.

Vercambre, M.-N.l., M.-C. Boutron-Ruault, K. Ritchie, F.o. Clavel-Chapelon, & C. Berr. 2009. Long-term association of food and nutrient intakes with cognitive and functional decline: a 13-year follow-up study of elderly French women, *British Journal of Nutrition*, *102* (03), 419–427.

Voutilainen, S., T. Nurmi, J. Mursu, & T.H. Rissanen. 2006. Carotenoids and cardiovascular health, *American Journal of Clinical Nutrition*, *83* (6), 1265–1271.

Wald, D.S., A. Kasturiratne, & M. Simmonds. 2010. Effect of Folic Acid, with or without Other B Vitamins, on Cognitive Decline: Meta-Analysis of Randomized Trials, *American Journal of Medicine*, *123* (6), 522–527.e2.

Wald, D.S., M. Law, & J.K. Morris. 2002. Homocysteine and cardiovascular disease: evidence on causality from a meta-analysis, *British Medical Journal*, *325* (7374), 1202.

Wengreen, H.J., C. Neilson, R. Munger, & C. Corcoran. 2009. Diet Quality Is Associated with Better Cognitive Test Performance among Aging Men and Women, *Journal of Nutrition*, *139* (10), 1944–1949.

Wengreen, H.J., R.G. Munger, C.D. Corcoran, P. Zandi, K.M. Hayden, M. Fotuhi, et al. 2007. Antioxidant intake and cognitive function of elderly men and women: The cache county study, *Journal of Nutrition Health and Aging*, *11* (3), 230–237.

Wilkins, C.H., S.J. Birge, Y.I. Sheline, & J.C. Morris. 2009. Vitamin D Deficiency Is Associated With Worse Cognitive Performance and Lower Bone Density in Older African Americans, *Journal of the National Medical Association*, *101* (4), 349–354.

Wimo, A., B. Winblad, H. Aguero Torres, & E. von Strauss. 2003. The magnitude of dementia occurrence in the world, *Alzheimer Disease and Associated Disorders*, *17* (2), 63–67.

Witte, A.V., M. Fobker, R. Gellner, S. Knecht, & A. Floel. 2009. Caloric restriction improves memory in elderly humans, *Proceedings of the National Academy of Sciences of the United States of America*, *106* (4), 1255–1260.

Yaffe, K., T.E. Clemons, W.L. McBee, & A.S. Lindblad. 2004. Impact of antioxidants, zinc, and copper on cognition in the elderly - A randomized, controlled trial, *Neurology*, *63* (9), 1705–1707.

Yurko-Mauro, K., D. McCarthy, D. Rom, E.B. Nelson, A.S. Ryan, A. Blackwell, et al. 2010. Beneficial effects of docosahexaenoic acid on cognition in age-related cognitive decline, *Alzheimers Dementia*, *6* (6), 456–464.

Zajacova, A., J.B. Dowd, & S.A. Burgard. 2011. Overweight Adults May Have the Lowest Mortality-Do They Have the Best Health?, *American Journal of Epidemiology*, *173* (4), 430–437.

11

Inflammation and Cognitive Decline

RÓISÍN GALLINAGH SMITH, MB BCH, STEPHEN TODD, MD, AND

PETER A. PASSMORE, MD

Introduction

The link between neuroinflammation and cognitive dysfunction is the subject of increasing medical and biochemical research interest. Conventional wisdom held that the brain had immune privilege, but this is now known to be untrue. Researchers are uncovering more about the brain's own inflammatory cascade and the possible damaging effects of this. Certain neurodegenerative diseases with an inflammatory component, such as Alzheimer's disease (AD), Parkinson's disease, and Amyotrophic Lateral Sclerosis (ALS), are associated with cognitive decline. Conditions with inflammatory effects such as cardiovascular disease and metabolic syndrome are also linked to cognition decline (these are the subject of separate chapters 3 and 6 this book). Furthermore, central nervous system (CNS) and systemic infections have been shown to contribute to acceleration of AD. Some, but not all, evidence suggests that nonsteroidal anti-inflammatory drugs (NSAIDS) may be protective against the development of AD. It is unclear whether inflammation is the key cause of cognitive decline or whether it is a secondary effect of this process. Neuroinflammation is a broad term and consists of the interplay of complex pathways that are both destructive and restorative. Gaining balance between inflammation and a quiescent state is key. Teasing out crucial aspects of the inflammatory process aids our understanding of causes and progression of cognitive decline. This chapter will review core aspects of the inflammatory hypothesis including neuropathological features of AD, relevant genetics, the neuroinflammatory cytokine cascade, oxidative stress, disruption in blood–brain barrier (BBB), inflammatory risk factors, and the role of anti-inflammatory treatments. Reference will be made to relevant studies pertaining to cognition.

Neuropathological Features of Alzheimer's Disease

Alzheimer's disease is defined clinically by loss of cognitive function and is a fatal neurodegenerative disease (Bertram & Tanzi, 2009). It is typified by the presence of extracellular accumulation of amyloid-β (Aβ) plaques and the intracellular presence of hyperphosphorylated tau proteins in the form of neurofibrillary tangles (NFTs), associated with microvascular damage and inflammation (Bertram et al., 2010). Amyloid plays a key role in the development of AD (Wang et al., 2006). Aβ arises from amyloid precursor protein (APP), and this is a normal occurring process. The APP gene is located on chromosome 21. Abnormal breakdown of APP as a result of cleavage by β-secretase and γ-secretase yields peptide fragments or oligomers (Small et al., 2010). Deposition of Aβ in the form of oligomers can lead to impaired synapse communication, contribute to oxidative stress, impair cellular glucose metabolism, and induce gliosis and, ultimately, lead to cognitive decline (Wang et al, 2006).

Low-density lipoprotein receptor-related protein 1 (LRP1) is involved in the efflux of Aβ from the brain to the blood across the BBB (Owen et al., 2010). Post mortem analysis of AD brains has shown that Aβ impairs its own efflux from the brain by oxidation and damage of its transporter (Owen et al., 2010). This contributes to increased Aβ deposition and to the cycle of neuroinflammation, resulting in cognitive impairment in AD. A study comparing the rate of CSF Aβ clearance in AD, and controls showed that clearance was approximately 30% slower in 12 individuals with AD than in 12 cognitively normal individuals (Mawuenyega et al., 2010). This suggests that slower clearance of the protein, rather than overproduction or both, may be reasons for the accumulation of protein in the AD brain.

Genetics

Alzheimer's disease can be broadly divided into early onset (<60 years), often familial AD (EOAD) and late onset (>60 years), nonfamilial AD (LOAD). Three genes are associated with EOAD and follow autosomal inheritance pattern. Mutations of these include APP and presenillin 1 and 2 (PSEN1 and 2), (Bertram et al., 2010).

The apolipoprotein E (APOE) ϵ4 allele increases the risk of developing LOAD. As a susceptibility gene, inheritance of the gene does not necessarily mean that an individual will develop the disease. It is estimated that APOE ϵ4 accounts for 50% of the genetic effect (Pericak-Vance et al., 2000). Recently, genome-wide association studies (GWAS) have significantly contributed to the identification of additional causative genes. Approximately two dozen AD loci have been identified as a result of these studies (Harold et al., 2009; Lambert et al., 2009).

Many of these loci are genes that are involved in inflammation and lipid-related regulation. Further analysis of these genes of small effect, which are just below the significance level, show that two key pathways involved are those relating to both cholesterol and inflammation (Jones et al., 2010).

Microglia

Microglial cells are the CNS macrophages, and their activation is the hallmark of neuroinflammation (Kaushik et al., 2010). They actively process tissue and their involvement can either be neuroprotective or neurotoxic (Walter & Neumann, 2009). Activation occurs via toll-like receptors (TLRs) (Sloane et al., 2010). Once activated, they can take up MHC class I/II proteins; express receptors for interleukin (IL)-1, IL-12, IL-16, IL-23 and tumor necrosis factor (TNF); instigate a proinflammatory cascade; and, ultimately, undertake phagocytosis. Byproducts such as destructive matrix metalloproteinases (MMPs) and free radicals are implicated in neuronal death.

Microglial cells in brain can interact with signals from the periphery (Dilger & Johnson, 2008). It is proposed that this is achieved through the following means: passive diffusion of cytokines from blood to brain via circumventricular organs to hypothalamic neurons, energy-dependent pathways involving transporter in intact BBB, peripherally stimulated BBB inflammatory cytokine release, and endothelial secretion of cytokines and transmission of peripheral immune signals via the autonomic system.

Systemic T cells, upon binding with microglia, are also involved in cascade of pathological events. Although this may be a protective response, excessive production of peripheral cytokines can inflict neuronal damage and add to acute brain injury and cerebral ischemia (Dilger & Johnson, 2008). In an effort to compensate for this, microglia express anti-inflammatory factors such as transforming growth factor (TGF)-β and IL-10 as well as being involved in the recruitment of neurons and astrocytes (Rock et al., 2004).

Microglia and Cognitive Decline

Cognitive decline is associated with chronic microglial activation (Zlokovic, 2008, Perry et al., 2010). Relating this to AD, it is hypothesized that damage to neurons is a result of chronic exposure to various exogenous factors (e.g., head injury) or endogenous risk factors (e.g., oxidative stress, lipid disorders, Aβ deposits) with concomitant upregulation of glial cells and inflammatory process (Maccioni et al., 2009). The results of these converge in the final common pathway of tau hyperphosphorylation (Fernandez et al., 2008). This process escalates the inflammatory process and neuronal cell death, culminating in progressive irreversible tissue damage (Maccioni et al., 2009).

The evidence of microglial activation associated with plaques in AD is extensive, but research is mainly derived from animal studies. Aβ can recruit and activate microglia. In turn, activated microglia have both primary and secondary functions as they are linked with formation of amyloid plaques and associated phagocytosis thereof (McNaull et al., 2010). Activation of inflammatory cascades can be beneficial in preventing neuronal damage. However, persistent activation of microglia may give rise to chronic inflammation and additional tissue damage with neurotoxic consequences (Neumann et al., 2009).

Complement: Interaction Central Nervous System and Periphery

The role of the complement system is to recognize and kill invading pathogens such as bacteria and viruses and preserve normal "self" cells (Van Beek et al., 2003). A fine balance is required between the effects of complement stimulation and prevention of host damage (Mastellos et al., 2005). There are three complement systems—the classical, lectin, and alternative pathways. All three share the common step of activating the central component C3 but differ according to the nature of recognition. The cellular source of complement within brain is represented by neurons, glial cells, and vascular endothelium (Mastellos et al., 2005).

Expression of complement from the three pathways in the brain is generally low (Stahel et al., 1998). There is some indication that there may be active two-way communication between the brain and the peripheral system by means of TLRs regarding pathogenic invasion and host-derived ligands (Downes & Crack, 2010). Toll-like receptors can have a beneficial or detrimental outcome on CNS diseases (Cameron & Landreth, 2010), and failure to modulate against complement mediated damage can lead to neuronal death.

Blood–Brain Barrier

The BBB is a membrane structure, comprised of specialized endothelial cells and, in combination with astrocytes, pericytes, extracellular matrix, and neurons, is referred to as the "neurovascular unit" (NVU) (Hawkins & Davis, 2005). The BBB serves to protect the delicate CNS from the peripheral system. The presence of "tight junctions" (TJs) between endothelial cells regulates BBB permeability and is involved in regulation and transport of paracellular molecules (Balbuena et al., 2011). Tight junctions proteins are subject to changes in expression, post-translational modification and protein–protein interactions under differing physiological conditions such as inflammation (Huber et al., 2001). Inflammatory mediators (such as complement, bradykinin, IL-1β, and TNF-α) caused by infection or trauma can cause increased BBB permeability (Annane, 2009). This can range from subtle increases in BBB permeability to edema of the brain, all of which could impair cognition and contribute to neurodegeneration. From a therapeutic stance, it is surmised that options for treatment could lie in the tightening of the TJs or agents to reduce the expression of adhesion molecules (Simka, 2009).

Systemic Infection and Memory

A prospective study examining the effects of naturally occurring upper respiratory tract infection on cognition, mood, and emotional processing found deficits in accuracy of episodic or working memory or speed of performance on attention tasks (Bucks et al., 2008). Holmes et al. (2009) studied the effects of acute and chronic systemic inflammation in relation to cognitive decline in AD patients ($n = 275$). Those who experienced measured systemic inflammatory events (based on caregiver history and interview) showed a twofold increase in rate of cognitive decline compared with those who did not experience a systemic inflammatory event. Further, high baseline levels of TNF-α were also associated with a fourfold rate in cognitive decline over a 6-month period (Holmes et al., 2009). It is thus suggested that those with vulnerable brains are more susceptible to deterioration in cognition when there are elevated pro-inflammatory cytokines.

Neural Arc and Inflammation

The inflammatory reflex of the vagus nerve consists of an afferent sensory neural arc that detects infection and inflammation and an efferent motor neural arc that can modulate immune responses (Das, 2011). Enhancing the activity of this immune-mediated neural circuit confers protection against damage by inhibiting cytokine release during infection, autoimmunity, shock, and other inflammatory conditions (Das, 2011). Acetylcholine (ACh), the principal vagal neurotransmitter, inhibits the production of pro-inflammatory cytokines through a mechanism dependent on the α7 nicotinic ACh receptor subunit (α7nAChR) (Das, 2011). Enhancement of this immune neural circuit can be undertaken through application of electrodes to stimulate the vagus nerve and protects against damaging inflammation in experimental autoimmune, rheumatic conditions (Das, 2011). Acetylcholinesterase inhibitors commonly used in the treatment of AD enhance cholinergic neurotransmission. A Cochrane Review revealed their efficacy in mild to moderate AD (Birks, 2006). It is also postulated that they have a preventative suppression of neuroinflammation through the cholinergic inflammatory pathway (Tabet, 2006).

Inflammatory Markers and Cognitive Decline

The evidence suggests involvement of a number of different inflammatory processes in the brain that may affect memory. The influence may range from cognitive decline, development of mild cognitive impairment (MCI), and conversion from MCI to dementia through to development of both AD and vascular dementia (VaD). As a result, the association among inflammatory markers, cognitive decline, and dementia has attracted increasing interest. The most commonly used inflammatory marker is C-Reactive Protein (CRP), which is associated with atherosclerosis as well as being a predictor for vascular events and outcome from these (Idicula et al., 2009). However, the utility of CRP as a tool in global risk assessment has some important limitations because of its poor specificity in coexisting inflammatory conditions (Hackam et al., 2003). Other markers that have been studied include cytokines and fibrinogen.

In terms of cognitive decline, a number of studies exist. The features of the various studies are shown in Table 11.1. Cross-sectional associations between raised levels of peripherally circulating markers of systemic inflammation and reduced cognitive ability in individuals without dementia have already been established. It is unclear whether these markers are predictive of cognitive decline in older age or whether they may have a causal role in the development of cognitive decline. To date, results for CRP are conflicting. In a large cohort from the The Womens Health Study, there was no evidence of a link between high sensitivity CRP (hsCRP) and cognitive decline (Weuve et al., 2006). In a cross-sectional analysis of older populations in the Rotterdam Study (mean follow-up: 4.6 years) and the Leiden 85-plus Study (maximal follow-up: 5 years), the authors concluded that CRP and IL-6 were only moderately associated with cognitive function and decline and tended to be stronger in carriers of the APOE ε4 allele (Schram et al., 2007). Among 1,284 participants in the Longitudinal Aging Study Amsterdam serum inflammatory protein α1-antichymotrypsin was associated with cognitive decline in older persons, whereas CRP and IL-6 were not (Dik et al., 2005). The MacArthur Studies of Successful Aging showed that those in the highest IL-6 tertile were significantly more likely to experience cognitive decline after adjustment for confounders (Weaver et al., 2002). In a small cohort from the Maastricht Ageing Study, CRP levels at baseline correlated negatively with performance on the Word Learning tests over the 6-year

Table 11.1 **Studies Involving Inflammation and Cognitive Decline, Mild Cognitive Impairment (MCI) and Dementia**

Author	Study details	Age	Study design	Follow-up (years)	Outcome	Results
Teunissen et al., 2002	Maastricht Aging Study n = 65	54 (10)	Longitudinal study	6	Cognitive decline: Letter–Digit Coding, Stroop, Word Learning	Baseline CRP levels correlated negatively with performance on the Word Learning tests
Schmidt et al., 2002	Honolulu Asia Aging Study n = 1050	54.2 (4.5)	Nested case–control	25	Dementia: (CASI, IQCODE, CERAD battery)	hsCRP (upper 3 quartiles) had a threefold significantly increased risk for all dementias combined, AD, and VaD compared to lowest quartile. Risk increased with increasing quartile for VaD.
Weaver et al., 2002	Mac Arthur Studies of Successful Aging n =779	70–79	Longitudinal follow-up	2.5 & 7		relationship between elevated baseline plasma IL-6 and risk for subsequent cognitive decline
Yaffe et al., 2003	Health Aging and Body Composition Study n = 3031	74	Prospective cohort study	2	Cognitive decline: 3MS	IL-6 and CRP, but not TNF-α associated with cognitive decline
Ravaglia et al., 2007	Conselice Study of Brain Aging n = 804	73.6 ± 6.3	Prospective population study	4	AD and VaD	high CRP and high IL6 associated with risk of VaD
Engelhart et al., 2004	Rotterdam Study n = 727	71.7 (9)	Case cohort	5–8	Dementia, AD, VaD	IL-6 associated with dementia and AD, CRP associated with VaD

(continued)

Table 11.1 **(Continued)**

Author	Study details	Age	Study design	Follow-up (years)	Outcome	Results
Yaffe et al., 2004	Health Aging and Body Composition Study n = 2632	2632 73.6 (2.9)	Prospective cohort study	4	Cognitive decline: 3MS	After stratifying for inflammation, those with metabolic syndrome and high inflammation had an increased likelihood of cognitive impairment compared with those without metabolic syndrome
Dik et al., 2005	Longitudinal Aging Study Amsterdam n = 1284	62–85 71.8 (4.2)	Prospective cohort study	3	Cognitive decline: MMSE, Auditory Verbal Learning, Raven's Colored Progressive Matrices, Coding Task	CRP, IL-6 not associated with cognitive decline
Weuve et al., 2006	Womens Health Study n = 4231	60–90	Prospective study	4.4–7.8	Cognitive decline:Telephone Interview for Cognitive Status, Immediate and delayed recalls East Boston Memory Test, Delayed recall of the 10-word list, Test of Category Fluency.	HsCRP not associated with cognitive function
Komulainen et al., 2007	Risk Factor Survey Finland n = 97	60–70	Population based follow-up	12	Cognitive decline: MMSE, Word Recall Test, Stroop, Letter Digit Substitution Test	hsCRP predicts poorer memory in elderly women. No association of hsCRP with MMSE or cognitive speed
Rafnasson et al., 2007	Edinburgh Artery Study n = 452	73.1 (5)	Prospective cohort study	4	Cognitive decline: Wechsler Logical Memory Test, Raven's Standard Progressive Matrices, Verbal Fluency Test, Wechsler Digit Symbol Test	Fibrinogen independently predicted 4-year decline in nonverbal reasoning

Study	Sample	Age	Design	Follow-up (years)	Cognitive measures	Findings
Schram et al., 2007	Rotterdam n = 2433 Leiden 85+ study n = 440	70.2 (5.7) 85	Population based cohorts	4.6 5	Cognitive decline: MMSE, abbreviated Stroop test part 3, Letter Digit Substitution Task (both). Word Fluency (Rdam), 12-Picture Learning test (Leiden)	Higher levels of CRP & IL-6 cross sectionally associated with worse global cognition and executive function (Rdam). Higher IL-6 levels related to a steeper annual decline in memory function in longitudinal analysis (Leiden)
Gimeno et al., 2008	Whitehall II study n = 4362	35–55	Prospective cohort	6	Cognition, cognitive decline: short-term verbal memory, Alice Heim 4-I, Mill Hill vocabulary test, verbal fluency	Higher CRP & IL-6 in midlife moderately associated with lower cognitive status. CRP minor associations with cognitive decline
Haan et al., 2008	Sacramento Area Latino Study on Aging n = 1445	60–101	Prospective cohort	5	Dementia: Verbal Episodic Memory test, 3MSE, NINCDS ADRDA	APOE4 +ve: CRP associated with lower rates of combined dementia/CIND APOE4 −ve: no effect of CRP on dementia/CIND
Laurin et al., 2009	Honolulu-Asia Aging Study n = 691	77 (4.1)	Prospective cohort	31	Cognitive decline and dementia: CASI, NINCDS ADRDA	Difference in decline between those in the lowest compared to highest quartile of hs-CRP. Differences no longer significant after incident dementia cases removed from analysis.
Marioni et al., 2009	Aspirin for Asymptomatic Atherosclerosis Trial n = 2312	50–80	Prospective cohort study	5	Cognitive decline: Auditory Verbal Learning Test, Raven's Standard Progressive Matrices, Digit Symbol Test, Verbal Fluency Test, Trail-Making Test, Part B	Raised levels of CRP & fibrinogen, predicted poorer subsequent cognitive ability and were associated with age-related cognitive decline in several domains

(continued)

Table 11.1 (Continued)

Author	Study details	Age	Study design	Follow-up (years)	Outcome	Results
Roberts et al., 2009	The Mayo Clinic Study of Aging n = 1969	70–89	Cross-sectional		MCI: WAIS-R, WMS-R, Trail Making Test B, Digit Symbol Substitution Test, Boston Naming Test and Category Fluency, Logical Memory-II, Visual Reproduction-II Auditory Verbal Learning Test, Picture Completion and Block Design	Plasma CRP associated with prevalent MCI and with non-amnestic MCI but not with amnestic MCI
Schuitemaker et al., 2009	n = 212	58–78	Cross-sectional		MCI (Petersen) AD (NINCDS ADRDA)	CSF and serum CRP levels significantly higher in MCI compared to AD after adjustment for age, APOE ε4 genotype and cardiovascular diseases
Xu et al., 2009	n = 168	71.6 (7.4)	Prospective cohort	2	Cognitive decline and dementia in MCI: MMSE	High CRP associated with cognitive decline, dementia and VaD
Noble et al., 2010	WHICAP II n = 1331	76.1 (71.5–81.0)	Cross-sectional		Selective Reminding Test, Benton Visual Retention Test, Rosen– Drawing Test, Benton Visual Retention Test, BostonNaming Test, Controlled Oral Word Association Test, Category Fluency Test, Color Trails Test 1, Similarities subtest from the Wechsler Adult Intelligence Scale– Revised, Color Trails Test 2	highest hsCRP tertile had higher adjusted odds of impaired memory and greater odds of visuospatial impairment Higher hsCRP not associated with executive or language impairment.

Study	Cohort	Age	Follow-up	Study design	Cognitive assessment / MCI criteria	Findings
Roberts et al., 2010	The Mayo Clinic Study of Aging n = 1969	70–89		Cross-sectional	MCI: WAIS-R, WMS-R, Trail Making Test B, Digit Symbol Substitution Test, Boston Naming Test and Category Fluency, Logical Memory-II, Visual Reproduction-II, Auditory Verbal Learning Test, Picture Completion and Block Design	High CRP (highest tertile vs lowest tertile) associated with na-MCI but not with a-MCI, after adjusting for sex, age, years of education. Combination of MetS and high CRP (compared to no MetS and lowest CRP tertile) associated with na-MCI but not with a-MCI
Trollor et al., 2010	Sydney Memory and Ageing Study n = 710	70–90		Cross-sectional	MCI (Winblad criteria)	Findings suggest an association between specific inflammatory markers (TNF-α, SAA) and MCI subtypes
Dlugaj et al., 2012	Heinz Nixdorf Recall Study n = 296	50–80	5	Population-based case–control study	MCI	Baseline hsCRP levels significantly associated with MCI and amnestic MCI. At follow-up, the fourth hsCRP quartile associated with MCI, amnestic MCI and non-amnestic MCI.
Jefferson et al., 2011	Framingham Offspring study n = 1878	60 ± 9, 35–85	6.3 ± 1	Population cohort study, longitudinal and cross-sectional analysis	Cognitive decline: Logical memory delayed, Visual reproduction delayed, Trail making test A&B, Boston naming test-30 item, Hooper visual organization test, Similarities subtest, WRAT-3 reading subtest	Largely negative, but suggest specific inflammatory markers may have limited associations with poorer cognition (CRP, TNF-α) and reading performance (TNF-α)

follow-up period (Teunissen et al., 2003). Increased CRP was associated with lower clock drawing scores in another study (Ravaglia et al., 2003). In the Health Aging and Body Composition study those with metabolic syndrome and high inflammation had significantly greater 4-year decline on the modified Mini-Mental State Examination (3MS) (Yaffe et al., 2004). In a study of older women, hsCRP predicted poorer memory 12 years later (Komulainen et al., 2007). The Whitehall II study showed that raised levels of CRP and IL-6 were associated with lower cognitive status but not cognitive decline (Gimeno et al., 2008). Cross-sectional analysis of a population-based community study in New York of more than 1,300 participants from a longitudinal study of aging without dementia showed that those in the highest hsCRP tertile had significantly higher adjusted odds of impaired memory than those in the lowest tertile (Noble et al., 2010). A recent cross-sectional analysis of Framingham Offspring showed that specific inflammatory markers may have limited associations with poorer cognition and reading performance (Jefferson et al., 2011). The majority of the studies would suggest a prospective role for inflammatory processes in cognitive decline.

A role for plasma fibrinogen in age-associated cognitive decline has been suggested (Rafnasson et al., 2007). In a further study of participants in the Aspirin for Asymptomatic Atherosclerosis Trial, the same group reported that increased circulating levels of CRP, fibrinogen, and elevated plasma viscosity predicted poorer subsequent cognitive ability and were associated with age-related cognitive decline in several domains (Marioni et al., 2009).

With regard to MCI, there are a few studies suggesting a role of inflammatory mediators. Plasma CRP was associated with prevalent MCI and with non-amnestic MCI in elderly, non-demented persons (70–89 years) in a population-based setting. These findings suggest the involvement of inflammation in the pathogenesis of MCI (Roberts et al., 2009). High CRP (highest tertile vs. lowest tertile) was significantly associated with non-amnestic MCI but not with amnestic MCI, after adjusting for sex, age, and years of education (Roberts et al., 2010). There were also associations between specific inflammatory markers and MCI in the Sydney Memory and Aging Study (TNF-α, serum amyloid A). There were also differences in some MCI subtypes (Trollor et al., 2010). A nested case–control study examined the relation of hsCRP and MCI at different time-points. High-sensitivity CRP levels were measured 5 years before (baseline) and at the time of neuropsychological testing in 148 MCI cases (106 amnestic, 42 non-amnestic and 148 matched controls identified from a prospective population-based cohort study of 4,359 participants ages 50–80 years). In the fully adjusted model, baseline hsCRP levels were significantly associated with both MCI and amnestic MCI. At follow-up, the fourth hsCRP quartile was associated with MCI, amnestic MCI (OR = 3.73, 95% CI, 1.52–9.17), and non-amnestic MCI. Elevated hsCRP levels, even detected

5 years before diagnosis, are associated with an at least twofold increased probability of MCI. These findings suggest that inflammation plays an important role in the development and presence of MCI (Dlugaj et al., 2012).

Suggestions that inflammatory markers were associated with both AD and vascular VaD have been made (Schmidt et al., 2002). In the Honolulu Asia Aging Study, men in the upper three quartiles of hsCRP had a threefold significantly increased risk for all dementias combined, AD, and VCI independent of vascular risk factors (Schmidt et al., 2002).

There is an increasing awareness of the interaction between cerebrovascular disease and AD. The exact nature of those links is not clear. There is a considerable literature on inflammation, atherosclerosis, and cerebrovascular disease. Cerebrovascular disease could be a confounding factor for the link between inflammation and cognitive ability. In the study where CRP and fibrinogen were found to be associated with cognitive decline, these were still significant when baseline cardiovascular disease was included in the analysis (Marioni et al., 2009). In a recent study, CRP and plasminogen activator inhibitor-1 (PAI-1) levels were associated with white matter (WM) integrity loss in corticosubcortical pathways and association fibers of frontal and temporal lobes, independently of age, sex, and vascular risk factors. Plasminogen activator inhibitor-1 was also related to lower speed and visuomotor coordination. None of the biomarkers were related to gray matter volume changes. The findings suggest that inflammation and dysregulation of the fibrinolytic system may be involved in the pathological mechanisms underlying the WM damage seen in cerebrovascular disease and subsequent cognitive impairment (Miralbell et al., 2012).

Antibiotics in Alzheimer's Disease

Because of the potential role of inflammation, there has been some focus on use of antibiotics. Rifamycins can inhibit the aggregation of Aβ in vitro and interfere with fibril formation (Matsuzaki et al., 2007). Tetracyclines such as minocycline have also been studied because they have anti-amyloid properties and tau inhibition properties as well as anti-inflammatory factors (Garwood et al., 2010). Minocycline can modulate microglia and thus interfere with cytokine and inflammatory mediator release and is also anti-apoptotic (Noble et al., 2009). Animal studies have shown promise (Hunter et al., 2004, Ryu et al., 2004). A phase 2 study showed significantly less cognitive decline in mild to moderate AD patients treated with doxycycline and rifampicin compared to those who received placebo (Loeb et al., 2004), but this was not confirmed in a larger follow-up study (Molloy, presentation at EUGMS 2010).

Anti-Inflammatory Agents

The possible role of inflammation in cognitive decline and dementia has resulted in a closer examination of the role of anti-inflammatory medication. It is useful to consider the epidemiological evidence and the evidence for prevention and for treatment, including the duration of treatment, the influence of any confounders such as age and APOE genotype, and the type of agent studied. Table 11.2 shows epidemiological studies.

In an early review of 17 studies of arthritis and anti-inflammatory agents, seven case–control studies with arthritis as the risk factor yielded an overall odds ratio of 0.556 ($p < 0.0001$), whereas four case–control studies with steroids yielded odds ratios of 0.656 ($p = 0.049$), and three case–control studies with nonsteroidal anti-inflammatory drugs (NSAIDs) yielded an odds ratio of 0.496 ($p = 0.0002$). When NSAIDs and steroids were combined into a single category of anti-inflammatory drugs, the odds ratio was 0.556 ($p < 0.0001$). The authors suggested that anti-inflammatory drugs may have a protective effect against AD (McGeer et al., 1996). Further studies showed similar results and seemed to suggest that a longer duration of treatment had more of an effect (Stewart et al., 1997; In't Veld et al., 2001).

Pooled data from nine studies involving 14,654 subjects have confirmed that the protective effects depend on the duration of NSAID use with relative risks of 0.95 among short-term (<1 month), 0.83 among intermediate-term (1–24 months), and 0.27 among long-term (>24 months) users (Etminan et al., 2003). A systematic review of seven prospective cohort studies found that for those reporting duration of use of 2 years or more the combined risk estimate for developing AD was 0.42 compared to 0.74 for those in whom any lifetime NSAID exposure was reported (Szekely et al., 2004). The retrospective study of Vlad et al. (2008) showed a form of "dose–response" effect in terms of duration of therapy in that those on treatment for longer had a more reduced risk of AD. Some of the prospective studies were negative, perhaps because of this "duration" effect, but all the retrospective studies showed a reduced risk ratio for AD (Landi et al., 2003).

These epidemiological findings stimulated the design of prospective trials to examine whether anti-inflammatory agents could affect progression of AD and indeed prevent development of AD. Table 11.3 shows the results of the placebo-controlled trials of treatment in established AD. An early small study showed benefits for indomethacin (Rogers et al., 1993). However, all other trials did not show benefit and in fact there were some studies with adverse results. The conclusion, therefore, is that there is no benefit from use of anti-inflammatory agents in established AD. One explanation for the negative results in a dementia population is that the neuroprotective effects of such drugs occur before dementia symptoms are clinically obvious (Small et al., 2008).

Table 11.2 **Summary of the Main Prospective and Retrospective Epidemiological Studies of Non-Steroidal Anti-Inflammatory Drugs and Alzheimer's Disease**

Study	Study sample size	Duration NSAID use	AD cases	Risk ratio(95% Confidence interval)
Prospective studies				
Stewart et al., 1997	1,686	≥2 yr	81	0.40(0.19–0.84)
		<2 yr		0.65(0.33–1.29)
in't Veld et al., 2001	6,989	≥2 yr	4	0.2(0.05–0.83)
		1–23 months	210	0.83(0.62–1.11)
		<1 month	88	0.95(0.70–1.29)
Zandi et al., 2002	3,227	>2 yr	104	0.45(.0.17–0.97)
		≤2 yr		0.75(0.38–1.34)
Cornelius et al., 2004	1,301	NA	164	0.61(0.32–1.15)
Szekely et al., 2008	3,229	NA	321	0.63(0.45–0.88)
Arvanitakis et al., 2008	1,019	NA	209	1.19(0.87–1.62)
Breitner et al., 2009	2,736	NA	356	1.57(1.10–2.23)
Retrospective studies				
Landi et al., 2003	2,708	NA	269	0.43(0.23–0.82)
Yip et al., 2005	1034	>6 months	61	0.64(0.38–1.05)
Vlad et al., 2008	246,199	>5 yr	49,349	0.76(0.68–0.85)
		>4 to ≤5 yr		0.76(0.69–0.84)
		>3 to ≤4 yr		0.90(0.84–0.97)
		>2 to ≤3 yr		0.93(0.88–0.99)
		>1 to ≤2 yr		0.90(0.86–0.94)
		≤1 yr		0.98(0.95–1.00)

Studies have also focused on conversion from MCI to dementia. A 4-year, double-blind, placebo-controlled study with rofecoxib in 1,457 patients with MCI showed that the annual conversion rate to AD was significantly higher in patients treated with rofecoxib (25 mg/day) than in those treated with placebo (6.4% vs. 4.5%, $p = 0.011$) (Thal et al., 2005). Another double-blind, placebo-controlled trial in MCI patients was conducted with triflusal,

Table 11.3 **Double-Blind, Randomized, Placebo-Controlled Trials of Anti-Inflammatory Agents in Patients With Mild-to-Moderate Alzheimer's Disease**

Study	Drug	Dose (mg)	Treatment duration (months)	Number	Outcome
Rogers et al., 1993	Indomethacin	100-150	6	44	Beneficial
Scharf et al., 1999	Diclofenac	50	6	41	Neutral
Aisen et al., 2000	Prednisone	10	12	138	Neutral/detrimental
Sainati et al., 2000	Celecoxib	400	12	285	Neutral
Van Gool et al., 2001	Hydroxychloroquine	200–400	18	168	Neutral
Aisen et al., 2002	Nimesulide	200	3	40	Neutral
Bain et al., 2002	Dapsone	100	12	201	Neutral
Aisen et al., 2003	Rofecoxib	25	12	351	Neutral
Aisen et al., 2003	Naproxen	440	12	351	Neutral/detrimental
Reines et al., 2004	Rofecoxib	25	12	692	Neutral
Soininen et al., 2007	Celecoxib	400	12	425	Neutral
de Jong et al., 2008	Indomethacin	100	12	51	Neutral
Wilcock et al., 2008	Tarenflurbil	800-1600	12	210	Neutral
Green et al., 2009	Tarenflurbil	1600	18	1684 (mild AD)	Neutral/detrimental
Pasqualetti et al., 2009	Ibuprofen	800	12	132	Neutral
Wilcock, 2009	Tarenflurbil	1600	18	840 (mild AD)	Neutral

a non-selective NSAID (Gómez-Isla et al., 2008). Two hundred and fifty-seven subjects were enrolled and followed-up for an average of 13 months. Compared to placebo, there was a significant lower rate of conversion to AD in the triflusal group (hazard ratio = 2.10; 95% confidence interval, 1.10–4.01; $p = 0.024$). The trial was prematurely halted, therefore these results should be interpreted with caution and require further confirmation. Another 18-month, double-blind, placebo-controlled study of celecoxib in 88 subjects with mild, self-reported, memory complaints but with normal memory performance score (Small et al., 2008) reported significant differences in favor of the celecoxib on executive functioning ($p = 0.03$) and language/semantic memory ($p = 0.02$). There was a very high attrition rate in this study (48 of 88 subjects), therefore these results should be viewed with caution.

Another logical approach was to examine whether anti-inflammatory approaches would prevent dementia in those at risk. The Alzheimer's Disease Anti-inflammatory Prevention Trial (ADAPT) was a primary prevention trial in cognitively normal older people at risk of AD. Subjects were randomized to receive naproxen (220 mg twice a day), celecoxib (200 mg twice a day) or placebo. The trial was stopped early because of issues that emerged with COX-2 inhibitors, although each group received treatment for 733 days. Naproxen was associated with a significantly increased risk for AD (ADAPT Research Group, 2007). Cognitive decline was also significantly worse with celecoxib (ADAPT Research Group, 2008). The long-term follow-up in this study is interesting, as it showed no negative effects of either anti-inflammatory but, in fact, showed that there was a later reduction in AD incidence among asymptomatic enrollees who were given naproxen (Breitner et al., 2011). The authors concluded that NSAIDs have an adverse effect in later stages of AD pathogenesis, whereas asymptomatic individuals treated with conventional NSAIDs such as naproxen experience reduced AD incidence, but only after 2 to 3 years. Treatment effects differ at various stages of disease, which is consistent with data from both trials and epidemiological studies. Not all studies have found that NSAID use is associated with a decreased risk of AD. A meta-analysis of 25 case–control and cohort studies found that the benefit of NSAIDs in preventing dementia was 50% in studies with prevalent dementia cases, reduced to 20% in studies with incident dementia cases, and was absent in studies where cognitive decline was used as endpoint (de Craen et al., 2005). Authors have concluded that most of the reported beneficial effects of NSAIDs may result from recall bias, prescription bias, and publication bias. In a study in 1,019 older Catholic clergy followed for up to 12 years, there was no relationship between NSAID use and incident AD, change in cognitive performance, or AD neuropathology (Arvanitakis et al., 2008). The fact that clinical data and pathological data were used in this study strengthens the findings.

It is perhaps worth reflecting on the role of the APOE allele and age in these studies. These have been reviewed by Imbimbo et al. (2010). Nonsteroidal anti-inflammatory drug users with one or more APOE ε4 alleles consistently have a greater AD risk reduction (In't Veld et al., 2001; Cornelius et al., 2004; Yip et al., 2005; Hayden et al., 2007; Szekely et al., 2008). Several studies have suggested that the risk reduction with NSAIDs decreases with age (In't Veld et al., 2001; Zandi et al., 2002; Szekely et al., 2008). A population-based cohort study (the Adult Changes in Thought study) in 2,736 elderly subjects (median: 74.8 years at enrollment) without dementia at baseline followed for up to 12 years unexpectedly found that NSAID users had a significantly increased incidence of AD, with adjusted hazard ratios of 1.17 for moderate users and 1.57 for heavy users (Breitner et al., 2009). To explain these unexpected findings, authors hypothesized that NSAID exposure may delay the onset of AD, with younger cohorts showing a reduced frequency of disease and older cohorts being enriched for cases that would otherwise have appeared earlier.

Immunotherapy

Vaccination was the first treatment approach to affect the AD process in animal models (Schenk et al., 1999). Peripheral injections of monoclonal antibodies against Aβ have had similar effects on Aβ load, indicating that the therapeutic effect of the vaccine is based primarily on generation of a humoral response (Bard et al., 2000). There may be a number of mechanisms involved: targeting brain deposits of Aβ causing disruption; dissolution of Aβ fibrils; preventing reassembly of Aβ and inhibiting toxicity; microglial activation; creation of a peripheral-sink effect, where removal of excess circulatory soluble Aβ draws soluble Aβ from the brain; hydrolysis of Aβ; and neutralization of neurotoxic oligomers (Wisniewski & Konietzko, 2008).

Immunization can involve active and passive approaches. The earliest active vaccination trial (AN-1792) was stopped in Phase II because of development of meningoencephalitis in approximately 6% of the vaccinated patients (Nicoll et al., 2003). Post mortem analysis of 12 subjects in the AN-1792 trial, including 2 who suffered meningoencephalitis, provided data in support of the hypothesis that there is clearance of deposited Aβ as assessed solely by histochemical analysis of Aβ (Holmes et al., 2008). Passive approaches using humanized monoclonal antibodies targeting Aβ and intravenous immunoglobulin (IVIG) are being actively tested in humans. The most advanced of these involves bapineuzumab, a humanized monoclonal antibody that targets the amino-terminus of Aβ and is capable of binding monomeric, oligomeric, and fibrillar Aβ. Initial studies were negative, although there were differential responses according to APOE genotype. Follow-up studies are ongoing. These monoclonal approaches are associated with development of vasogenic edemas. Several small, early phase studies have reported improvement in cognition, decreases in CSF Aβ and increases in plasma Aβ following IVIG administration to AD patients (Relkin et al., 2009). Studies with IVIG are ongoing. These studies are likely to provide further insight into disease mechanisms and to help refine therapeutic approaches.

Conclusion

There are a number of interactive pathways that can contribute to neuroinflammation. Effective immune response in the CNS is required for maintaining a healthy brain. A chronic or exaggerated inflammatory response is detrimental to the brain and can lead to irreversible damage and cognitive decline. These effects could be mediated in part by cerebrovascular disease. There appears to be a consistent relationship between higher CRP levels and MCI. It appears as though long-term exposure to anti-inflammatory agents can reduce cognitive decline and AD but that once AD is established, anti-inflammatory agents have no benefit.

References

ADAPT Research Group. Lyketsos CG, Breitner JC, Green RC, Martin BK, Meinert C, Piantadosi S, et al. Naproxen and celecoxib do not prevent AD in early results from a randomized controlled trial. *Neurology* 2007;68:1800–1808.

ADAPT Research Group. Martin BK, Szekely C, Brandt J, Piantadosi S, Breitner JC, Craft S, et al. Cognitive function over time in the Alzheimer's Disease Antiinflammatory Prevention Trial (ADAPT): results of a randomized controlled trial of naproxen and celecoxib. *Arch. Neurol.* 2008;65:896–905.

Aisen PS, Davis KL, Berg JD, Schafer K, Campbell K, Thomas RG, Weiner MF, Farlow MR, Sano M, Grundman M, Thal LJ. A randomized controlled trial of prednisone in Alzheimer's disease. Alzheimer's Disease Cooperative Study. *Neurology* 2000; 54(3): 588–593.

Aisen PS, Schmeidler J, & Pasinetti GM. Randomized pilot study of nimesulide treatment in Alzheimer's disease. *Neurology* 2002;58:1050–1054.

Aisen PS, Schafer KA, Grundman M, et al. Effects of rofecoxib or naproxen vs placebo on Alzheimer disease progression: a randomized controlled trial. *JAMA.* 2003;289: 2819–2826.

Annane D. Sepsis-associated delirium: the pro and con of C5a blockade. *Critical Care.* 2009;13:135.

Arvanitakis Z, Grodstein F, Bienias JL, Schneider JA, Wilson RS, Kelly JF, et al. Relation of NSAIDs to incident AD, change in cognitive function, and AD pathology. *Neurology* 2008;70:2219–2225.

Balbuena P, Li W, & Ehrich M. Assessments of tight junction proteins occludin, claudin 5 and scaffold proteins ZO1 and ZO2 in endothelial cells of the rat blood–brain barrier: Cellular responses to neurotoxicants malathion and lead acetate. *NeuroToxicology* 2011;32:58–67.

Bard F, Cannon C, Barbour R, et al. Peripherally administered antibodies against amyloid beta-peptide enter the central nervous system and reduce pathology in a mouse model of Alzheimer disease. *Nat Med.* 2000;6:916–919.

Bertram L & Tanzi R. Alzheimer disease. "New light on an old CLU." *Nature Reviews Neurology* 2009;6:11–13.

Bertram L, Lill CM, & Tanzi R. *The genetics of Alzheimer disease: back to the future*. *Neuron* 2010;*68*:270–228.

Beydoun MA, Beydoun HA, & Wang Y. Obesity and central obesity as risk factors for incident dementia and its subtypes: a systematic review and meta-analysis. *Obesity Reviews* 2008;*9*:204–214.

Birks J. Cholinesterase inhibitors for Alzheimer's disease. *Cochrane Database of Systematic Reviews* 2006, Issue 1. Art. No.: CD005593. DOI: 10.1002/14651858.CD005593

BreitnerJC, Haneuse SJ, Walker R, Dublin S, Crane PK, Gray SL, et al. Risk of dementia and AD with prior exposure to NSAIDs in an elderly community-based cohort. *Neurology* 2009;*72*:1899–1905.

Breitner JC, Baker LD, Montine TJ, Meinert CL, Lyketsos CG, Ashe KH, Brandt J, Craft S, Evans DE, Green RC, Ismail MS, Martin BK, Mullan MJ, Sabbagh M, Tariot PN; ADAPT Research Group. Extended results of the Alzheimer's disease anti-inflammatory prevention trial. *Alzheimers Dementia* 2011; 7:402–411.

Bucks RS, Gidron Y, Harris P, Teeling J, Wesnes KA, & Perry VH. Selective effects of upper respiratory tract infection on cognition, mood and emotion processing: a prospective study. *Brain Behaviour and Immunology* 2008;*22*:399–407.

Cameron B & Landreth GE. Inflammation, Microglia and Alzheimer's Disease. *Neurobiol Dis.* 2010;*37*:503–509.

Cornelius C, Fastbom J, Winblad B, & Viitanen M. Aspirin, NSAIDs, risk of dementia, and influence of the apolipoprotein E ε4 allele in an elderly population. *Neuroepidemiology* 2004;*23*:135–143.

Das UN. Can vagus nerve stimulation halt or ameliorate rheumatoid arthritis and lupus? *Lipids in Health and Disease* 2011;*10*:19 doi:10.1186/1476-511X-10-19.

de Craen AJ, Gussekloo J, Vrijsen B, & Westendorp RG. Metaanalysis of nonsteroidal antiinflammatory drug use and risk of dementia. *Am. J. Epidemiol.* 2005;*161*:114–120.

de Jong D, Jansen R, Hoefnagels W, Jellesma-Eggenkamp M, Verbeek M, Borm G, Kremer B. No effect of one-year treatment with indomethacin on Alzheimer's disease progression: a randomized controlled trial. *PLoS One* 2008; 3(1): e1475.

Dik MG, Jonker C, Hack CE, Smit JH, Comijs HC, & Eikelenboom P. Serum inflammatory proteins and cognitive decline in older persons. *Neurology* 2005;*64*:1371–1377.

Dilger RN & Johnson RW. Aging, microglial cell priming, and the discordant central inflammatory response to signals from the peripheral immune system. *Journal of Leukocyte Biology* 2008;*84*:932–939.

Dlugaj M, Gerwig M, Wege N, Siegrist J, Mann K, Bröcker-Preuß M, et al. Elevated Levels of High-Sensitivity C-Reactive Protein are Associated with Mild Cognitive Impairment and its Subtypes: Results of a Population-Based Case-Control Study. *Journal of Alzheimer's Disease*; 2012; *28*:503–514.

Downes CE & Crack PJ. Neural injury following stroke: are Toll-like receptors the link between the immune system and the CNS? *British Journal of Pharmacology* 2010; *160*:1872–1888.

Engelhart MJ, Geerlings MI, Meijer J, Kiliaan P, Amanda RA, van Swieten TJC, et al. Inflammatory Proteins in Plasma and the Risk of Dementia The Rotterdam Study. *Archives of Neurology*. 2004; *61*: 668–672.

Etminan M, Gill S, & Samii A. (2003). Effect of non-steroidal anti-inflammatory drugs on risk of Alzheimer's disease: systematic review and metaanalysis of observational studies. *BMJ* 327, 128–132.

Fernandez JA, Leone R, Kuljisa RO, & Maccioni RB. The damage signals hypothesis of Alzheimer's disease pathogenesis. *Journal of Alzheimers Disease* 2008;*14*:329–333.

Garwood CJ, Cooper JD, Hanger DP, & Noble W. Anti-inflammatory impact of minocycline in a mouse model of tauopathy. *Frontiers in Neurodegeneration Psychiatry* 2010;*12*:136.

Gimeno D, Marmot MG, & Singh-Manoux A. Inflammatory markers and cognitive function in middle aged adults: the Whitehall II study. *Psychoneuroendocrinology* 2008;*33*:1322–1334.

Gómez-Isla T, Blesa R, Boada M, Clarimón J, Del Ser T, Domenech G, et al. A randomized, double-blind, placebo controlled-trial of triflusal in mild cognitive impairment: the TRIMCI study. *Alzheimer Dis. Assoc.Disord.*2008; *22*:21–29.

Green RC, Schneider LS, Amato DA, Beelen AP, Wilcock G, Swabb EA, et al. Effect of taren-flurbil on cognitive decline and activities of daily living in patients with mild Alzheimer disease: a randomized controlled trial. *Journal of the American Medical Association.* 2009;*16*:2257–2264.

Haan MN, Aiello AE, West NA, & Jagust WJ. 12. C-reactive protein and rate of dementia in carriers and non carriers of Apolipoprotein APOE4 genotype. Neurobiol Aging. 2008;*29*:1774–1782

Hackam DG & Sonia S. Emerging Risk Factors for Atherosclerotic Vascular Disease. A Critical Review of the Evidence. *Journal of the American Medical Association* 2003;*290*:932–940.

Harold D, Abraham R, Hollingworth P, et al. Genome –wide association study identifies variants at CLU and PICALM associated with Alzheimer's disease. *Nature Genetics* 2009;*41*:1088–1093.

Hawkins BT & Davis TP. The blood-brain barrier/neurovascular unit in health and disease. *Pharmacological Reviews.* 2005;*57*:173–185.

Hayden KM, Zandi PP, Khachaturian AS, Szekely CA, Fotuhi M, Norton MC, et al. Cache County Investigators. Does NSAID use modify cognitive trajectories in the elderly? The Cache County study. *Neurology* 2007;*69*:275–282.

Höglund K & Blennow K. Effect of HMG-CoA reductase inhibitors on beta-amyloid peptide levels: implications for Alzheimer's disease. *CNS Drugs* 2007;*21*:449–462.

Holmes C, Boche D, Wilkinson D, Yadegarfar G, Hopkins V, Bayer A, et al. Long-term effects of Abeta42 immunisation in Alzheimer's disease: follow-up of a randomised, placebo-controlled phase I trial. *Lancet.* 2008;*372*:216–223.

Holmes C, Cunningham C, Zotova E, Woolford J, Dean C, Kerr S, et al. Systemic inflammation and disease progression in Alzheimer disease. *Neurology* 2009;*73*:768–774.

Huber JD, Egleton RD, & Davis TD. Molecular physiology and pathophysiology of tight junctions in the blood–brain barrier. *Trends in Neurosciences* 2001;*24*: 719–725.

Hunter CL, Bachman D, & Granholm A-C. Minocycline prevents cholinergic loss in a mouse model of Down's syndrome. *Annals of Neurology.* 2004;*56*: 675–688.

Idicula TT, Brogger J, Naess H, Waje-Andreassen U, & Thomassen L. Admission C-reactive protein after acute ischemic stroke is associated with stroke severity and mortality: The Bergen stroke study. *BMC Neurology* 2009;*9*:1–9.

Imbimbo BP, Solfrizzi V, & Francesco P. Are NSAIDS useful to treat Alzheimers disease or mild cognitive impairment? *Frontiers in Aging Neuroscience* 2010;*2*:1–13.

Int'Veld BA, Ruitenberg A, Hofman A, et al. Non-steroidal anti-inflammatory drugs and the risk of Alzheimer's disease. *N Engl J Med* 2001;*345*:1515–1521.

Jefferson A, Massaro JM, Beiser AS, Seshadri S, Larson MG, Wolf PA, et al. Inflammatory markers and neuropsychological functioning: the Framingham Heart Study. *Neuroepidemiology* 2011;*37*:21–30.

Jones L, Holmans PA, Hamshere ML, et al. Genetic evidence implicates the immune system and cholesterol metabolism in the aetiology of Alzheimer's disease. *PLoS One.* 2010;*5*:e13950.

Kálmán J & Janka Z. Cholesterol and Alzheimer's Disease. *Orv Hetil* 2005;*146*: 1903–1911.

Kaushik DK, Gupta M, Das S, & Basu A. Krüppel-like factor 4, a novel transcription factor regulates microglial activation and subsequent neuroinflammation. *Journal of Neuroinflammation* 2010;*7*:68 doi:10.1186/1742-2094-7-68.

Komulainen P, Lakka TA, Kivipelto M, Hassinen M, Penttila IM, Helkala EL, et al. Serum high sensitivity C-reactive protein and cognitive function in elderly women. *Age Ageing* 2007;*36*:443–448.

Lambert,JC., Heath S, Even G, et al. Genome-wide association study identifies variants at CLU and CR1 associated with Alzheimer's disease. *Nature Genetics* 2009;*41*:1094–1099.

Landi F, Cesari M, Onder G, et al. Non-steroidal anti-inflammatory drug (NSAID) use and Alzheimer disease in community-dwelling elderly patients. *Am J Geriatr Psychiatry* 2003;*11*:179–1185.

Laurin D, David Curb J, Masaki KH, White LR, & Launer LJ. Midlife C-reactive protein and risk of cognitive decline: a 31-year follow-up. *Neurobiol Aging.* 2009;*30*:1724–1727.

Lin YH, Lee JK, Huang Hl, Huang KC, & Chen MF. Plasma leptin levels and digital pulse volume in obese patients without metabolic syndrome—a pilot study. *Clinica Chimica Acta* 2010;*412*:730–734.

Loeb MB, Molloy WD, Smieja M, et al. A Randomized, Controlled Trial of Doxycycline and Rifampin for Patients with Alzheimer's' Disease. *Journal of the American Geriatrics Society* 2004;*52*:381–387.

McGeer PL, Schulzer M, & McGeer EG. Arthritis and anti-inflammatory agents as possible protective factors for Alzheimer's disease: a review of 17 epidemiologic studies. *Neurology* 1996;*47*:425–432.

McGuinness B, Craig D, Bullock R, & Passmore P (2009) Statins for the prevention of dementia. *Cochrane Database of Systematic Reviews* 2009, Issue 2. Art. No.: CD003160. DOI: 10.1002/14651858.CD003160.pub2

McNaull BBA, Todd S, McGuinness B, & Passmore AP. Inflammation and anti-inflammatory strategies for Alzheimers disease: a review' *Gerontology* 2010;*56*:3–14.

Maccioni RB, Rojo LE, Fernández JA, & Kuljis R. The role of neuroimmunomodulation in Alzheimer's disease. *Annals of the New York*. Academy of Sciences 2009; *1153*: 240–246.

Maase I, Bordet R, Deplanque D, Al Khedr A, Richard F, Libersa C, & Pasquier F. Lipid lowering agents are associated with a slower cognitive decline in Alzheimer disease. *Journal of Neurology, Neurosurgery and Psychiatry* 2005;*76*:1624–1629.

Marioni R, Marioni MSC, Stewart MC, Murray GD, Deary I, Fowkes GR, et al. Peripheral Levels of Fibrinogen, C-Reactive Protein, and Plasma Viscosity Predict Future Cognitive Decline in Individuals Without Dementia. *Psychosomatic Medicine* 2009;*71*:901–906.

Martin BK, Szekely C, Brandt J, Piantadosi S, Breitner JC, Craft S, et al. Cognitive function over time in the Alzheimer's Disease Anti-inflammatory Prevention Trial (ADAPT): results of a randomized, controlled trial of naproxen and celecoxib. *Archives of Neurology*. 2008;*65*:896–905.

Mastellos D, Germenis AE, & Lambris JD. Complement: An Inflammatory Pathway Fulfilling Multiple Roles at the Interface of Innate Immunity and Development. *Current Drug Targets—Inflammation & Allergy* 2005; *4*:125–127.

Matsuzaki K, Noguch T, Wakabayashi M, Ikeda K, Okada T, Ohashi Y, et al. Inhibitors of amyloid beta-protein aggregation mediated by GM1-containing raft-like membranes. *Biochim Biophys Acta.* 2007;*68*:122–130.

Mawuenyega KG, Sigurdson W, Ovod V, Munsell L, Kasten T, Morris JC, et al. Decreased clearance of CNS B amyloid in Alzheimers disease. *Science*.2010; *330*:1774.

Miralbell J, Sorianoa JJ, Spulberb G, et al. Structural brain changes and cognition in relation to markers of vascular dysfunction. *Neurobiology of Aging* 2012; *33*;1003.e9-17.

Neumann H, Kotter M, & Franklin RJM. Debris clearance by microglia: an essential link between degeneration and regeneration. *Brain* 2009;*132*:288–95.

Noble W, Garwood C, & Hanger DP. Minocycline as a potential therapeutic agent in neurodegenerative disorders characterised by protein misfolding. *Prion* 2009;*3*:78–83.

Noble JM, Manly JJ, Schupf N, Tang MX, Mayeux R, & Luchsinger JA. . Association of C-reactive protein with cognitive impairment. *Arch. Neurol.* 2010;*67*:87–92.

Nicoll JA, Wilkinson D, Holmes C, Steart P, Markham H, & Weller RO. Neuropathology of human Alzheimer disease after immunization with amyloid-beta peptide: a case report. *Nat Med.* 2003;*9*:448–452.

Owen JB, Sultana R, Aluise CD, Erickson MA, Price TO, Bu G, et al. Oxidative modification to LDL receptor-related protein 1 in hippocampus from subjects with Alzheimer disease: Implications for Aβ accumulation in AD brain. *Free Radical Biology and Medicine*2010;*49*:1798–1803.

Panza F, FrisardiV, Imbimbo BP, D'Onofrio G, Pietrarossa G, Seripa D, et al. Drug Evaluation Bapineuzumab: anti-β-amyloid monoclonal antibodies for the treatment of Alzheimer's disease'. *Immunotherapy* 2010;*2*:767–782.

Pasqualetti P, Bonomini C, Dal Forno G, Paulon L, Sinforiani E, Marra C, et al. A randomized controlled study on effects of ibuprofen on cognitive progression of Alzheimer's disease. *Aging Clinical and Experimental Research* 2009;*21*:102–110.

Pericak-Vance MA, Grubber J, Bailey LR, Hedges D, West S, Santoro L, et al. Identification of novel genes in late onset Alzheimers disease. *Experimental Gerontology* 2000;*359*:1343–1352.

Perry VH, Nicoll JA, & Holmes C. Microglia in neurodegenerative disease. *Nature Reviews Neurology.* 2010;6:193–201.

Poirier J. Apolipoprotein E and Alzheimer's disease. A role in amyloid catabolism. *Annals of the New York Academy of Sciences* 2000;*924*:81–90.

Puglielli L, Konopka G, Pack-Chung E, MacKenzie I, Laura A, Berezovska O, et al. Acyl-coenzyme A: cholesterol acyltransferase modulates the generation of the amyloid β-peptide. *Nature Cell Biology* 2001;3:905–912.

Rafnasson S, Deary I, Smith FB, Whiteman M, Rumley A, Lowe GD, et al. Cognitive decline and markers of inflammation and hemostasis: The Edinburgh Artery Study. *J The American Geriatrics Society* 2007;55:700–707.

Ravaglia G, Forti P, Maioli F, Arnone G, Pantieri G, Cocci C, et al. The clock-drawing test in elderly Italian community dwellers: associations with sociodemographic status and risk factors for vascular cognitive impairment. *Dementia and Geriatric Cognitive Disorders* 2003;16:287–295.

Ravaglia G, Forti P, Maioli F, Chiappelli M, Montesi F, Tumini E, et al. Blood inflammatory markers and risk of dementia: The Conselice Study of Brain Aging. *Neurobiology of Aging* 2007;28;1810–1820.

Reines SA, Block GA, Morris JC, et al. Rofecoxib: no effect on Alzheimer's disease in a 1-year, randomized, blinded, controlled study. *Neurology.* 2004;*62*:66–71.

Relkin NR, Szabo P, Adamiak B, Burgut T, Monthe C, Lent RW, et al. 18-Month study of intravenous immunoglobulin for treatment of mild Alzheimer disease. *Neurobiol Aging* 2009; *30*:1728–1736.

Roberts RO, Geda YE, Knopman DS, Boeve BF, Christianson TJ, Pankratz VS, et al. Association of C-Reactive Protein with mild cognitive impairment. *Alzheimers Dement.* 2009;5:398–405.

Roberts RO, Geda YE, Knopman DS, Cha RH, Boeve BF, Ivnik RJ, et al. Metabolic syndrome, inflammation, and nonamnestic mild cognitive impairment in older persons: a population-based study. *Alz Dis Assoc Disord* 2010;24:11–18.

Rock RB, Gekker G, Hu S, Sheng WS, Cheeran ML, James R, et al. Role of Microglia in Central Nervous System Infections. *Clinical Microbiology Reviews* 2004;17:942–964.

Rogers J, Kirby LC, Hempelman SR, Berry DL, McGee PL, Kaszniak AW, et al. Clinical trial of indomethacin in Alzheimer's disease. *Neurology* 1993;*43*:1609–1611.

Ryu JK, Franciosi S, Sattayaprasert P, Kim SU, & McLarnon JG. Minocycline inhibits neuronal death and glial activation induced by beta-amyloid peptide in rat hippocampus. *Glia* 2004;48:85–90.

Sainati S, Ingram D, Talwalker S, & Geis G. Results of a double-blind, randomized, placebo-controlled study of celecoxib in the treatment of progression of Alzheimer's disease. Presented at: The Sixth International Stockholm-Springfield Symposium of Advances in Alzheimer's Therapy; April 5-8, 2000; Stockholm, Sweden.

Scharf S, Mander A, Ugoni A, et al. A double-blind, placebo-controlled trial of diclofenac/misoprostol in Alzheimer's disease. *Neurology.* 1999;*53*:197–201.

Schenk D, Barbour R, Dunn W, et al. Immunization with amyloid-β attenuates Alzheimer-disease-like pathology in the PDAPP mouse. *Nature* 1999;*400*:173–177.

Schram MT, Euser SM, de Craen AJM, Witteman JC, Frolich M, Hofman A, et al. Systemic markers of inflammation and cognitive decline in old age. *J Am Geriatr Soc* 2007;55:708–716.

Schmidt R, Schmidt H, Curb JD, Masaki K, White LR, & Launer LJ. Early inflammation and dementia: a 25-year follow-up of the Honolulu-Asia Aging Study. *Ann. Neurol.* 2002;*52*:168–174.

Schuitemaker A, Dik MG, Veerhuis R, Scheltens P, Schoonenboom NS, Hack CE, et al. Inflammatory markers in AD and MCI patients with different biomarker profiles. *Neurobiol Aging.* 2009;*30*:1885–1889.

Silverman JM, Beeri MS, Schmeidler J, Rosendorff C, Angelo G, Mavris R, et al. C reactive protein and memory function suggest antagonistic pleiotropy in very old non demented subjects. *Age and Ageing* 2009;*38*:237–241.

Simka M. Blood brain barrier compromise with endothelial inflammation may lead to auto-immune loss of myelin during multiple sclerosis. *Current Neurovascular Research*, 2009, 6:1–8.

Sloane JA, Blitz D, Margolin Z, & Vartanian T. A clear and present danger: endogenous ligands of toll like receptors. *Neuromolecular Medicine* 2010;12:149–163.

Small DH, Klaver DW, & Foa L. Presenilins and the γ-secretase:still a complex problem. *Molecular Brain* 2010;3; Published online 2010 February 5. doi: 10.1186/1756-6606-3-7.

Small GW, Bookheimer SY, Thompson PM, et al. Current and future uses of neuroimaging for cognitively impaired patients. *Lancet Neurol* 2008;7:161–172.

Soininen H, West C, Robbins J, Niculescu L. Long-term efficacy and safety of celecoxib in Alzheimer's disease. Dement Geriatr Cogn Disord 2007; 23(1): 8–12.

Sparks DL, Kuo Yu-Min, Roher A, Martin T, & Lukas RJ. Alterations of Alzheimer's Disease in the Cholesterol-fed Rabbit, Including Vascular Inflammation: Preliminary Observations. *Annals of the New York Academy of Sciences* 2000;903: 335–4.

Stahel P, Morganti-Kossman MC, & Kossmann T. The role of the complement system in trau-matic brain injury. *Brain Research Reviews* 1998;27:243–256.

Stewart, WF, Kawas C, Corrada M, & Metter EJ. Risk of Alzheimer's disease and duration of NSAID use. *Neurology*1997; 48: 626–632.

Szekely CA, Thorne JE, Zandi PP, Ek M, Messias E, Breitner JC, et al. Nonsteroidal anti-infl ammatory drugs for the prevention of Alzheimer's disease: a systematic review. *Neuroepidemiology* 2004;23:159–169.

Szekely CA, Breitner JC, Fitzpatrick AL, Rea TD, Psaty BM, Kuller LH, et al. NSAID use and de-mentia risk in the Cardiovascular Health Study: role of APOE and NSAID type. *Neurology* 2008;70:17–24.

Tabet N. Acetylcholinesterase inhibitors for Alzheimer's disease: anti-inflammatories in acetyl-choline clothing. *Age Ageing* 2006;35:336–338.

Teunissen CE, van Boxtel MPJ, Bosma H, Bosmans E, Delanghe J, De Bru C, et al. Inflammation markers in relation to cognition in a healthy aging population. *Journal of Neuroimmunology* 2003;134 :142–150.

Thal LJ, Ferris SH, Kirby L, et al. A randomized, double-blind, study of rofecoxib in patients with mild cognitive impairment. *Neuropsychopharmacology*. 2005; 30:1204–1215.

Trollor JN, Smith E, Baune BT, Kochan NA, Campbel L, Samaras K, et al. Systemic inflam-mation is associated with MCI and its subtypes: the Sydney Memory and Aging Study. *Dementia and Geriatric Cognitive Disorders*. 2010;30:569–578.

Van Beek J, Elward K, & Gasque P. Activation of complement in the central nervous system: roles in neurodegeneration and neuroprotection. *Annals of the New York Academy of Sciences*. 2003; 992:56–71.

Van den Kommer TN, Dik MG, Comijs HC, Jonker C, & Deeg D. The role of lipoproteins and inflammation in cognitive decline: Do they interact? *Neurobiology of Aging* 2010; http://dx.doi.org/10.1016/j.neurobiolaging.2010.05.024.

Van Gool WA, Weinstein HC, Scheltens P, Walstra GJ. Effect of hydroxychloroquine on progres-sion of dementia in early Alzheimer's disease: an 18-month randomised, double-blind, placebo-controlled study. Lancet 2001; 358(9280): 455–460.

van Oijen M, Witteman JC, Hofman A, Koudstaal PJ, & Breteler MM. Fibrinogen is as-sociated with an increased risk of Alzheimer disease and vascular dementia. *Stroke*. 2005;36:2637–2641.

Varvel NH, Bhaska K, Kounnas MZ, Wagner SL, Yang Yan T, Lamb BT, et al. NSAIDs prevent, but do not reverse, neuronal cell cycle reentry in a mouse model of Alzheimer disease *Journal of Clinical Investigation* 2009;119:3692–3702.

Vlad SC, Miller DR, Kowall NW, et al. Protective effects of NSAIDs on the development of Alzheimer disease. *Neurology* 2008;70:1672–1677.

Walter L & Neumann H. Role of microglia in neuronal degeneration and regeneration. *Seminars in Immunopathology* 2009;31:513–525.

Wang DS, Dickson DW, & Malter JS. β-Amyloid Degradation and Alzheimer's Disease. *Journal of Biomedicine and Biotechnology* 2006;58:406.

Weuve J, Ridker PM, Cook NR, Buring JE, & Grodstein F. High-sensitivity C-reactive protein and cognitive function in older women. *Epidemiology* 2006;17:183–189.

Wilcock GK, Black SE, Hendrix SB, Zavitz KH, Swabb EA, Laughlin MA; Tarenflurbil Phase II Study Investigators. Efficacy and safety of tarenflurbil in mild to moderate Alzheimer's disease: a randomised phase II trial. *Lance Neurol* 2008; 7(6): 483–493.

Weaver JD, Huang M-H, Albert M, et al. Interleukin-6 and risk of cognitive decline. MacArthur Studies of Successful Aging. *Neurology* 2002;59:371–378.

Wilcock GK, Black SE, Balch AH, Amato DA, Beelen AP, Schneider L S, et al. Safety and efficacy of tarenflurbil in subjects with mild Alzheimer's disease: results from an 18-month international multi-center Phase 3 trial. *Alzheimers and Dementia.* 2009;5(Suppl. 1), P86 (Abstract O1-04-07).

Wisniewski T & Konietzko U. Amyloid-β immunisation for Alzheimer's disease. *Lancet Neurol.* 2008;7:805–811.

Xue Qing-Shan, Sparks DL, & Streit WJ. Microglial activation in the hippocampus of hyper-cholesterolemic rabbits occurs independent of increased amyloid production. *Journal of Neuroinflammation* 2007;4:20.

Yaffe K, Lindquist K, Penninx BW, Simonsick EM, Pahor M, Kritchevsky S, et al.Inflammatory markers and cognition in well-functioning African-American and white elders. *Neurology* 2003;61:76–80.

Yaffe KA, Kanaya K, Lindquist K, Simonsick EM, Harris T, Shorr RI, et al. The metabolic syndrome, inflammation, and risk of cognitive decline. *JAMA* 2004;292:2237–2242.

Yip AG, Green RC, Huyck M, Cupples LA, & Farrer LA. MIRAGE Study Group. Nonsteroidal anti-inflammatory drug use and Alzheimer's disease risk: the MIRAGE Study. *BMC Geriatr.* 2005;5:2.

Zandi PP, Anthony JC, Hayden KM, Mehta K, Mayer L, & Breitner JC. Reduced incidence of AD with NSAID but not H2 receptor antagonists: the Cache County Study. *Neurology* 2002;59:880–886.

Zlokovic B. The blood brain barrier in health and chronic neurodegenerative disorders. *Neuron* 2008;57:178–201.

12

HIV Infection and Aging: An Emerging Chronic Medical Illness

LAUREN WENDELKEN, MS AND VICTOR VALCOUR, MD

Introduction and Demographics

In the spectrum of chronic diseases, Human Immunodeficiency Virus (HIV) is a relative newcomer. The first case of Acquired Immune Deficiency Syndrome (AIDS), which results from infection with HIV, was described in 1981 (Gottlieb, 1981; Quagliarello, 1982). At the time, there were no known treatments for the disease, and infection with HIV led to the development of AIDS within 3 to 5 years as a result of immune suppression and opportunistic infection. The U.S. government quickly recognized the threat of a viral epidemic and invested millions of dollars in research, which led to introduction of the first antiretroviral treatment (ART) in 1986: azidothymidine, or AZT.

Treatment with AZT greatly reduced the mortality of AIDS (Richman et al., 1987; Stambuk et al., 1989). However, not all patients responded to the treatment. Single drug therapy did not halt disease progression, and roughly one-fourth to one-third of patients developed anemia resulting from AZT toxicity in bone marrow. New advances ensued, leading to four principle classes of antiretroviral medications, which, when used together, can suppress the virus to undetectable levels in blood.

Today, it is estimated that more than 1 million individuals in the United States are living with a diagnosis of HIV (Lansky et al., 2010). Most are treated with a combination therapy of three medications, termed highly active antiretroviral therapy (HAART). In the years since the advent of HAART, the population has shifted from a predominantly young demographic (91% younger than 45 years old in 1996) to an older, aging population, with approximately one-half of HIV-infected individuals currently older than age 45 years (Fig. 12.1). It is estimated that by 2015, half of all people living with HIV/AIDS will be older than age 50 years (Stoff et al., 2004). Although the majority of older cases have aged with

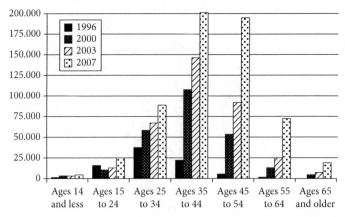

Figure 12.1 Shifting demographics of the HIV population. Reproduced with kind permission from Springer Science+Business Media B.V.

HIV, a growing proportion of new HIV infections occur in older adults who tend to lack sufficient information on safe sexual practices (Zablotsky & Kennedy, 2003; Waysdorf, 2002). In 2005, 15% of reported new infections occurred in individuals older than age 50 years (CDC, 2009).

Thus, over the last three decades, HIV has evolved from a relatively rapid terminal disease to a long-term chronic illness affecting greater numbers of older individuals. Even with large reductions in the rate of mortality and improved health outcomes, a significant portion of the HIV+ population continues to suffer from HIV-associated neurocognitive disorders (HAND). Researchers estimate the HAART-era prevalence of HAND at 50% (Heaton et al., 2010; Woods et al., 2009). In the United States, the current trend toward growing numbers of aged HIV patients has led to concern for increased risk for development of age-related neurodegenerative diseases, principally Alzheimer's disease (AD), as well as concern for the effects of comorbid cerebrovascular disease, leading to new focused resources devoted to addressing these important issues.

HIV Pathology and Central Nervous System Infection

HIV enters the body most often through sexual contact or needle sharing among IV drug users, and without proper HAART treatment, HIV can be passed from a mother to her infant at birth, termed vertical transmission. Although current HAART therapies have reduced the vertical transmission rates to less than 2% in the United States, more than 2.5 million children worldwide are now living with HIV as a chronic illness (UNAIDS, 2010), and many of these children are growing into young adulthood with cognitive and behavioral symptoms (Hazra et al., 2010).

The HIV virus targets cells expressing the cell surface protein CD4, which is found in T cells, monocytes, macrophages, and dendritic cells. The HIV envelope protein gp120 binds the extracellular portion of CD4, which allows subsequent interaction with a cell surface co-receptor, preferably CCR5 or CXCR4, which in turn allows the viral particle to invade the CD4+ cell (*see* Ellis et al., 2007, for review).

Infection of CD4+ T cells results in cellular activation, HIV viral replication, and subsequent cell death, leading to massive and precipitous drops in total body CD4+ cells, particularly in gut-associated lymphoid tissue, and a more gradual decline of CD4+ lymphocytes in plasma. The depletion of CD4+ cells leads to immunodeficiency and susceptibility to opportunistic infection. Normal CD4+ levels are greater than 500 cells/μL, and current guidelines call for initiation of ART when CD4+ levels drop below 350 cells/μL; although current trends suggest initiation may move to a higher threshold (OARAC, 2011). AIDS is diagnosed when CD4+ counts drop below 200 cells/μL, or if an opportunistic infection occurs (CDC, 2008).

HIV has been shown to cross the blood–brain barrier (BBB) and enter the central nervous system (CNS) as early as 8 days after infection (Ellis et al., 2007; Gonzalez-Scarano & Martin-Garcia, 2005; Valcour et al., 2012). The most likely explanation for this crossing is the Trojan horse hypothesis, whereby infected monocytes cross the BBB and differentiate to become perivascular macrophages (Fig. 12.2). Infected macrophages have been shown to modify the permeability of the BBB via secreted proteins that induce upregulation of adhesion molecules in the endothelial cells lining CNS vasculature (Gonzalez-Scarano & Martin-Garcia, 2005). This results in increased trafficking of monocytes across the BBB, thereby amplifying infection in the CNS. Lacking the CD4 receptor, neurons are not a direct target of HIV infection.

Infection of the CNS can result in encephalitis, the neuropathological fingerprint of brain inflammation (Ellis et al., 2007; Gonzalez-Scarano & Martin-Garcia, 2005). HIV encephalitis (HIVE) is characterized by perivascular accumulation of macrophages, the presence of multinucleated giant cells, and white matter thinning (Fischer-Smith et al., 2004). Studies prior to HAART suggested that inflammation in the CNS correlated more strongly with cognitive impairment and dementia than did the presence of virus (McArthur et al., 2003). Histological indicators of HIVE have been noted throughout the brain, with greater involvement of the basal ganglia and central white matter, and to a lesser extent the neocortical grey matter, brain stem, and cerebellum (Anthony & Bell, 2008). However, it is important to note that HIVE does not appear to be the pathological correlate of HAND in patients treated with HAART (Everall et al., 2009).

There have been few neuropathological studies in the HAART era, such that the neuropathology of HAND in the absence of frank HIVE has not been well characterized, although imaging studies have shown a correlation between white

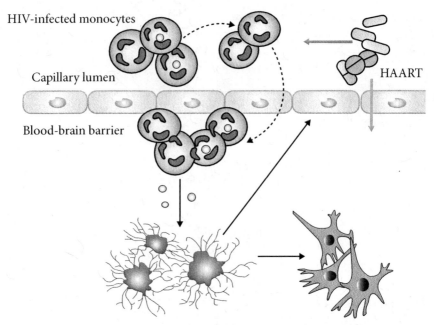

Figure 12.2 HIV likely enters the brain via infected immune cells. Antiretroviral medications have mixed ability to penetrate and be effective in cerebrospinal fluid and likely in brain tissue. Permission granted/ Curr HIV/AIDS Rep. 2011;8(1):54–61. Pathogenesis of HIV in the central nervous system. Valcour V, Sithinamsuwan P, Letendre S, Ances B.

matter loss and cognitive decline in HIV (Ragin et al., 2004; Thompson et al., 2006). Cerebral atrophy has been linked to lower CD4+ levels and higher viral loads, indicating an interaction with immune health (Thompson et al., 2005; Cardenas et al., 2009). Neuroimaging has confirmed early pathological findings of greater involvement of deep grey structures and white matter, with atrophy in AIDS patients more pronounced in the basal ganglia and cortical white matter (Chiang et al., 2007). Other studies have revealed generalized CNS atrophy, which increases with age and persists despite HAART (Cardenas et al., 2009).

The Clinical Presentation of HIV-Associated Neurocognitive Disorders

HIV-associated neurocognitive diagnoses were redefined in 2007 and range from asymptomatic neurocognitive impairment (ANI) to mild neurocognitive disorder (MND), to HIV-associated dementia (HAD) (Table 12.1) (Antinori et al., 2007). Asymptomatic neurocognitive impairment (ANI) is diagnosed in individuals who show impairment in two domains by cognitive testing but do not

Table 12.1 **Diagnostic Criteria for HAND**

Diagnosis	Criteria
Asymptomatic cognitive impairment (ANI)	Impairment in at least two cognitive domains by NP testing (<1 SD); no functional impairment
Mild neurocognitie disorder (MND)	Impairment in at least two cognitive domains by NP testing (<1 SD); mild interference with daily functioning
HIV-associated dementia (HAD)	Severe impairment in at least two domains by NP testing (<2 SD); marked impact on daily functioning

report any difficulties in accomplishing daily functional activities. Individuals with MND show impairment in at least two domains by cognitive testing and struggle with activities of daily living, typically mildly, whereas those with HAD demonstrate severe impairment in two or more domains by cognitive testing and report a marked impact on their ability to perform daily activities (*see* Foley et al., 2008, for review).

Patients with HAND may report that they have trouble completing tasks that involve a series of steps, or they may be more easily distracted. They may also report problems with balance and motor coordination and often evidence difficulty with learning, such as memorizing lists of words (Ances & Ellis, 2007). Early signs of CNS involvement are mental slowing with impaired retrieval of information, gait disturbances with reports of falling or tripping, decreased manual dexterity, and general signs of apathy or depression (McArthur et al., 2003). In cognitive testing, HAND generally manifests as psychomotor slowing, problems with attention and concentration, executive dysfunction, and impairment of working memory, with sparing of semantic and visuospatial abilities (Ances & Ellis, 2007; Cysique et al., 2006).

A few studies have been conducted to determine whether the profile of cognitive impairment in HIV has changed with the advent of HAART. Heaton et al. (2011) conducted an analysis of NP performance of HIV patients in the HAART versus pre-HAART era and discovered a decreasing prevalence of deficits in motor function, speed of information processing, and verbal fluency and increasing prevalence of deficits in the domains of learning and executive functioning in the HAART era. Since the introduction of HAART therapy, several groups have reported a reduction in the overall incidence of the most severe form of cognitive impairment, HAD. In the Multi-Center AIDS Cohort Study (MACS), researchers observed a 50% reduction in HAD incidence between 1990 and 1998, from 21.1% in 1990 to 10.5% in 1998 (Sacktor et al., 2001). In the

HAART-era CHARTER study, researchers reported HAD in only 2% of their cohort, but 44% demonstrated milder forms of cognitive impairment (Heaton et al., 2010). This group ultimately concluded that the rate of all-form cognitive impairment remains unchanged since before the use of antiretroviral medications, a sobering finding that suggests current approaches inadequately protect against brain injury (Heaton et al., 2011). Critically, the CHARTER study noted that most impaired subjects did not endorse symptoms and were thus designated to have ANI.

It is important to note that in contrast to most dementia syndromes, HAND is not a linearly progressive disorder. The NEAD Cohort, for example, reported both progression to dementia and recovery from demented to non-demented status in similar proportions of the patient population over a 6-month period (McArthur et al., 2003). Similarly, the Hawaii Aging with HIV Cohort noted a bidirectional change in cognitive diagnoses over a period of 12 months (Antinori et al., 2007). Although cognitive impairments have been shown to improve with a reduction in viral load (Sacktor et al., 2003; Cysique & Brew, 2009), one study reported a 53% probability of persistent cognitive deficits over a 3-year period, despite HAART treatment (Tozzi et al., 2007). This group found that both lower education and greater baseline impairment were associated with persistent deficits.

Depression is notably prevalent in the HIV population, with infected individuals being two to seven times more likely to meet the criteria for depression than non-infected individuals (Hinkin et al., 2001). Depression has been implicated in increased risk for progression to AIDS, declines in CD4 count, and increased mortality (Baldewicz et al., 2004). Apathy, which manifests as a reduction in general activity and goal-directed behavior, is also commonly reported in HIV patients. In a study conducted by Tate et al. (2003), researchers reported 80% prevalence of depression and 26% prevalence of apathy in their cohort. Apathy is correlated with smaller nucleus accumbens volumes (Paul et al., 2005) and reductions in white matter integrity in the corpus callosum (Hoare et al., 2010). It is essential to understand that behavioral disturbances (i.e., apathy and depression) may be part of the disease and may be exacerbated by chronic illness or social isolation. However, depression has also been associated with over-reporting of symptoms, thus mood disturbances must be taken into account when assessing the likelihood of cognitive impairment (Thames et al., 2011).

Although the frequency of cognitive impairment has not changed with the advent of HAART, severe disease (HAD) is relatively rare. Nevertheless, functional consequences may occur even in cases of milder impairment. Patients with HAND tend to have trouble with prospective memory that is, remembering to execute a task (Woods et al., 2009). This deficit can have serious implications for both everyday life (employment, bill management, etc.) and medical management. Lack of adherence to medication therapies has been linked to cognitive impairment. In one cohort of HAART-treated individuals with pre-dominantly mild to moderate impairment, impaired individuals were twice as likely to exhibit low adherence compared to unimpaired individuals, and more complex regimens were associated with lower adherence in the impaired group (Hinkin et al., 2002). The link between adherence and HAND creates a feedback loop wherein poor adherence and cognitive impairment are mutually exacer-bated. Unlike other diseases that are resilient to small errors in adherence, in HIV even small oversights can have tremendous impact on viral resistance and ultimate medication failure.

Deficits in attention, speed of information processing, and motor slow-ing can have a variety of functional consequences, including interfering with driving ability. Marcotte et al. (1999) directly investigated this issue using a computer-based driving simulator. Using number of accidents as the outcome measure, they showed that mildly to moderately impaired HIV+ patients failed the simulation at a much higher rate than a group of cognitively normal HIV+ controls. Another group used attentional performance to classify the risk status of a group of HIV+ individuals and found that 93% of those considered high risk also reported a recent history of automobile accidents (Marcotte et al., 2006).

Diagnostic criteria for HAND rely on identifying disturbances in perfor-mance of functional activities, which can be difficult to accurately assess in HIV patients. Relying on self-report or even subjective proxy reporting may have major limitations in HIV populations as in others where insight is affected. In our experience, HIV patients often offer proxy informants who have less reliable information resulting from lack of social or physical proximity, and patients may lack insight into their own impairment or harbor fears of the stigma associated with an additional diagnosis. Further, there is a trend toward underemployment in the HIV population because of physical morbidity, resulting in a floor effect that presents challenges to assessing real-world daily functioning. As a conse-quence, the reported rates of ANI may be overestimates.

Mechanisms of Central Nervous System Injury in the Setting of Highly Active Antiretroviral Therapy

The leading hypotheses for continued brain vulnerability in the setting of HAART relate to an inability to fully suppress inflammation. Although neurons are not directly infected by HIV, CNS inflammation, microglial dysregulation, and pro-ductive viral infection may result in cognitive deficits. The loss of staining for pre- and post-synaptic markers on autopsy in the striatum and hippocampus, indicative of synaptodendritic loss or injury, has been correlated with cognitive impairment in HIV (Ellis et al., 2007; Moore et al., 2006). Chronic or repetitive cycles of low-grade inflammation may be responsible for the synaptodendritic disruption observed.

Another emerging explanation for continued inflammation rests on latent CNS infection or low-level seeding by peripheral monocytes and possibly low-levels of viral replication. HIV has been shown to infect astrocytes—glial cells that express CD4 and CXCR4—although there is no in vivo evidence that this infection produces new virions (Wiley, 1986; Hult et al., 2008). Although highly productive viral infection (i.e., viral replication and release of new HIV virions) in the CNS is unlikely (Hult et al., 2008), lower level infection may result in mild inflammation and cognitive disturbance.

Antiretroviral regimens with greater CNS penetrance have been hypothesized to impart better clinical outcomes. A CNS penetration-effectiveness (CPE) ranking system based on antiretroviral properties has been developed to provide an estimate of anticipated overall effectiveness of a medication in the cerebrospinal fluid (CSF) as a surrogate for the brain. However, researchers have investigated this possibility with contradictory outcomes. There have been fairly consistent data demonstrating the predictive impact of this score on CSF levels of HIV RNA in a small subset of individuals who do not fully suppress CSF virus despite suppression in plasma. One study demonstrated a correlation between CPE score and global improvement in NP performance in patients who were impaired at baseline, but in a different study of patients who were not impaired, they saw improvement only in fine motor functioning (Tozzi et al., 2009). In contrast, a pivotal randomized study designed to investigate this issue and conducted with the AIDS Clinical Trials Group demonstrated paradoxical NP improvement in patients who began drug regimens with lower rather than higher CPE-ranking (Marra et al., 2009). The CHARTER cohort also failed to demonstrate a positive correlation between CPE rank and cognitive functioning in their baseline cross-sectional analyses (Heaton et al., 2010), raising important questions about the utility of this ranking system to direct treatment in subjects doing well on HAART. Given the central role of monocytes in CNS disease, others have started to consider the potential CNS impact of drugs that efficiently target HIV in monocytes (Valcour et al., 2010). This target is particularly challenging because monocytes may emerge from the bone marrow with infection and may remain quiescent, making them a difficult target for viral eradication by current antiretroviral medications.

A number of clinical factors have been linked to the development of HAND. For example, researchers have found a correlation between severity of HIV and cognitive status (Hardy et al., 1999) and between viral load in plasma and CSF and performance on neuropsychological testing (Becker et al., 2004; Cherner et al., 2004). In both the Northeastern AIDS Dementia (NEAD) Cohort and the AIDS Clinical Trials Group ALLRT cohort, researchers reported a 30% prevalence of cognitive impairment in individuals with CD4 counts below 200 cells/μL (McArthur et al., 2003). These data confirm that in the era of HAART, current immunological status remains important, as does control of HIV in plasma. In several cohorts, including the ALLRT cohort, researchers reported a strong correlation between a lifetime CD4 nadir of less than 200 cells/μL and HAND development (Robertson et al., 2007). In general, CD4 nadir count has proved to be a better marker of impairment than has duration of infection. This should not be surprising, as individuals who were infected with HIV in the late 1970s and early 1980s who are still alive today are likely to have important survival tendencies that may protect from CNS disease, rendering a simple measure of duration of disease less meaningful in this population.

Other comorbid conditions must also be considered. Many HIV patients are co-infected with Hepatitis C, a virus that has been shown to enter the CNS. Hepatitis C can cause neurotoxicity and has been correlated with deficits in cognitive performance (Hult et al., 2008). Syphilis is often identified in HIV patients and can impact the CNS with negative cognitive consequences (Marra, 2004). Further, illicit drug use is prevalent among the general HIV population, with a variety of potential deleterious effects. HIV+ drug users are more likely to demonstrate poor medication adherence, leading to periods of poorly controlled infection (McArthur et al., 2003). In addition, drug users face additional CNS complications that may exacerbate HIV-related neuropathology (Hult et al., 2008).

Medications used in HAART therapies have a variety of side effects, including increased risk for cardiovascular disease and metabolic disturbances such as insulin resistance, and one drug in particular—efavirenz—is directly associated with clinical CNS effects (Volberding & Deeks, 2010). Thus, medications used to control the HIV virus may themselves have deleterious direct or secondary effects on cognition. In fact, one study reported cognitive improvement in stable HIV patients who interrupted ART treatment for up to 96 weeks, providing suggestive evidence for a possible negative impact of antiretroviral therapy on cognitive functioning (Robertson et al., 2010). Despite this one finding, there is universal agreement that cognitive impairment in HIV should be treated with HAART. Medications used to treat numerous comorbid illnesses in HIV similarly carry the propensity for cognitive effects, particularly medications used to treat pain associated with illnesses such as HIV-associated neuropathy.

Screening for HIV-Associated Neurocognitive Disorders in the Clinic

Although lengthy neuropsychological testing may provide the most accurate diagnostic information, exams that can be administered in the clinical setting are vital. These should include assessment of mood and behavior as well as thorough neurological examination. There has been some debate over the best screening measures to use in clinical settings and, to date, there are no universally accepted approaches. Because HAND has been shown to have a frontal-subcortical profile (Heaton et al., 1995), tests such as the Mini-Mental State Examination (MMSE), designed to detect more "classic" cortical dementias, are not particularly sensitive to HAND. A group of researchers developed the 5-minute HIV Dementia Scale (HDS), which identified HAD with 84% sensitivity (Power et al., 1995). However, the HDS showed poor sensitivity to milder forms of cognitive impairment, thus rendering it unhelpful for detecting ANI or MND-type impairment (Skinner et al., 2009). Limited data show promise for the Montreal Cognitive Assessment test (MoCA), which requires approximately 10 minutes to administer and thus may prove to be a useful screening tool in the clinical setting (Koski et al., 2011).

Carey et al. (2004) attempted to determine which tests within a neuropsychological battery were most sensitive to HAND and found that the Hopkins Verbal Learning Test-Revised (HVLT-R) Total Recall, the Grooved Pegboard Test nondominant hand, and the Weschler Adult Intelligence Scale (WAIS-III) Digit Symbol subtest showed the greatest sensitivity to HIV+ cognitively impaired individuals. These tests tap domains of verbal learning and memory (HVLT-R), motor function (Grooved Pegboard), and speed of information processing (WAIS-III Digit Symbol). Unfortunately, these tests are too long to administer in clinical settings as screening tools. Researchers also rely on the Trail Making Test part B to assess psychomotor slowing in HAND, and in the research setting such tests have been used to detect change with intervention.

Cognitive Impact of Aging With HIV

Older adults with HIV are at an increased risk for developing cognitive impairment. During the pre-HAART era, several epidemiological studies identified age as a robust risk factor for HAND (Janssen et al., 1992; Chiesi et al., 1996). Investigations of HAART-era patterns of impairment have remarked on similarities between cognitive deficits seen in HAND and those observed in typical aging, such as deficits in attention, concentration, learning, memory, psychomotor ability, and speed of processing (Hardy & Vance, 2009). This led researchers to hypothesize a synergistic risk for cognitive impairment with HIV status and increasing age; although this has not been universally observed (Valcour et al., 2011; Cysique et al., 2011).

Some research suggests enhanced cognitive vulnerability in the older HIV population. For example, researchers at the HIV Neurobehavioral Research Center (HNRC) reported an interaction between age and CSF HIV levels, where older individuals with detectable CSF HIV RNA had twice the rate of impairment than their older counterparts with undetectable CSF HIV RNA, whereas this relationship was absent in the younger cohort (Cherner et al., 2004). In addition, they found that 76% of older patients not receiving HAART compared to 57% of older patients on HAART met impairment criteria, whereas the rates in younger patients were unaffected by HAART status (54% vs. 52%). Further, in the Hawaii Aging with HIV cohort, cognitive vulnerability associated with having at least one apolipoprotein ε4 allele was identified in older, but not younger, adults (Valcour et al., 2004). Several groups have noted delayed diagnosis in newly infected older adults, which allows a longer window of opportunity for the virus to cause early CNS damage (Castilla et al., 2002; Ferro & Salit, 1992; Mugavero et al., 2007; Nogueras et al., 2006).

In studies with HIV cohorts older than age 50 years, researchers have found that older groups perform worse on neuropsychological measures than younger subjects, and that HIV+ subjects perform worse than age-matched HIV-negative controls (Becker et al., 2004; Cherner et al., 2004). In the Hawaii Aging with HIV cohort, increasing age was shown to be a robust risk factor for cognitive impairment, with 44.7% of the older group compared to 26.3% of the younger group qualifying for a diagnosis of MND (Valcour et al., 2004). One fMRI study investigated the link between age and brain function and found that both increasing age and HIV were correlated with decreased cerebral blood flow (Ances et al., 2010).

Comorbid illnesses such as cardiovascular disease, cerebrovascular disease, and metabolic dysfunction (i.e., high cholesterol and diabetes) may also affect cognitive functioning and are more likely to be present in older individuals (Becker et al., 2009). Clinical epidemiological data support the argument for increased risk of cardiovascular disease in HIV, with researchers reporting an increased risk for stroke in AIDS patients (Cole et al., 2004) and a significant rise in HIV patients hospitalized for stroke between 1997 and 2006 (Ovbiagele & Nath, 2011). Older HAD patients are also more likely to have comorbid diabetes mellitus than their non-HAD counterparts (Valcour et al. 2005), and this may affect cognition.

Older adults tend to have a longer overall duration of infection and exposure to antiretroviral medications, two potentially confounding or contributing conditions (Cherner et al., 2004; Valcour et al., 2004). Older patients are also more likely to have been exposed to more toxic or higher doses of antiretroviral medications used in the 1990s, such as AZT, which was shown to cross over the BBB (Yarchoan & Broder, 1987). In addition, protective factors may exist, as many older individuals survived the era prior to HAART; they may harbor survivorship tendencies whereby unrecognized host or viral factors contribute to long-term survival. The issue of survivorship in the older HIV population may be a cohort phenomenon not present in the aging populations that will emerge over the next decade, who will be more likely to have received less toxic therapies in the early years of their disease. Thus, mild vulnerabilities currently observed in older HIV+ patients may become more pronounced in future cohorts, as the older HIV population shifts to an entirely post-HAART demographic.

Further, there is significant concern that even in the absence of HAND, the inflammatory processes implicated in HIV CNS pathology might lead to increased vulnerability to other age-related dementias such as AD (Alisky, 2007; Anthony et al., 2006). In AD, the hallmark pathological correlates are extracellular neuritic plaques primarily composed of amyloid-β, a metabolite of amyloid precursor protein (APP), and intracellular neurofibrillary tangles, composed of hyperphosphory-lated tau protein. Researchers have pointed to reports of increased APP expression in HIV brains as evidence for a potential interaction with AD pathology (Green et al., 2005, Alisky, 2007) and as a possible indication of increased susceptibility to early onset AD. Anthony et al. (2006) presented evidence for increased tau deposition in HAART-treated HIV patients relative to age-matched controls, although they reported no correlation between tau levels and cognitive status.

However, as yet there is no clear evidence for a neuropathological link between HIV and AD, and no evidence of higher rates of early onset AD in the HIV population. It is likely that current published reports contain insufficient numbers of sufficiently old HIV patients in the range where AD would be common enough to detect increased rates. As the HIV population advances over the ages of 60 years and 70 years, there will be a greater potential to test for a possible increased risk, and it will become increasingly important to monitor older HIV individuals for not only HAND development but also AD.

Treatment Options and Moving Forward

The HIV population is incredibly heterogeneous and becoming even more so. In particular, the older HIV+ populations is composed of various subpopulations, including those who survived the pre-HAART era, those who have always had access to HAART treatment, and those infected later in life who often lack sufficient awareness to seek early treatment. Further, only about half are likely to develop HIV-related cognitive impairment. Comorbidities are frequent and commonly contribute to cognitive impairment (Heaton et al., 2010).

HIV-specific treatment strategies have been disappointing in terms of their ability to effectively treat HAND. Highly active antiretroviral therapy is universally accepted as the cornerstone of treatment, and methods to maximize medication adherence and viral suppression are critical. Although limited data support use of antiretroviral therapies with better CPE in focused settings, particularly in HAART-naïve subjects with HAND or in rare cases of new onset subacute impairment in treated individuals often associated with detectable virus in CSF despite suppression in plasma ("CNS escape"), the data do not provide sufficient evidence to support a universal approach in patients currently doing well on HAART or in those who report an insidious cognitive syndrome present over a period of years. Future research may present evidence for monocyte-directed strategies.

Although older HIV patients may face an increased risk for neurodegenerative disorders, there are currently no treatment trials using cholinesterase inhibitors or other AD drugs in HIV. The use of the NMDA-receptor antagonist memantine in HIV patients has had generally disappointing results (Zhao et al., 2010).

In the absence of highly effective interventional studies, empiric approaches must be considered. The overall benefits of physical exercise, which has received much attention in preventative efforts for AD (Yaffe, 2010), and management of cerebrovascular risk factors must be considered, even if not clinically proven in the setting of HIV. Patients who engage in illicit drug use are more vulnerable to cognitive decline, and interventions targeted at stopping or reducing these behaviors could prove beneficial. In addition, medication adherence must be emphasized and intervention strategies must be considered in those individuals who struggle with adherence. Cognitive and social engagement coupled with approaches aimed at minimizing depression is also likely to be important.

It remains critical to assess for treatable conditions including vitamin deficiencies, thyroid function abnormalities, and liver disease, as well as infections that may pose additional risks to the CNS, particularly hepatitis C and syphilis. Centers with expertise in neuroAIDS can provide added support for clinicians who encounter atypical cases, particularly more rapidly progressive cases or those with new-onset motor abnormalities, where in-depth investigations may be required. As older HIV patients face multiple risks for cognitive impairment in addition to HIV burden, it will become increasingly important to utilize testing strategies that are sensitive to HIV-specific cognitive impairment and that allow differential diagnoses that take into account various risk factors, including possible development of age-related neurodegenerative disorders.

The HIV epidemic in the United States has now entered its fourth decade. With a cure for disease remaining elusive, management of HIV as a chronic condition has emerged as the mainstay of care. Consideration for cognitive syndromes has become increasingly important, particularly as this population ages. Research is needed to fill major gaps in our existing knowledge of these HIV-related CNS disorders and may simultaneously inform underlying mechanisms for other cognitive disorders thought to be driven by a common theme of neuroinflammation.

References

(CDC), Centers for Disease Control and Prevention. (2008). Revised surveillance case definitions for HIV infection among adults, adolescents, and children aged <18months and for HIV infection and AIDS among children aged 18 months to <13 years. Department of Health and Human Services. Atlanta: Morbidity and Mortality Weekly Report.

(CDC), Centers for Disease Control and Prevention. (2009). HIV/AIDS Surveillance Report, 2007. Department of Health and Human Services. Atlanta.

(UNAIDS), Joint United Nations Programme on HIV/AIDS. (2010). Global Report: UNAIDS Report on the Global AIDS Epidemic 2010. United Nations. Geneva, Switzerland.

Alisky, J. M. (2007). The coming problem of HIV-associated Alzheimer's disease. *Med Hypotheses* 69 (5):1140–1143.

Ances, B. M., & R. J. Ellis. (2007). Dementia and neurocognitive disorders due to HIV-1 infection. *Semin Neurol* 27 (1):86–92.

Ances, B. M., F. Vaida, M. J. Yeh, C. L. Liang, R. B. Buxton, S. Letendre, et al. (2010). HIV infection and aging independently affect brain function as measured by functional magnetic resonance imaging. *J Infect Dis* 201 (3):336–340.

Anthony, I. C., & J. E. Bell. (2008). The Neuropathology of HIV/AIDS. *Int Rev Psychiatry* 20 (1):15–24.

Anthony, I. C., S. N. Ramage, F. W. Carnie, P. Simmonds, & J. E. Bell. (2006). Accelerated Tau deposition in the brains of individuals infected with human immunodeficiency virus-1 before and after the advent of highly active anti-retroviral therapy. *Acta Neuropathol* 111 (6):529–538.

Antinori, A., G. Arendt, J. T. Becker, B. J. Brew, D. A. Byrd, M. Cherner, et al. (2007). Updated research nosology for HIV-associated neurocognitive disorders. *Neurology* 69 (18):1789–1799.

Baldewicz, T. T., J. Leserman, S. G. Silva, J. M. Petitto, R. N. Golden, D. O. Perkins, et al. (2004). Changes in neuropsychological functioning with progression of HIV-1 infection: results of an 8-year longitudinal investigation. *AIDS Behav* 8 (3):345–355.

Becker, J. T., L. Kingsley, J. Mullen, B. Cohen, E. Martin, E. N. Miller, et al. (2009). Vascular risk factors, HIV serostatus, and cognitive dysfunction in gay and bisexual men. *Neurology* 73 (16):1292–1299.

Becker, J. T., O. L. Lopez, M. A. Dew, & H. J. Aizenstein. (2004). Prevalence of cognitive disorders differs as a function of age in HIV virus infection. *AIDS* 18 Suppl 1:S11–S18.

Cardenas, V. A., D. J. Meyerhoff, C. Studholme, J. Kornak, J. Rothlind, H. Lampiris, et al. (2009). Evidence for ongoing brain injury in human immunodeficiency virus-positive patients treated with antiretroviral therapy. *J Neurovirol* 15 (4):324–333.

Carey, C. L., S. P. Woods, J. D. Rippeth, R. Gonzalez, D. J. Moore, T. D. Marcotte, et al. (2004). Initial validation of a screening battery for the detection of HIV-associated cognitive impairment. *Clin Neuropsychol* 18 (2):234–248.

Castilla, J., P. Sobrino, L. De La Fuente, I. Noguer, L. Guerra, & F. Parras. (2002). Late diagnosis of HIV infection in the era of highly active antiretroviral therapy: consequences for AIDS incidence. *AIDS* 16 (14):1945–1951.

Cherner, M., R. J. Ellis, D. Lazzaretto, C. Young, M. R. Mindt, J. H. Atkinson, et al. (2004). Effects of HIV-1 infection and aging on neurobehavioral functioning: preliminary findings. *AIDS* 18 (Suppl 1):S27–S34.

Chiang, M. C., R. A. Dutton, K. M. Hayashi, O. L. Lopez, H. J. Aizenstein, A. W. Toga, et al. (2007). 3D pattern of brain atrophy in HIV/AIDS visualized using tensor-based morphometry. *Neuroimage* 34 (1):44–60.

Chiesi, A., S. Vella, L. G. Dally, C. Pedersen, S. Danner, A. M. Johnson, et al. (1996). Epidemiology of AIDS dementia complex in Europe. AIDS in Europe Study Group. *J Acquir Immune Defic Syndr Hum Retrovirol* 11 (1):39–44.

Cole, J. W., A. N. Pinto, J. R. Hebel, D. W. Buchholz, C. J. Earley, C. J. Johnson, et al. (2004). Acquired immunodeficiency syndrome and the risk of stroke. *Stroke* 35 (1):51–56.

Cysique, L. A., & B. J. Brew. (2009). Neuropsychological functioning and antiretroviral treatment in HIV/AIDS: a review. *Neuropsychol Rev* 19 (2):169–185.

Cysique, L. A., P. Maruff, & B. J. Brew. (2006). The neuropsychological profile of symptomatic AIDS and ADC patients in the pre-HAART era: a meta-analysis. *J Int Neuropsychol Soc* 12 (3):368–382.

Cysique L.A., P. Maruff, M.P. Bain, E. Wright, & B.J. Brew. (2011). HIV and age do not substantially interact in HIV-associated neurocognitive impairment. *J Neuropsychiatry Clin Neurosci* 23: 83–89.

Ellis, R., D. Langford, & E. Masliah. (2007). HIV and antiretroviral therapy in the brain: neuronal injury and repair. *Nat Rev Neurosci* 8 (1):33–44.

Everall, I., F. Vaida, N. Khanlou, D. Lazzaretto, C. Achim, S. Letendre, et al. (2009). Cliniconeuropathologic correlates of human immunodeficiency virus in the era of antiretroviral therapy. *J Neurovirol* 15 (5-6):360–370.

Ferro, S., & I. E. Salit. (1992). HIV infection in patients over 55 years of age. *J Acquir Immune Defic Syndr* 5 (4):348–353.

Fischer-Smith, T., S. Croul, A. Adeniyi, K. Rybicka, S. Morgello, K. Khalili, et al. (2004). Macrophage/microglial accumulation and proliferating cell nuclear antigen expression in the central nervous system in human immunodeficiency virus encephalopathy. *Am J Pathol* 164 (6):2089–2099.

Foley, J., M. Ettenhofer, M. Wright, & C. H. Hinkin. (2008). Emerging issues in the neuropsychology of HIV infection. *Curr HIV/AIDS Rep* 5 (4):204–211.

Gonzalez-Scarano, F., & J. Martin-Garcia. (2005). The neuropathogenesis of AIDS. *Nat Rev Immunol* 5 (1):69–81.

Gottlieb, M. S., R. Schroff, H. M. Schanker, J. D. Weisman, P. T. Fan, R. A. Wolf, et al. (1981). Pneumocystis carinii pneumonia and mucosal candidiasis in previously healthy homosexual men: evidence of a new acquired cellular immunodeficiency. *N Engl J Med* 305 (24):1425–1431.

Green, D. A., E. Masliah, H. V. Vinters, P. Beizai, D. J. Moore, & C. L. Achim. (2005). Brain deposition of beta-amyloid is a common pathologic feature in HIV positive patients. *AIDS* 19 (4):407–411.

Hardy, D., C. Hinkin, P. Satz, P. Stenquist, W. van Gorp, & L. Moore. (1999). Age Differences and Neurocognitive Performance in HIV-Infected Adults. *New Zealand Journal of Psychology* 28 (2):94–101.

Hardy, D. J., & D. E. Vance. (2009). The neuropsychology of HIV/AIDS in older adults. *Neuropsychol Rev* 19 (2):263–272.

Hazra, R., G. K. Siberry, & L. M. Mofenson. (2010). Growing up with HIV: children, adolescents, and young adults with perinatally acquired HIV infection. *Annu Rev Med* 61:169–185.

Heaton, R. K., D. B. Clifford, D. R. Franklin, Jr., S. P. Woods, C. Ake, F. Vaida, et al. (2010). HIV-associated neurocognitive disorders persist in the era of potent antiretroviral therapy: CHARTER Study. *Neurology* 75 (23):2087–2096.

Heaton, R. K., D. R. Franklin, R. J. Ellis, J. A. McCutchan, S. L. Letendre, S. Leblanc, et al. (2011). HIV-associated neurocognitive disorders before and during the era of combination antiretroviral therapy: differences in rates, nature, and predictors. *J Neurovirol* 17 (1):3–16.

Heaton, R. K., I. Grant, N. Butters, D. A. White, D. Kirson, J. H. Atkinson, et al. (1995). The HNRC 500—neuropsychology of HIV infection at different disease stages. HIV Neurobehavioral Research Center. *J Int Neuropsychol Soc* 1 (3):231–251.

Hinkin, C. H., S. A. Castellon, J. H. Atkinson, & K. Goodkin. (2001). Neuropsychiatric aspects of HIV infection among older adults. *J Clin Epidemiol* 54 (Suppl 1):S44–S52.

Hinkin, C. H., S. A. Castellon, R. S. Durvasula, D. J. Hardy, M. N. Lam, K. I. Mason, et al. (2002). Medication adherence among HIV+ adults: effects of cognitive dysfunction and regimen complexity. *Neurology* 59 (12):1944–1950.

Hoare, J., J. P. Fouche, B. Spottiswoode, J. A. Joska, R. Schoeman, D. J. Stein, et al. (2010). White matter correlates of apathy in HIV-positive subjects: a diffusion tensor imaging study. *J Neuropsychiatry Clin Neurosci* 22 (3):313–320.

Hult, B., G. Chana, E. Masliah, & I. Everall. (2008). Neurobiology of HIV. *Int Rev Psychiatry* 20 (1):3–13.

Janssen, R. S., O. C. Nwanyanwu, R. M. Selik, & J. K. Stehr-Green. (1992). Epidemiology of human immunodeficiency virus encephalopathy in the United States. *Neurology* 42 (8):1472–1476.

Koski, L., M. J. Brouillette, R. Lalonde, B. Hello, E. Wong, A. Tsuchida, et al. (2011). Computerized testing augments pencil-and-paper tasks in measuring HIV-associated mild cognitive impairment(*). *HIV Med* 12 (8):472–480.

Lansky, A., J. T. Brooks, E. DiNenno, J. Heffelfinger, H. I. Hall, & J. Mermin. (2010). Epidemiology of HIV in the United States. *J Acquir Immune Defic Syndr 55* (Suppl 2):S64–S68.

Marcotte, T. D., R. K. Heaton, T. Wolfson, M. J. Taylor, O. Alhassoon, K. Arfaa, et al. (1999). The impact of HIV-related neuropsychological dysfunction on driving behavior. The HNRC Group. *J Int Neuropsychol Soc 5* (7):579–592.

Marcotte, T. D., D. Lazzaretto, J. C. Scott, E. Roberts, S. P. Woods, & S. Letendre. (2006). Visual attention deficits are associated with driving accidents in cognitively-impaired HIV-infected individuals. *J Clin Exp Neuropsychol 28* (1):13–28.

Marra, C. M. (2004). Syphilis and human immunodeficiency virus: prevention and politics. *Arch Neurol 61* (10):1505–1508.

Marra, C. M., Y. Zhao, D. B. Clifford, S. Letendre, S. Evans, K. Henry, et al. (2009). Impact of combination antiretroviral therapy on cerebrospinal fluid HIV RNA and neurocognitive performance. *AIDS 23* (11):1359–1366.

McArthur, J. C., N. Haughey, S. Gartner, K. Conant, C. Pardo, A. Nath, et al. (2003). Human immunodeficiency virus-associated dementia: an evolving disease. *J Neurovirol 9* (2):205–221.

Moore, D. J., E. Masliah, J. D. Rippeth, R. Gonzalez, C. L. Carey, M. Cherner, et al. (2006). Cortical and subcortical neurodegeneration is associated with HIV neurocognitive impairment. *AIDS 20* (6):879–887.

Mugavero, M. J., C. Castellano, D. Edelman, & C. Hicks. (2007). Late diagnosis of HIV infection: the role of age and sex. *Am J Med 120* (4):370–373.

Nogueras, M., G. Navarro, E. Anton, M. Sala, M. Cervantes, M. Amengual, et al. (2006). Epidemiological and clinical features, response to HAART, and survival in HIV-infected patients diagnosed at the age of 50 or more. *BMC Infect Dis 6*:159.

Ovbiagele, B., & A. Nath. (2011). Increasing incidence of ischemic stroke in patients with HIV infection. *Neurology 76* (5):444–450.

Panel on Antiretroviral Guidelines for Adults and Adolescents, Office of AIDS Research Advisory Council (OARAC). (2011). Guidelines for the use of antiretroviral agents in HIV-1 infected adults and adolescents. edited by D. o. H. a. H. Services.

Paul, R. H., A. M. Brickman, B. Navia, C. Hinkin, P. F. Malloy, A. L. Jefferson, et al. (2005). Apathy is associated with volume of the nucleus accumbens in patients infected with HIV. *J Neuropsychiatry Clin Neurosci 17* (2):167–171.

Power, C., O. A. Selnes, J. A. Grim, & J. C. McArthur. (1995). HIV Dementia Scale: a rapid screening test. *J Acquir Immune Defic Syndr Hum Retrovirol 8* (3):273–278.

Quagliarello, V. (1982). The Acquired Immunodeficiency Syndrome: current status. *Yale J Biol Med 55* (5-6):443–452.

Ragin, A. B., P. Storey, B. A. Cohen, L. G. Epstein, & R. R. Edelman. (2004). Whole brain diffusion tensor imaging in HIV-associated cognitive impairment. *AJNR Am J Neuroradiol 25* (2):195–200.

Richman, D. D., M. A. Fischl, M. H. Grieco, M. S. Gottlieb, P. A. Volberding, O. L. Laskin, et al. (1987). The toxicity of azidothymidine (AZT) in the treatment of patients with AIDS and AIDS-related complex. A double-blind, placebo-controlled trial. *N Engl J Med 317* (4):192–197.

Robertson, K. R., M. Smurzynski, T. D. Parsons, K. Wu, R. J. Bosch, J. Wu, et al. (2007). The prevalence and incidence of neurocognitive impairment in the HAART era. *AIDS 21* (14):1915–1921.

Robertson, K. R., Z. Su, D. M. Margolis, A. Krambrink, D. V. Havlir, S. Evans, et al. (2010). Neurocognitive effects of treatment interruption in stable HIV-positive patients in an observational cohort. *Neurology 74* (16):1260–1266.

Sacktor, N., R. H. Lyles, R. Skolasky, C. Kleeberger, O. A. Selnes, E. N. Miller, et al. (2001). HIV-associated neurologic disease incidence changes:: Multicenter AIDS Cohort Study, 1990-1998. *Neurology 56* (2):257–260.

Sacktor, N., R. L. Skolasky, P. M. Tarwater, J. C. McArthur, O. A. Selnes, J. Becker, et al. (2003). Response to systemic HIV viral load suppression correlates with psychomotor speed performance. *Neurology 61* (4):567–569.

Skinner, S., A. J. Adewale, L. DeBlock, M. J. Gill, & C. Power. (2009). Neurocognitive screening tools in HIV/AIDS: comparative performance among patients exposed to antiretroviral therapy. *HIV Med 10* (4):246–252.

Stambuk, D., M. Youle, D. Hawkins, C. Farthing, D. Shanson, R. Farmer, et al. (1989). The efficacy and toxicity of azidothymidine (AZT) in the treatment of patients with AIDS and AIDS-related complex (ARC): an open uncontrolled treatment study. *Q J Med 70* (262):161–174.

Stoff, D. M., J. H. Khalsa, A. Monjan, & P. Portegies. (2004). Introduction: HIV/AIDS and Aging. *AIDS 18* Suppl 1:S1–S2.

Tate, D., R. H. Paul, T. P. Flanigan, K. Tashima, J. Nash, C. Adair, et al. (2003). The impact of apathy and depression on quality of life in patients infected with HIV. *AIDS Patient Care STDS 17* (3):115–120.

Thames, A. D., B. W. Becker, T. D. Marcotte, L. J. Hines, J. M. Foley, A. Ramezani, et al. (2011). Depression, cognition, and self-appraisal of functional abilities in HIV: an examination of subjective appraisal versus objective performance. *Clin Neuropsychol 25* (2):224–243.

Thompson, P. M., R. A. Dutton, K. M. Hayashi, A. Lu, S. E. Lee, J. Y. Lee, et al. (2006). 3D mapping of ventricular and corpus callosum abnormalities in HIV/AIDS. *Neuroimage 31* (1):12–23.

Thompson, P. M., R. A. Dutton, K. M. Hayashi, A. W. Toga, O. L. Lopez, H. J. Aizenstein, et al. (2005). Thinning of the cerebral cortex visualized in HIV/AIDS reflects CD4+ T lymphocyte decline. *Proc Natl Acad Sci U S A 102* (43):15,647–15,652.

Tozzi, V., P. Balestra, R. Bellagamba, A. Corpolongo, M. F. Salvatori, U. Visco-Comandini, et al. (2007). Persistence of neuropsychologic deficits despite long-term highly active antiretroviral therapy in patients with HIV-related neurocognitive impairment: prevalence and risk factors. *J Acquir Immune Defic Syndr 45* (2):174–182.

Tozzi, V., P. Balestra, M. F. Salvatori, C. Vlassi, G. Liuzzi, M. L. Giancola, M. et al. (2009). Changes in cognition during antiretroviral therapy: comparison of 2 different ranking systems to measure antiretroviral drug efficacy on HIV-associated neurocognitive disorders. *J Acquir Immune Defic Syndr 52* (1):56–63.

Valcour, V., T. Chalermchai, N. Sailasuta, M. Marovich, S. Lerdlum, D. Suttichom, et al. (2012). Central Nervous System Viral Invasion and Inflammation During Acute HIV Infection. *J Infect Dis. 206*(6):275–282.

Valcour, V. G., C. M. Shikuma, B. T. Shiramizu, A. E. Williams, M. R. Watters, P. W. Poff, et al. (2005). Diabetes, insulin resistance, and dementia among HIV-1-infected patients. *J Acquir Immune Defic Syndr 38* (1):31–36.

Valcour, V. G., B. T. Shiramizu, & C. M. Shikuma. (2010). HIV DNA in circulating monocytes as a mechanism to dementia and other HIV complications. *J Leukoc Biol 87* (4):621–626.

Valcour, V., R. Paul, J. Neuhaus, & C. Shikuma. (2011). The Effects of Age and HIV on Neuropsychological Performance. *J Int Neuropsychol Soc 17* (1):190–195.

Valcour, V., C. Shikuma, B. Shiramizu, M. Watters, P. Poff, O. A. Selnes, et al. (2004). Age, apolipoprotein E4, and the risk of HIV dementia: the Hawaii Aging with HIV Cohort. *J Neuroimmunol 157* (1-2):197–202.

Valcour, V., C. Shikuma, B. Shiramizu, M. Watters, P. Poff, O. Selnes, et al. (2004). Higher frequency of dementia in older HIV-1 individuals: the Hawaii Aging with HIV-1 Cohort. *Neurology 63* (5):822–827.

Volberding, P. A., & S. G. Deeks. (2010). Antiretroviral therapy and management of HIV infection. *Lancet 376* (9734):49–62.

Waysdorf, S. L. (2002). The aging of the AIDS epidemic: emerging legal and public health issues for elderly persons living with HIV/AIDS. *Elder Law J 10* (1):47–89.

Wiley, C. A., R. D. Schrier, J. A. Nelson, P. W. Lampert, & M. B. Oldstone. (1986). Cellular localization of human immunodeficiency virus infection within the brains of acquired immune deficiency syndrome patients. *Proc Natl Acad Sci U S A 83* (18):7089–7093.

Woods, S. P., D. J. Moore, E. Weber, & I. Grant. (2009). Cognitive neuropsychology of HIV-associated neurocognitive disorders. *Neuropsychol Rev 19* (2):152–168.

Yaffe, K. (2010). Biomarkers of Alzheimer's disease and exercise: one step closer to prevention. *Ann Neurol 68* (3):275–276.

Yarchoan, R., & S. Broder. (1987). Development of antiretroviral therapy for the acquired immunodeficiency syndrome and related disorders. A progress report. *N Engl J Med 316* (9):557–564.

Zablotsky, D., & M. Kennedy. (2003). Risk factors and HIV transmission to midlife and older women: knowledge, options, and the initiation of safer sexual practices. *J Acquir Immune Defic Syndr 33* (Suppl 2):S122–S130.

Zhao, Y., B. A. Navia, C. M. Marra, E. J. Singer, L. Chang, J. Berger, et al. (2010). Memantine for AIDS dementia complex: open-label report of ACTG 301. *HIV Clin Trials 11* (1):59–67.

13

Postoperative Delirium and Cognitive Decline

JACQUELINE M. LEUNG, MD, MPH AND TIFFANY L. TSAI, BA

Introduction

After surgery, changes in cognitive status may present in the form of frank delirium or cognitive decline, or both. While delirium is a well-known and frequent complication in the postoperative setting, postoperative cognitive decline (POCD) is also becoming increasingly recognized as a common outcome after major surgery (Williams-Russo et al., 1995; Moller et al., 1998; Johnson et al., 2002; Rasmussen et al., 2003). Following major noncardiac surgery, 7% to 26% of patients have POCD (Modena et al., 1997; Moller et al., 1998; Johnson et al., 2002; Rasmussen et al., 2003), and 10% to 60% of patients have delirium (Parikh & Chung, 1995). Among hospitalized medical patients, delirium occurs at a rate of 14% to 50%. Delirium has significant adverse effects on patient outcomes, including higher risk of subsequent cognitive decline, functional impairment, and increased long-term mortality (Ansaloni et al., 2010; Bickel et al., 2008; Kat et al., 2008; Robinson et al., 2009; Koebrugge et al., 2009).

Postoperative cognitive decline and delirium represent unique conditions and should not be used interchangeably. Delirium describes an acute confusional state featuring disturbances in attention and decreased awareness of the environment (Lipowski, 1987; Inouye et al., 1990). In contrast, POCD refers to subtle declines in cognitive functioning that can occur in the absence of delirium often detected through cognitive testing. Postoperative cognitive decline has been defined in a consensus statement as "a spectrum of postoperative central nervous system (CNS) dysfunction both acute and persistent...including brain death, stroke, subtle neurologic signs and cognitive impairment" (Murkin et al., 1995). Unlike delirium, POCD is not recognized in the International Classification of Diseases and is not listed as a diagnosis in the Diagnostic and Statistical Manual of Mental Disorders (DSM). The term POCD is used mostly in literature to represent a decline in a variety of cognitive domains, including memory, executive functioning, and speed of processing. A typical patient with POCD is oriented but exhibits significant declines from his or her own baseline level of performance on one or more cognitive domains (Blumenthal et al., 1995; Mackensen & Gelb, 2004; Wu et al., 2004).

In contrast, delirium symptoms fluctuate during the course of the day, and the patient often is disoriented. In addition, hallucinations and inappropriate communication or behavior may be observed. The definition of delirium combines key clinical symptoms and signs with required contextual items; diagnosis is based on characteristic symptoms rather than a pathognomonic feature. Delirium typically occurs in individuals with preexisting cognitive impairment and occurs in the setting of precipitating illness, surgery, or drug effects. Therefore, delirium occurs under a complex clinical picture with varying causation and treatment strategies. Most of the publications on delirium utilize the DSM, Third or Fourth Edition (American Psychiatric Association, 1994), or a derived version such as the Confusion Assessment Method (Inouye et al., 1990). Both POCD and delirium should be distinguished from dementia, which describes a chronic and often insidious decline in cognitive function with significant functional impairment.

In this chapter, we will summarize the current findings and research on POCD and delirium.

Delirium

HOSPITALIZED NONSURGICAL ELDERS

Delirium is a serious problem for hospitalized geriatric patients. It may be caused by an underlying medical illness, but often the exact etiology is not identifiable (Brauer et al., 2000). The course of delirium can vary considerably and depends on the resolution of the causative factors. The development of delirium is thought to be a multifactorial process in which there is a complex interrelationship between baseline patient vulnerability and precipitating factors or insults (Inouye & Charpentier, 1996). In elderly persons who were hospitalized for nonsurgical reasons, identified vulnerability factors included advanced age, cognitive impairment or dementia, functional impairment, depression, preexistent high number of and severity of comorbid conditions, chronic renal insufficiency, dehydration, malnutrition, and sensory impairment (Williams et al., 1985; Foreman, 1989; Gustafon, Berggren, & Brannstron, 1988; Rogers et al., 1989; Rockwood, 1989; Francis, Martin, & Kapoor 1990; Schor et al., 1992; Elie et al., 1998). Precipitating factors that were identified in the nonsurgical setting included sleep disorders, sensory deprivation or overload, and psychological stress such as that resulting from bereavement or relocation to an unfamiliar environment, the use of physical restraints, more than three medications added, use of bladder catheter, and any iatrogenic event (Lipowski, 1989; Inouye & Charpentier, 1996).

GERIATRIC SURGICAL PATIENTS

Table 13.1 summarizes the most important geriatric risk factors for postoperative delirium and cognitive decline.

In the perioperative period, the precipitating risk factors for the development of postoperative delirium in older patients include an unfamiliar environment, the stress of surgery, and exposure to medications that have the potential for profound effects on the CNS, such as opioids used in the treatment of postoperative pain.

Table 13.1 **eriatric Risk Factors of Postoperative Cognitive Decline or Delirium**

Postoperative cognitive decline	*Postoperative delirium*
Increasing age (Moller et al., 1998; Ancelin et al., 2001)	Increasing age (Gustafson et al., 1988; Marcantonio et al., 1994; Marcantonio et al,. 2000; Litaker et al., 2001)
Prior cognitive impairment (Ancelin et al., 2001)	Prior cognitive impairment (Gustafson et al., 1988; Marcantonio et al., 1994; Marcantonio et al., 2000; Litaker et al., 2001; Morrison et al., 2003)
Depression (Ancelin et al., 2001)	Depression (Gustafson et al., 1988; Galanakis et al., 2001; Leung, Sands, et al., 2005)
Low education level (<12 years) (Moller et al., 1998; Ancelin et al., 2001)	Poor functional status (Marcantonio et al., 1994; Marcantonio et al., 2000; Litaker et al., 2001)
Heart failure on hospital admission (Morrison et al., 2003)	Abnormal blood pressure (Morrison et al., 2003)
	Abnormal serum electrolytes or glucose (Marcantonio et al., 1994; Zakriya et al., 2002) (Marcantonio et al., 1994; Zakriya et al., 2002)
	Self-reported alcohol abuse (Williams-Russo et al., 1992; Marcantonio et al., 1994; Litaker et al., 2001)
	Narcotic use prior to admission (Litaker et al., 2001)

In surgical patients, successful interventions of postoperative delirium are limited. In one study of elderly patients admitted for emergency surgical repair of hip fracture, patients were randomly assigned to an intervention (a "proactive geriatrics consultation") or the usual care (Marcantonio et al., 2001). Delirium occurred in 32% of the intervention patients and in 50% of the usual-care patients. However, the length of hospital stay did not differ significantly between the two groups. Two other studies on hip fracture patients showed similar beneficial results in reducing the incidence of postoperative delirium when a "specialized geriatric ward" was utilized versus a conventional orthopedic ward (Lundstrom et al., 2007) or when an evidence-based clinical pathway was used (Beaupre et al., 2006). Other interventions such as prophylactic treatment with pharmacologic agents did not prevent the occurrence of delirium. For example, haloperidol did not prevent delirium but did reduce its severity and duration as well as the duration of hospital stay (Kalisvaart et al., 2005). This result suggests that haloperidol was effective in the treatment of delirium when it occurred but was ineffective in preventing its occurrence. Similarly, rivastigmine was shown to be ineffective in preventing postoperative delirium in elderly patients undergoing elective cardiac surgery (Gamberini et al., 2009). A more recent randomized clinical trial showed that olanzapine reduced the incidence of postoperative delirium in patients undergoing joint replacement (Larsen et al., 2010). However, in this study, a mixture of chart review and assessment by research assistants were used. Also, heterogeneous methods of delirium measurements were used, including the use of the Mini-Mental State Examination (MMSE), which has practice and ceiling effects and is not designed to detect delirium. As a result, a confirmatory study is necessary to validate this finding.

In the surgical setting, limited data exist as to whether specific intra-operative management precipitates postoperative delirium. Several areas that are of interest include drugs, anesthetic techniques, and management. We recently identified pain as an independent predictor of postoperative delirium (Vaurio et al., 2006) and thus a potentially important and modifiable precipitating factor for adverse cognitive outcomes. These results were corroborated by another study of older patients undergoing major elective noncardiac surgery (Lynch et al., 1998) that also showed that higher postoperative pain scores at rest were associated with an increased risk of delirium in the postoperative period. In addition, patients with postoperative delirium not only had higher pain levels but also received more intravenous opioids postoperatively than those without delirium (Leung, Sand, et al., 2005). These results suggest that in addition to pain, the CNS effects of opioids may cause or contribute to the development of postoperative delirium and cognitive decline. Therefore, pain management may be an area to target for intervention to improve cognitive outcomes for the geriatric surgical patients.

In a pilot randomized clinical trial, we tested the hypothesis that gabapentin as an add-on agent in the treatment of postoperative pain reduced the occurrence of postoperative delirium (Leung et al., 2006). The reduction in delirium appeared to be secondary to the opioid-sparing effect of gabapentin. This initial result provides a basis for future investigations on alternative pain therapy for at-risk patients to reduce postoperative delirium, such as non-opioid adjuvants or techniques to optimize postoperative pain control.

Although previous studies have demonstrated that certain drugs may be associated with postoperative delirium (Larson et al., 1987), there have been no prospective randomized clinical trials to determine whether the elimination of certain drugs used in the perioperative period will actually lead to a reduction in the incidence of postoperative delirium. A sensible guideline is to avoid "polypharmacy" when treating elderly patients because delirium has been demonstrated to be related to the number of medications prescribed in nonsurgical patients (Larson et al., 1987; Inouye & Charpentier, 1996).

Controversy persists as to whether any anesthetic technique (regional vs. general) has an impact on incident postoperative delirium. Earlier studies suggested an association between general anesthesia and a higher incidence of postoperative delirium compared to epidural anesthesia (Hole, Terjesen, & Brevik, 1980; Berggren et al., 1987). However, recent studies concluded that there was no relationship between anesthetic techniques and the magnitude or pattern of postoperative delirium (Williams-Russo et al., 1995; Moller et al., 1998; O'Hara et al., 2000). The influence of intra-operative hypotension on postoperative delirium has also been evaluated. To date, no single anesthetic technique has been identified to be superior for the elderly surgical patients in minimizing postoperative delirium.

Finally, a recent study showed that longer duration of fluid fasting preoperatively was independently associated with postoperative delirium (Radtke et al., 2010). Although dehydration has been linked to impaired cognitive performance in both young and older subjects (Phillips et al., 1984; Wilson & Morley, 2003), a study in older subjects who had bowel preparation-induced dehydration showed no change in cognitive function compared with those who had no bowel preparation (Ackland et al., 2008). Because the duration and magnitude of hydration are critical factors affecting cognitive function, future studies examining the role of dehydration and cognitive performance should consider whether there is a critical level of water deficit affecting cognition.

Overall, the pathophysiology of delirium still remains to be defined as the syndrome likely occurs as a result of multiple risk factors and heterogeneous stressors present in different clinical settings. It is possible that this geriatric syndrome ultimately may require a multicomponent therapy rather than a single pharmacologic agent for treatment. Until more definitive clinical studies become available, minimizing the number of medications used, avoiding hypoxemia and extremes of hypocarbia or hypercarbia, and providing adequate postoperative pain control appear to be the best approaches in minimizing the occurrence of postoperative delirium in geriatric surgical patients.

Postoperative Cognitive Decline

Because older age has been consistently demonstrated as a strong preoperative risk factor of POCD (Moller et al., 1998; Monk et al., 2008), the incidence of POCD is expected to increase as the population of older surgical patients grows. Recent studies have shown that POCD has the potential to impact daily functioning (Phillips-Bute et al., 2006), cause premature departure from the labor market (Steinmetz et al., 2009), and decrease the ability to self-care after hospital discharge (Steinmetz et al., 2009). However, POCD itself remains a poorly defined clinical syndrome, and its incidence depends on the researcher's approach to defining POCD and several other methodological factors that have not been standardized across studies.

ASSESSMENT OF POSTOPERATIVE COGNITIVE DECLINE

Assessment of POCD requires cognitive testing, as cognitive changes present subtly and patients' self-reported perceptions of cognitive impairment are frequently discrepant with the results of cognitive testing (Newman et al., 1989; Moller et al., 1998; Johnson et al., 2002). Test selection is influenced by numerous practical and theoretical considerations. For example, evaluations are affected by time constraints, language fluency, and often in the case of repeated cognitive measurements and decreased patient interest.

Overall, studies still lack agreement over which cognitive domains are more vulnerable to the effects of surgery and anesthesia and thus should be targeted for testing. A recent study suggested that attention and cognitive speed were more vulnerable to the surgical experience in patients who showed cognitive deficits based on preoperative cognitive tests (Silverstein et al., 2007). Jankowski et al. (2011) reported that preoperative short-term memory was an independent risk factor for postoperative delirium in older noncardiac surgical patients, whereas other studies suggested that executive function and depression independently predicted postoperative delirium in noncardiac surgical patients (Smith et al., 2009; Greene et al., 2009). Given the current difficulty in comparing POCD data across studies, establishing a consensus on a standard test battery would benefit this growing field of research by allowing the pooling of data and increasing the statistical power of meta-analyses.

The timing of assessments after surgery has been also heterogeneous. In previous studies, cognitive function was measured beginning 1 day to as long as

5 years after surgery. Postoperative cognitive decline can be broadly divided into acute (within 1 week after surgery), intermediate (within 3 months), and late or long-term (1–2 years) changes based on information from previous studies. However, the exact significance of detecting POCD at these various time-points is unclear. The time interval at which a diagnosis of POCD holds the greatest clinical significance has not been determined, nor have any studies invalidated the importance of conducting assessments at a specific time-point.

Early assessments of POCD likely capture a different phenomenon than what late assessments of POCD capture, and each are accompanied by a unique set of issues. Surgery-related factors may affect test performance in the immediate postoperative period, including acute pain (Duggleby & Lander, 1994; Heyer et al., 2000; Wang et al., 2007), the use of drugs (Sands, Katz, & Doyle, 1993; Ersek et al., 2004), nausea, limited mobility, and fatigue. Thus, it has been argued that patients should not be evaluated for POCD until at least 1 week postoperatively (Murkin et al., 1995; Hanning, 2005; Rasmussen, Stygall, & Newman, 2009). Recent evidence has suggested this delay might be arbitrary, as negative outcomes were associated with POCD detected in the first week after surgery. In a 2008 study of patients undergoing noncardiac surgery, POCD detected at hospital discharge (mean duration of stay < 7 days) was associated with an increased risk of death within the first 3 months after surgery (Monk et al., 2008).

Postoperative cognitive decline assessments that occur in the immediate postoperative period are important for elucidating the relationship between POCD and delirium. Because POCD and delirium both feature deficits in attention, whether they are related events on a continuum or are distinct conditions remains unclear (Fig. 13.1). Recently, Monk et al. (2008) found that patients who were delirious after major noncardiac surgery were also more likely to have POCD at hospital discharge. In terms of longer-term POCD, Jankowski et al. (2011) found that postoperative delirium in older patients undergoing noncardiac surgery did not predict POCD at 3 months after surgery. As most cases of

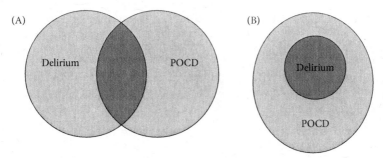

Figure 13.1 otential relationship between POCD and postoperative delirium. (A) Delirium and POCD may be distinct entities with some overlapping features. (B) Delirium and POCD may exist on a continuum.

delirium occur in the early postoperative period, an improved understanding of the relationship between POCD and delirium will be derived from additional studies that perform neurocognitive testing and delirium assessment simultaneously within the first several days after surgery.

PATHOLOPHYSIOLOGY OF POSTOPERATIVE COGNITIVE DECLINE

Because the exact pathophysiology of POCD remains undefined, potential interventions of POCD have not been identified. Previous studies on POCD have focused on investigating the risk factors associated with early POCD. Baseline characteristics of patients that have been shown to be associated with POCD included preoperative cognitive status (McDonagh et al., 2010), increasing age and lower levels of education (Moller et al., 1998), and the avoidance of alcohol intake (Johnson et al., 2002). Conversely, Hudetz et al. (2007) identified history of alcohol abuse as a risk factor for POCD at 2 weeks after surgery in middle-aged and older patients.

In addition to predisposing risk factors, numerous potential precipitating risk factors for POCD have been reported, including the duration of anesthesia, a second operation, postoperative infections, and pulmonary complications (Moller et al., 1998). In cardiac surgery, the use of cardiopulmonary bypass has been implicated as one of the precipitating factors (Selnes et al., 1999; Newman et al., 2006). During cardiopulmonary bypass, cannulation of the aortic root may result in cerebral microemboli, which could lead to POCD (Pugsley et al. 1994). In addition, a profound systemic inflammatory response occurs with cardiopulmonary bypass, which may contribute to POCD (Mathew et al., 2004). A systemic review by van Dijk et al. (2000) evaluated 12 cohort studies and 11 intervention studies and found 22.5% of patients with a cognitive deficits 2 months after coronary artery bypass graft surgery. However, despite the earlier reports that POCD was prevalent after cardiac surgery (Selnes et al., 1999; Newman et al., 2006), studies in patients who underwent cardiac surgery without the use of cardiopulmonary bypass did not demonstrate a lower incidence of POCD, despite a smaller embolic load in the middle cerebral artery measured by Doppler in patients undergoing off-pump surgery (Jensen et al., 2008; Liu et al., 2009). More recently, Evered et al. (2011) studied older patients undergoing coronary angiography under sedation, total hip joint replacement surgery under general anesthesia, or coronary artery bypass graft under general anesthesia. Despite the different invasiveness of these procedures and types of anesthesia, the investigators reported similar rates of POCD at 3 months across all groups of patients, suggesting that surgery type, including cardiopulmonary bypass and anesthesia type, may not contribute substantially to the development of POCD. Another important methodological consideration is that most studies of cognitive outcomes after coronary artery bypass graft surgery lack a control group. Therefore, although POCDs are clearly noted, it is not clear whether the changes are specifically related to the cardiac procedure itself, rather than other etiologies.

In terms of the potential influence of anesthetics, in experimental settings involving animals, general anesthetics have produced neurotoxicity and subsequent cognitive impairment in young and aged animals, but whether these changes are reproducible in clinical studies has not been determined (Culley, Xie, & Crosby, 2007). The effect of the type of anesthesia on the occurrence of POCD is inconclusive. Initial results from ISPOCD group (Johnson et al., 2002) did not show that the type of anesthesia (general vs. regional) affected the incidence of POCD. A subsequent study by the same group (Rasmussen et al., 2003) showed a trend toward a decreased incidence of POCD at 7 days after surgery in patients who received regional anesthesia compared to those who received general anesthesia (12.5% vs. 19.7%). Unfortunately, the study was stopped prematurely before reaching the intended sample size to achieve statistical significance. The effect of hypotension on postoperative cognition was another focus of investigation because systemic hypotension may lead to brain hypoperfusion and subtle permanent cognitive dysfunction. In a randomized trial of hypotensive versus normotensive anesthesia in older patients undergoing elective primary hip replacement under epidural anesthesia, Williams-Russo et al. (1999) showed that after the operation, there was no significant difference in the incidence of early or long-term cognitive dysfunction between the two blood pressure management groups. Taken together, to date, no single anesthetic type or technique has been identified to be superior in minimizing POCD for older surgical patients.

The question of whether major surgery and anesthesia ultimately lead to long-term cognitive decline is controversial. In a population study, Dijkstra et al. (1998) reported that the number of operations and the total duration of anesthesia were related to the number of subject health-related complaints but did not predict cognitive performance or memory complaints. Several other studies that included assessments at more than 6 months after surgery similarly reported no decline in cognitive status from before surgery (Abildstrom et al., 2000; Billig, Stockton, & Cohen-Mansfield, 1996; Gilberstadt et al., 1968; Stockton, Cohen-Mansfield, & Billig, 2000; Goldstein, Fogel, & Young, 1996). However, two recent studies that included patients who had undergone noncardiac surgery reported that acute POCD was associated with increased mortality after surgery (for the first study, at 1 year; and for the second study, at 3 months) (Monk et al., 2008; Steinmetz et al., 2009). Also, in cardiac surgical patients, Newman et al. (2001) provided data showing that cognitive function at discharge was a significant predictor of long-term cognitive function. In contrast, a recent study by Avidan et al. (2009) provided results to the contrary. Thus, whether patients with early POCD actually have preexisting mild cognitive impairment and experience a steeper downward cognitive trajectory independent of the effect of anesthesia and surgery is a critical question that warrants further investigation.

Conclusion

The field of delirium and POCD has made considerable advances in the last decade. We have improved our recognition of delirium and begun to identify potential interventions to prevent delirium in older surgical patients. Similarly, in the field of POCD, studies have provided relatively clear evidence of the existence of POCD in the early postoperative period. Nonetheless, no studies have yet elucidated the possible pathophysiology for delirium or POCD after surgery. Future research on delirium and POCD should focus on predictors that are dynamic and modifiable. There is also a critical need for researchers to explore the delirium, POCD, and dementia interface. It remains to be determined whether delirium and POCD are related events on a continuum or are distinct conditions. Ultimately, understanding the pathophysiology of POCD and delirium may provide a clue as to how other neurodegenerative disease such as Alzheimer's disease may occur.

References

Abildstrom, H., L. S. Rasmussen, P. Rentowl, C. D. Hanning, H. Rasmussen, P. A. Kristensen, et al. (2000). Cognitive dysfunction 1-2 years after non-cardiac surgery in the elderly. ISPOCD group. International Study of Post-Operative Cognitive Dysfunction. *Acta Anaesthesiol Scand no. 44* (10):1246–1251.

Ackland, G. L., J. Harrington, P. Downie, J. W. Holding, D. Singh-Ranger, K. Griva, et al. (2008). Dehydration induced by bowel preparation in older adults does not result in cognitive dysfunction. *Anesth Analg no. 106* (3):924–929, table of contents. doi: 106/3/924 [pii] 10.1213/ane.0b013e3181615247.

American Psychiatric Association. (1994). *Diagnostic and statistical manual of mental disorders.* 4th ed. American Psychiatric Association, Arlington, VA.

Ancelin, M. L., G. de Roquefeuil, B. Ledesert, F. Bonnel, J. C. Cheminal, & K. Ritchie. (2001). Exposure to anaesthetic agents, cognitive functioning and depressive symptomatology in the elderly. *Br J Psychiatry no. 178*:360–366.

Ansaloni, L., F. Catena, R. Chattat, D. Fortuna, C. Franceschi, P. Mascitti, et al. (2010). Risk factors and incidence of postoperative delirium in elderly patients after elective and emergency surgery. *Br J Surg no. 97* (2):273–280. doi: 10.1002/bjs.6843.

Avidan, M. S., A. C. Searleman, M. Storandt, K. Barnett, A. Vannucci, L. Saager, et al. (2009). Long-term cognitive decline in elderly people was not attributable to non-cardiac surgery or major illness.*Anesthesiology no. 111* (5): 964–970.

Beaupre, L. A., J. G. Cinats, A. Senthilselvan, D. Lier, C. A. Jones, A. Scharfenberger, et al. (2006). Reduced morbidity for elderly patients with a hip fracture after implementation of a perioperative evidence-based clinical pathway. *Qual Saf Health Care no. 15* (5):375–379. doi: 15/5/375 [pii] 10.1136/qshc.2005.017095.

Berggren, D., Y. Gustafson, B. Eriksson, G. Bucht, L. –I. Hansson, S. Reiz, et al. (1987). Postoperative confusion after anesthesia in elderly patients with femoral neck fractures. *Anesth Analg no. 66*:497–504.

Bickel, H., R. Gradinger, E. Kochs, & H. Forstl. (2008). High risk of cognitive and functional decline after postoperative delirium. A three-year prospective study. *Dement Geriatr Cogn Disord no. 26* (1):26–31. doi: 000140804 [pii] 10.1159/000140804.

Billig, N, P Stockton, & J Cohen-Mansfield. (1996). Cognitive and affective changes after cataract surgery in an elderly population. *Am J Geriatr Psychiatry* no. 4:29–38.

Blumenthal, J. A., E. P. Mahanna, D. J. Madden, W. D. White, N. D. Croughwell, & M. F. Newman. (1995). Methodological issues in the assessment of neuropsychologic function after cardiac surgery. *Ann Thorac Surg* no. 59 (5):1345–1350.

Brauer, C., R. S. Morrison, S. B. Silberzweig, & A. L. Siu. (2000). The cause of delirium in patients with hip fracture. *Arch Intern Med* no. 160 (12):1856–1860.

Culley, D. J., Z. Xie, & G. Crosby. (2007). General anesthetic-induced neurotoxicity: an emerging problem for the young and old? *Curr Opin Anaesthesiol* no. 20 (5):408–413. doi: 10.1097/ ACO.0b013e3282efd18b00001503-200710000-00004 [pii].

Dijkstra, J. B., M. P. Van Boxtel, P. J. Houx, & J. Jolles. (1998). An operation under general anesthesia as a risk factor for age-related cognitive decline: Results from a large cross-sectional population study. *J Am Geriatr Soc* no. 46 (10):1258–1265.

Duggleby, W., & J. Lander. (1994). Cognitive status and postoperative pain: older adults. *J Pain Symptom Manage* no. 9 (1):19–27.

Elie, M., M. G. Cole, F. J. Primeau, & F. Bellavance. (1998). Delirium risk factors in elderly hospitalized patients. *J Gen Intern Med* no. 13 (3):204–212.

Ersek, M., M. M. Cherrier, S. S. Overman, & G. A. Irving. (2004). The cognitive effects of opioids. *Pain Manag Nurs* no. 5 (2):75–93.

Evered, L., D. A. Scott, B. Silbert, & P. Maruff. (2011). Postoperative cognitive dysfunction is independent of type of surgery and anesthetic. *Anesth Analg* no. 112 (5):1179–1185. doi: ANE.0b013e318215217e [pii] 10.1213/ANE.0b013e318215217e.

Foreman, M. D. (1989). Confusion in the hospitalized elderly: incidence, onset, and associated factors." *Res Nurs Health* no. 12 (1):21–29.

Francis, J., D. Martin, & W. N. Kapoor. (1990). A prospective study of delirium in hospitalized elderly. *Jama* no. 263 (8):1097–1101.

Galanakis, P., H. Bickel, R. Gradinger, S. Von Gumppenberg, & H. Forstl. (2001). Acute confusional state in the elderly following hip surgery: incidence, risk factors and complications. *Int J Geriatr Psychiatry* no. 16 (4):349–355.

Gamberini, M., D. Bolliger, G. A. Lurati Buse, C. S. Burkhart, M. Grapow, A. Gagneux, et al. (2009). Rivastigmine for the prevention of postoperative delirium in elderly patients undergoing elective cardiac surgery—a randomized controlled trial. *Crit Care Med* no. 37 (5):1762–1768. doi: 10.1097/CCM.0b013e31819da780.

Gilberstadt, H., R. Aberwald, S. Crosbie, H. Schuell, & E. Jimenez. (1968). Effect of surgery on psychological and social functioning in elderly patients. *Arch Intern Med* no. 122 (2):109–115.

Goldstein, M. Z., B. S. Fogel, & B. L. Young. (1996). Effect of elective surgery under general anesthesia on mental status variables in elderly women and men: 10-month follow-up. *Int Psychogeriatr* no. 8 (1):135–149.

Greene, N. H., D. K. Attix, B. C. Weldon, P. J. Smith, D. L. McDonagh, & T. G. Monk. (2009). Measures of executive function and depression identify patients at risk for postoperative delirium. *Anesthesiology* no. 110 (4):788–795.

Gustafon, Y., D. Berggren, & B. Brannstron. (1988). Acute confusional states in elderly patients treated for femoral neck fracture. *J Am Geriatr Soc* no. 36:525–530.

Gustafson, Y., D. Berggren, B. Brannstrom, G. Bucht, A. Norberg, L. I. Hansson, et al. (1988). Acute confusional states in elderly patients treated for femoral neck fracture. *J Am Geriatr Soc* no. 36 (6):525–530.

Hanning, C. D. (2005). Postoperative cognitive dysfunction. *Br J Anaesth* no. 95 (1):82–87.

Heyer, E. J., R. Sharma, C. J. Winfree, J. Mocco, D. J. McMahon, P. A. McCormick, et al. (2000). Severe pain confounds neuropsychological test performance. *J Clin Exp Neuropsychol* no. 22 (5):633–639.

Hole, A., T. Terjesen, & H. Brevik. (1980). Epidural versus general anaesthesia for total hip arthroplasty in elderly patients. *Acta Anaesthesiol Scand* no. 24:279–287.

Hudetz, J. A., Z. Iqbal, S. D. Gandhi, K. M. Patterson, T. F. Hyde, D. M. Reddy, et al. (2007). Postoperative cognitive dysfunction in older patients with a history of alcohol abuse. *Anesthesiology* no. 106 (3):423–430. doi: 00000542-200703000-00005 [pii].

Inouye, S. K., & P. A. Charpentier. (1996). Precipitating factors for delirium in hospitalized elderly persons: predictive model and interrelationship with baseline vulnerability. *JAMA* no. 275:852–857.

Inouye, S. K., C. H. van Dyke, C. A. Alessi, S. Balkin, A. P. Siegal, & R. I. Horwitz. (1990). Clarifying confusion: the confusion assessment method. *Ann Intern Med* no. 113:941–948.

Jankowski, C. J., M. R. Trenerry, D. J. Cook, S. L. Buenvenida, S. R. Stevens, D. R. Schroeder, et al. (2011). Cognitive and functional predictors and sequelae of postoperative delirium in elderly patients undergoing elective joint arthroplasty. *Anesth Analg* no. 112 (5):1186–1193. doi: ANE.0b013e318211501b [pii] 10.1213/ANE.0b013e318211501b.

Jensen, J., L. Hedin, C. Widell, P. Agnhom, B. Andersson, & M. Fu. (2008). Characteristics of heart failure in the elderly—a hospital cohort registry-based study. *Int J Cardiol* no. 125 (2):191–196. doi: S0167-5273(07)01618-X [pii] 10.1016/j.ijcard.2007.10.003.

Johnson, T., T. Monk, L. S. Rasmussen, H. Abildstrom, P. Houx, K. Korttila, et al. (2002). Postoperative cognitive dysfunction in middle-aged patients. *Anesthesiology* no. 96 (6):1351–1357.

Kalisvaart, K. J., J. F. de Jonghe, M. J. Bogaards, R. Vreeswijk, T. C. Egberts, B. J. Burger, et al. (2005). Haloperidol prophylaxis for elderly hip-surgery patients at risk for delirium: a randomized placebo-controlled study. *J Am Geriatr Soc* no. 53 (10):1658–1666.

Kat, M. G., R. Vreeswijk, J. F. de Jonghe, T. van der Ploeg, W. A. van Gool, P. Eikelenboom, et al. (2008). Long-term cognitive outcome of delirium in elderly hip surgery patients. A prospective matched controlled study over two and a half years. *Dement Geriatr Cogn Disord* no. 26 (1):1–8. doi: 000140611 [pii] 10.1159/000140611.

Koebrugge, B., H. L. Koek, R. J. van Wensen, P. L. Dautzenberg, & K. Bosscha. (2009). Delirium after abdominal surgery at a surgical ward with a high standard of delirium care: incidence, risk factors and outcomes. *Dig Surg* no. 26 (1):63–68. doi: 000194947 [pii] 10.1159/000194947.

Larsen, K. A., S. E. Kelly, T. A. Stern, R. H. Bode, Jr., L. L. Price, D. J. Hunter, et al. (2010). Administration of olanzapine to prevent postoperative delirium in elderly joint-replacement patients: a randomized, controlled trial. *Psychosomatics* no. 51 (5):409–418. doi: 51/5/409 [pii] 10.1176/appi.psy.51.5.409.

Larson, E. B., W. A. Kubull, D. Buchner, & B. V. Reifler. (1987). Adverse drug reactions associated with global cognitive impairment in elderly persons. *Ann Intern Med* no. 107:169–173.

Leung, J. M., L. P. Sands, M. Rico, K. L. Petersen, M. C. Rowbotham, J. B. Dahl, et al. (2006). Pilot clinical trial of gabapentin to decrease postoperative delirium in older patients. *Neurology* no. 67 (7):1251–1253. doi: 01.wnl.0000233831.87781.a9 [pii] 10.1212/01.wnl.0000233831.87781.a9.

Leung, J. M., L. P. Sand, L. Vaurio, & Y. Wang. (2005). Pathophysiology of postoperative delirium in geriatric surgical patients. *Anesthesiology*:A1461 (Abstract).

Leung, J. M., L. P. Sands, E. A. Mullen, Y. Wang, & L. Vaurio. (2005). Are preoperative depressive symptoms associated with postoperative delirium in geriatric surgical patients? *J Gerontology: Medical Sciences* no. 60A:1563–1568.

Lipowski, Z. J. (1987). Delirium (acute confusional states). *JAMA* no. 258:1789–1792.

———. (1989). Delirium in the elderly patient. *New Engl J Med* no. 320:578–582.

Litaker, D., J. Locala, K. Franco, D. L. Bronson, & Z. Tannous. (2001). Preoperative risk factors for postoperative delirium. *Gen Hosp Psychiatry* no. 23 (2):84–89. doi: S0163-8343(01)00117-7 [pii].

Liu, Y. H., D. X. Wang, L. H. Li, X. M. Wu, G. J. Shan, et al. (2009). The effects of cardiopulmonary bypass on the number of cerebral microemboli and the incidence of cognitive dysfunction after coronary artery bypass graft surgery. *Anesth Analg* no. 109 (4):1013–1022. doi: 109/4/1013 [pii] 0.1213/ane.0b013e3181aed2bb.

Lundstrom, M., B. Olofsson, M. Stenvall, S. Karlsson, L. Nyberg, U. Englund, et al. (2007). Postoperative delirium in old patients with femoral neck fracture: a randomized intervention study. *Aging Clin Exp Res* no. 19 (3):178–186. doi: 3697 [pii].

Lynch, E. P., M. A. Lazor, J. E. Gellis, J. Orav, L. Goldman, & E. R. Marcantonio. (1998). The impact of postoperative pain on the development of postoperative delirium. *Anesth Analg* no. 86:781–785.

Mackensen, G. B., & A. W. Gelb. (2004). Postoperative cognitive deficits: more questions than answers. *Eur J Anaesthesiol* no. 21 (2):85–88.

Marcantonio, E. R., J. M. Flacker, M. Michaels, & N. M. Resnick. (2000). Delirium is independently associated with poor functional recovery after hip fracture. *J Am Geriatr Soc* no. 48 (6):618–624.

Marcantonio, E. R., J. M. Flacker, R. J. Wright, & N. Resnick. (2001). Reducing delirium after hip fracture: a randomized trial. *JAGS* no. 49:516–522.

Marcantonio, E. R., L. Goldman, C. M. Mangione, L. R. Ludwig, B. Muraca, C. M. Haslauer, et al. (1994). A clinical prediction rule for delirium after elective noncardiac surgery. *JAMA* no. 271:134–139.

Mathew, J. P., S. K. Shernan, W. D. White, J. C. Fitch, J. C. Chen, L. Bell, et al. (2004). Preliminary report of the effects of complement suppression with pexelizumab on neurocognitive decline after coronary artery bypass graft surgery. *Stroke* no. 35 (10):2335–2339. doi: 10.1161/01.STR.0000141938.00524.8301.STR.0000141938.00524.83 [pii].

McDonagh, D. L., J. P. Mathew, W. D. White, B. Phillips-Bute, D. T. Laskowitz, M. V. Podgoreanu, et al. (2010). Cognitive function after major noncardiac surgery, apolipoprotein E4 genotype, and biomarkers of brain injury. *Anesthesiology* no. 112 (4):852–859. doi: 10.1097/ALN.0b013e3181d31fd7.

Modena, M. G., N. Muia, F. A. Sgura, R. Molinari, A. Castella, & R. Rossi. (1997). Left atrial size is the major predictor of cardiac death and overall clinical outcome in patients with dilated cardiomyopathy: a long-term follow-up study. *Clin Cardiol* no. 20:553–560.

Moller, J. T., P. Cluitmans, L. S. Rasmussen, P. Houx, H. Rasmussen, J. Canet, et al. (1998). Long-term postoperative cognitive dysfunction in the elderly: ISPOCD1 study. *Lancet* no. 351:857–861.

Monk, T. G., B. C. Weldon, C. W. Garvan, D. E. Dede, M. T. van der Aa, K. M. Heilman, et al. (2008). Predictors of cognitive dysfunction after major noncardiac surgery. *Anesthesiology* no. 108 (1):18–30. doi: 10.1097/01.anes.0000296071.19434.1e 00000542-200801000-00007 [pii].

Morrison, R. S., J. Magaziner, M. Gilbert, K. J. Koval, M. A. McLaughlin, G. Orosz, et al. (2003). Relationship between pain and opioid analgesics on the development of delirium following hip fracture. *J Gerontol A Biol Sci Med Sci* no. 58 (1):76–81.

Murkin, J. M., S. P. Newman, D. A. Stump, & J. A. Blumenthal. (1995). Statement of consensus on assessment of neurobehavioral outcomes after cardiac surgery. *Ann Thorac Surg* no. 59 (5):1289–1295. doi: 000349759500106U [pii].

Newman, M. F., J. L. Kirchner, B. Phillips-Bute, V. Gaver, H. Grocott, R. H. Jones, et al. (2001). Longitudinal assessment of neurocognitive function after coronary-artery bypass surgery. *N Engl J Med* no. 344 (6):395–402. doi: MJBA-440601 [pii].

Newman, M. F., J. P. Mathew, H. P. Grocott, G. B. Mackensen, T. Monk, K. A. Welsh-Bohmer, et al. (2006). Central nervous system injury associated with cardiac surgery. *Lancet* no. 368 (9536):694–703. doi: S0140-6736(06)69254-4 [pii] 10.1016/S0140-6736(06)69254-4.

Newman, S., L. Klinger, G. Venn, P. Smith, M. Harrison, and T. Treasure. (1989). Subjective reports of cognition in relation to assessed cognitive performance following coronary artery bypass surgery. *J Psychosom Res* no. 33 (2):227–233. doi: 0022-3999(89)90050-0 [pii].

O'Hara, D. A., A. Duff, J. A. Berlin, R. M. Poses, V. A. Lawrence, E. C. Huber, et al. (2000). The effect of anesthetic technique on postoperative outcomes in hip fracture repair. *Anesthesiology* no. 92:947–957.

Parikh, S. S., & C. Chung. (1995). Postoperative delirium in the elderly. *Anesth Analg* no. 80:1223–1232.

Phillips, P. A., B. J. Rolls, J. G. Ledingham, M. L. Forsling, J. J. Morton, M. J. Crowe, et al. (1984). Reduced thirst after water deprivation in healthy elderly men. *N Engl J Med* no. 311 (12):753–759.

Phillips-Bute, B., J. P. Mathew, J. A. Blumenthal, H. P. Grocott, D. T. Laskowitz, R. H. Jones, et al. (2006). Association of neurocognitive function and quality of life 1 year after coronary artery bypass graft (CABG) surgery. *Psychosom Med* no. *68* (3):369–375. doi: 68/3/369 [pii] 10.1097/01.psy.0000221272.77984.e2.

Pugsley, W., L. Klinger, C. Paschalis, T. Treasure, M. Harrison, & S. Newman. (1994). The impact of microemboli during cardiopulmonary bypass on neuropsychological functioning. *Stroke* no. *25* (7):1393–1399.

Radtke, F. M., M. Franck, M. MacGuill, M. Seekubg, A. Luetz, S. Westhoff, et al. (2010). Duration of fluid fasting and choice of analgesic are modifiable factors for early postoperative delirium. *European Journal of Anaesthesiology* no. *27* (5):411–416.

Rasmussen, L. S., T. Johnson, H. M. Kuipers, D. Kristensen, V. D. Siersma, P. Vila, et al. (2003). Does anaesthesia cause postoperative cognitive dysfunction? A randomised study of regional versus general anaesthesia in 438 elderly patients. *Acta Anaesthesiol Scand* no. *47* (3):260–266.

Rasmussen, L., J. Stygall, & S. P. Newman. (2009). Cognitive Dysfunction and Other Long-Term Complications of Surgery and Anesthesia. In R. D. Miller (ed.), *Miller's Anesthesia*, 2 v. (pp. xxii, 3084, I–89). Philadelphia, PA: Churchill Livingstone/Elsevier.

Robinson, T. N., C. D. Raeburn, Z. V. Tran, E. M. Angles, L. A. Brenner, & M. Moss. (2009). Postoperative delirium in the elderly: risk factors and outcomes. *Ann Surg* no. *249* (1):173–178. doi: 10.1097/SLA.0b013e31818e477600000658-200901000-00029 [pii].

Rockwood, K. (1989). Acute confusion in elderly medical patients. *J Am Geriatr Soc* no. *37* (2):150–154.

Rogers, M. P., M. H. Liang, L. H. Daltroy, H. Eaton, J. Peteet, E. Wright, et al. (1989). Delirium after elective orthopedic surgery: risk factors and natural history. *Int J Psychiatry Med* no. *19* (2):109–121.

Sands, L. P., I. R. Katz, & S. Doyle. (1993). Detecting subclinical change in cognitive functioning in older adults. Part I: Explication of the method. *Am J Geriatr Psychiatry* no. *1* (3):1–13.

Schor, J. D., S. E. Levkoff, L. A. Lipsitz, C. H. Reilly, P. D. Cleary, J. W. Rowe, et al. (1992). Risk factors for delirium in hospitalized elderly. *Jama* no. *267* (6):827–831.

Selnes, O. A., M. A. Goldsborough, L. M. Borowicz, & G. M. McKhann. (1999). Neurobehavioural sequelae of cardiopulmonary bypass. *Lancet* no. *353* (9164):1601–1606. doi: S0140-6736(98)07576-X [pii] 10.1016/S0140-6736(98)07576-X.

Silverstein, J. H., J. Steinmetz, A. Reichenberg, P. D. Harvey, & L. S. Rasmussen. (2007). Postoperative cognitive dysfunction in patients with preoperative cognitive impairment: which domains are most vulnerable? *Anesthesiology* no. *106* (3):431–435.

Smith, P. J., D. K. Attix, B. C. Weldon, N. H. Greene, & T. G. Monk. (2009). Executive function and depression as independent risk factors for postoperative delirium. *Anesthesiology* no. *110* (4):781–787.

Steinmetz, J., K. B. Christensen, T. Lund, N. Lohse, & L. S. Rasmussen. (2009). Long-term consequences of postoperative cognitive dysfunction. *Anesthesiology* no. *110* (3):548–555. doi: 10.1097/ALN.0b013e318195b569.

Stockton, P., J. Cohen-Mansfield, & N. Billig. (2000). Mental status change in older surgical patients. Cognition, depression, and other comorbidity. *Am J Geriatr Psychiatry* no. *8* (1):40–46.

van Dijk, D., A. M. Keizer, J. C. Diephuis, C. Durand, L. J. Vos, & R. Hijman. (2000). Neurocognitive dysfunction after coronary artery bypass surgery: a systematic review. *J Thorac Cardiovasc Surg* no. *120* (4):632–639. doi: 10.1067/mtc.2000.108901.

Vaurio, L., L. Sands, Y. Wang, E. A. Mullen, & J. M. Leung. (2006). The role of pain and medications on postoperative delirium. *Anesth Analg* no. *102*:267–273.

Wang, Y., L. P. Sands, L. Vaurio, A. Mullen, & J. M. Leung. (2007). The effects of postoperative pain and its management on postoperative cognitive dysfunction. *Am J Geriatr Psychiatry* no. *15*:50–59.

Williams, M. A., E. B. Campbell, W. J. Raynor, Jr., M. A. Musholt, S. M. Mlynarczyk, & L. F. Crane. (1985). Predictors of acute confusional states in hospitalized elderly patients. *Res Nurs Health* no. *8* (1):31–40.

Williams-Russo, P., N. E. Sharrock, S. Mattis, G. A. Liguori, C. Mancuso, M. G. Peterson, et al. (1999). Randomized trial of hypotensive epidural anesthesia in older adults. *Anesthesiology* no. *91*:926–935.

Williams-Russo, P., N. E. Sharrock, S. Mattis, T. P. Szatrowski, & M. E. Charlson. (1995). Cognitive effects after epidural vs general anesthesia in older adults. *JAMA* no. *274*:44–50.

Williams-Russo, P., B. L. Urquhart, N. E. Sharrock, & M. E. Charlson. (1992). Post-operative delirium: predictors and prognosis in elderly orthopedic patients. *J Am Geriatr Soc* no. *40*:759–767.

Wilson, M. M., & J. E. Morley. (2003). Impaired cognitive function and mental performance in mild dehydration. *Eur J Clin Nutr* no. *57* Suppl 2:S24–S29. doi: 10.1038/sj.ejcn.16018981601898 [pii].

Wu, C. L., W. Hsu, J. M. Richman, & S. N. Raja. (2004). Postoperative cognitive function as an outcome of regional anesthesia and analgesia. *Reg Anesth Pain Med* no. *29* (3):257–268.

Zakriya, K. J., C. Christmas, J. F. Wenz, Sr., S. Franckowiak, R. Anderson, & F. E. Sieber. (2002). Preoperative factors associated with postoperative change in confusion assessment method score in hip fracture patients. *Anesth Analg* no. *94* (6):1628–1632.

Disclosures

Pascale Barberger-Gateau, MD, PhD, has received funding for travel or speaker honoraria from Lesieur, Bausch & Lomb, Aprifel, Danone Institute, Canadian Association of Gerontology, the Jean Mayer Human Nutrition Research Center on Aging, Tufts University, Alzheimer's Association, Groupe Lipides et Nutrition, Institut Pasteur, Conseil Régional d'Aquitaine; serves on the editorial boards of Disability and Rehabilitation and the Journal of Alzheimer's disease; has received consultancy fees from Vifor Pharma; and receives research support from Danone, Institut Carnot LISA and Groupe Lipides et Nutrition.

Deborah E. Barnes is currently funded by the National Institute on Aging, Department of Veterans Affairs, Department of Defense, S. D. Bechtel Jr. Foundation, NARSAD, and UCB Pharma, Inc. None of the funders were involved with the writing or content of the material in this chapter.

Suzanne Craft has served as a consultant for GlaxoSmithKline, Takeda, and Zinfandel pharmaceuticals. Kurve Technology donated intranasal delivery devices to her studies.

Deborah Gustafson has nothing to disclose.

Tiffany L. Tsai has nothing to disclose.

Angela Jefferson's research is supported by K23-AG030962 (Paul B. Beeson Career Development Award in Aging); Alzheimer's Association IIRG-08-88733; R01-AG034962; R01-HL111516; and the Vanderbilt Memory & Alzheimer's Center. He serves on the editorial board for the Journal of Alzheimer's Disease and Archives of Clinical Neuropsychology. She also serves as a reviewer for federal and foundation grant reviews for the National Institute on Aging and the

Alzheimer's Association. She receives no compensation as a reviewer or member of the editorial or grant review boards.

Miia Kivipelto has not disclosed any conflicts of interest.

Manjulla Kurella-Tamura has nothing to disclose.

Lenore J. Launer has nothing to disclose.

Nicola Lautenschlager has nothing to disclose.

Jacqueline M. Leung has nothing to disclose.

José Alejandro Luchsinger's research is supported by the following grants: MD000206, AG026413, DK048404, AG028506, HD35897, AG037212, AG034189. He is an Associate Editor at the Journal of Alzheimer's Disease. He has received royalties from Springer for editing the book "Diabetes and the Brain". He has served in Advisory Boards for Nutricia, Inc.

Peter A. Passmore has nothing to disclose.

Alina Solomon has not disclosed any conflicts of interest.

Adam P. Spira received honoraria while serving as a clinical editor for the International Journal of Sleep and Wakefulness, Primary Care, which receives pharmaceutical company support.

Victor G. Valcour receives research funding from NIH and is a consultant for the International Antiviral Society, USA. Both provide travel support related to their projects.

Rachel Whitmer has not disclosed any conflicts of interest.

Index